100 *Best* Spas *of the* World

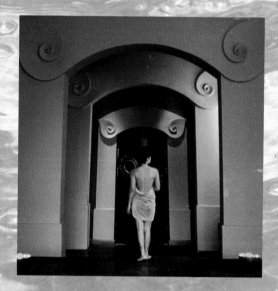

BERNARD BURT & PAMELA PRICE

SECOND EDITION

The Globe Pequot Press

GUILFORD, CONNECTICUT

Cover and interior design: Nancy Freeborn

Photo credits: Many thanks to the following people and organizations for providing photos: p. i © Luca Tettoni, The Regent Resort Chiang Mai; p. iii © Jane Lidz, The Golden Door; p. v Sheila Donnelly & Associates, Rajvilas; p. viii, xii Thalassa Spa at Anassa; p. 1 La Ventanas Al Paraiso; pp. 2-3 Canyon Ranch Health Resorts; p. 4 Mii' amo, a destination spa at Enchantment; pp. 6-7 Mraval; p. 8 The Boulders Resort & Golden Door Spa; p. 9 The Spa at Camelback Inn, Four Seasons Resort Scottsdale at Troon North, Sanctuary; p. 10 The Boulders Resort & Golden Door Spa; p. 11 Willow Stream Spa at The Fairmont Scottsdale Princess; p. 12 Marlove; p. 13 Cal-a-Vie; p. 14 Starwood Hotels; pp. 16-17 The Golden Door; pp. 18-19 The Oaks at Ojai; pp. 20-21 Ojai Valley Inn & Spa; pp. 22-23 The Palms at Palm Springs, The Spa Hotel & Casino; pp. 24-25 Renaissance Esmeralda Resort and Spa—Indian Wells, California; p. 26 Post Ranch Inn; pp. 28-29 Wyndham Peaks Resort & Golden Door Spa; pp. 30-31 The Spa at Mandarin Oriental, Miami; pp. 32-33 Marriott's Harbor Beach Resort & Spa; pp. 34-35 PGA National Resort & Spa; pp. 36-37 Grand Wailea Resort & Spa; pp. 38-39 © Thomas Barwick for Mauna Lani Resort; p. 40 Canyon Ranch Health Resorts; p. 42 Turnkey Brochures; pp. 44-45 Canyon Ranch Health Resorts; pp. 46-47 Elemis Spa at the Aladdin, StephenJohn Design for Elemis Spa at the Aladdin; pp. 48-49 The Grove Park Inn; pp. 50-51 Nemacolin Woodlands Resort & Spa; pp. 52-53 Green Valley Spa & Tennis Resort; pp. 54-55 Laura Davidson Public Relations; p. 56 The Greenbrier; p. 58 The American Club—Kohler Waters Spa; p. 60 Echo Valley Ranch & Spa, www.evranch.com; pp. 62-63 Banff Springs Hotel; pp. 64-65 © Roberto Lissia, Ste. Anne's Country Inn & Spa; pp. 66-67 © Don Weixi, The Hills Health Ranch; p. 68 Centre de Sante d'Eastman, Studio de la Montagne for Spa Eastman; pp. 70-71 Four Seasons Resort Punta Mita; pp. 72-73 Laura Davidson Public Relations; pp. 74-75 Las Ventanas Al Paraiso; pp. 76-77 Rancho La Puerta; p. 79 Thalassa Spa at Anassa; pp. 80-81 © 1997 Maxum, © by Rogner-Dorint, © Hundertwasser, Rogner-Bad Blumau; pp. 82-83 Le Meridien Limassol Spa & Resort; pp. 84-85 Grand Hotel Pupp; pp. 86-87 Naantali Spa Hotel & Resort; pp. 88-89 Institut de Thalassotherapie Louison Bobet at Hotel Miramar; pp. 90-91 Les Fermes de Marie; pp. 92-93 Guy Hervais, Les Pres d'Eugenie; pp. 94-95 Le Sources de Caudalie; pp. 96-97 Royal Parc Evian, Alice Marshall Public Relations, Victoria King Public Relations for Domaine du Royal Club Evian; pp. 98-99 Thalgo La Baule; pp. 100-101 Bad Woerishofen; pp. 102-103 © Rolf Gotwald Fotodesign, Brenner's Park-Hotel & Spa; pp. 104-105 Toscana Therme; pp. 106-107 Thermae Sylla Grand Hotel & Spa; pp. 108-110 Margitsziget Health Resort, Gellert Spa, Kiraly Baths, Angelo Cavalli; p. 111 Brian A. Gauvin; pp. 112-113 The Lodge & Spa at Inchydoney Island; pp. 114-115 Capri Beauty Farm at the Palace Hotel; pp. 116-117 Grand Hotel Terme Abano; pp. 118-119 Grotto Giusti Terme; pp. 120-121 Hawkins & Widness Public Relations International, Palazzo Arzaga Hotel—Saturnia Spa; pp. 122-123 Spa'Deus; pp. 124-125 Hotel Terme di Saturnia Resort; pp. 126-127 San Lawrenz Resort; pp. 128-129 Les Thermes Marins de Monte-Carlo; pp. 130-131 Marriott Vacation Club International; pp. 132-133 Sturebadet; pp. 134-135 Badrutt's Palace Hotel and Spa; pp. 136-137 Grand Hotels Bad Ragaz; pp. 138-139 Victoria-Jungfrau Grand Hotel; pp. 140-141 Champneys Health Resort & Spa; pp. 142-143 Chewton Glen Hotel, New Milton, England; pp. 144-145 Forest Mere Health Farm; pp. 146-147 The Spa at Mandarin Oriental situated at Mandarin Oriental Hyde Park, London; p. 148 Thermae Bath Spa; p. 150 Sheraton Grand Hotel and Spa; pp. 152-153 Turnberry Hotel, Golf Courses, and Spa; pp. 154-155 The Celtic Manor Resort; pp. 157-159 Rajvilas; pp. 160-161 Starwood Hotels; pp. 162-163 The Residence; p. 165 Movenpick Resort and Spa; pp. 166-167 Carmel Forest Spa Resort; pp. 168-169 PhotoDisc; pp. 170-171 Herods Vitalis; p. 173 Four Seasons Resort Bali at Jambaran Bay; pp. 174-175 Four Seasons Resort Bali at Jambaran Bay, Photographer Kevin Orpin for Four Seasons Resort Bali at Jambaran Bay; pp. 176-177 Le Meridien Nirwana Golf & Spa Resort; pp. 178-179 Inn Seiryuso; pp. 180-181 The Datai—Mandara Spa; p. 182 Banyan Tree Maldives Vabbinfaru; pp. 184-185 Banyan Tree Phuket; pp. 186-187 Chiva-Som International; pp. 188-189 Lou Hammond & Associates, The Oriental Hotel Bangkok; pp. 190-191 © Luca Tettoni, The Regent Resort Chiang Mai; pp. 193-194 Hawkins & Widness Public Relations, CuisinArt Resort & Spa; pp. 196-197 Mandara Spa, p. 196 © Macduff Everton, pp. 196-197 © Stewart Ferebee Photography; pp. 198-199 Sandy Lane; pp. 200-201 © Len Kaufman, Spring O'Brien & Co., Inc., Grand Lido Sans Souci Resort; pp. 202-203 Wyndham El Conquistador & Golden Door ™ Spa, Las Croabas, Puerto Rico; pp. 204-205 Marilyn Marx Public Relations, Le Sport; p. 208 Kurotel; pp. 210-211 Four Seasons Resort Carmelo; p. 212 Windstar Cruises; p. 213 Radisson Seven Seas Cruises; p. 214 Holland America, Seabourn Cruise Line; p. 215 Cunard Line; p. 216 Len Kaufman, Windstar Cruises. Spot art throughout: PhotoDisc.

ISBN 0-7627-2473-0

Manufactured in Canada
Second Edition/First Printing

WITH APPRECIATION TO
THE CAREGIVERS,
UNITING BODY AND SOUL
WITH ENERGY FROM THE HEART
—Bernard Burt

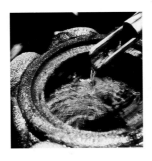

TO BERNARD BUBMAN
—Pamela Price

CONTENTS

Introduction. vii
Acknowledgments xii

NORTH AMERICA

UNITED STATES

Arizona
Canyon Ranch. 2
Mii' Amo at Enchantment Resort 4
Miraval 6
Scottsdale: Spa Town 8

California
Cal-a-Vie 12
The Century Plaza Hotel and Spa 14
The Golden Door. 16
The Oaks at Ojai 18
Ojai Valley Inn & Spa 20
Palm Springs Desert Resorts: Spa Town 22
The Post Ranch Inn 26

Colorado
Wyndham Peaks Resort & Golden Door Spa 28

Florida
Mandarin Oriental Hotel, Miami 30
Marriott's Harbor Beach Resort & Spa 32
PGA National Resort & Spa. 34

Hawaii
Grand Wailea Resort Hotel & Spa 36
Mauna Lani Spa at the Mauna Lani Resort. 38

Massachusetts
Canyon Ranch in the Berkshires 40
Cranwell Resort, Spa & Golf Club 42

Nevada
Canyon Ranch SpaClub at The Venetian 44
Elemis Spa at the Aladdin Hotel 46

North Carolina
The Grove Park Inn. 48

Pennsylvania
Nemacolin Woodlands Resort & Spa 50

Utah
Green Valley Spa & Tennis Resort 52
The Spa at Sundance 54

West Virginia
The Greenbrier. 56

Wisconsin
The American Club—Kohler Waters Spa 58

CANADA
Echo Valley Ranch & Spa 60
Fairmont Banff Springs Hotel—Willow Stream Spa. . . 62
Haldimand Hills Spa Village. 64
The Hills Health Ranch 66
Spa Eastman 68

MEXICO
Four Seasons Resort Punta Mita—Apuane Spa. 70
JW Marriott Cancun Resort & Spa 72
Las Ventanas al Paraiso. 74
Rancho La Puerta. 76

EUROPE

AUSTRIA
Rogner-Bad Blumau 80

CYPRUS
Le Meridien Limassol Spa & Resort 82

CZECH REPUBLIC
Grand Hotel Pupp—Harp Spa Clinic 84

FINLAND
Naantali Spa Hotel & Resort 86

FRANCE
Institut de Thalassotherapie Louison Bobet at
    Hotel Miramar–Crouesty 88
Les Fermes de Marie. 90
Les Prés d'Eugénie—La Ferme Thermale 92
Les Sources de Caudalie 94

Royal Parc Evian—Better Living Institute. 96
Thalgo La Baule Thalassotherapy Center 98

GERMANY
Bad Woerishofen: Spa Town 100
Brenner's Park-Hotel & Spa 102
Toskana Therme. 104

GREECE
Thermae Sylla Spa Wellness Hotel 106

HUNGARY
Budapest: Spa Town. 108

IRELAND
The Lodge & Spa at Inchydoney Island. 112

ITALY
Capri Beauty Farm at the Palace Hotel 114
Grand Hotel Terme Abano 116
Grotta Giusti Terme Spa Hotel. 118
Palazzo Arzaga Hotel—Saturnia Spa 120
Spa'Deus. 122
Terme di Saturnia Resort. 124

MALTA
Kempinski San Lawrenz Resort & Spa 126

MONACO
Les Thermes Marins de Monte-Carlo 128

SPAIN
Marriott Son Antem Golf Resort & Spa 130

SWEDEN
Sturebadet. 132

SWITZERLAND
Badrutt's Palace Hotel and Spa 134
Grand Hotels Bad Ragaz. 136
Victoria-Jungfrau Grand Hotel & Spa. 138

UNITED KINGDOM
England
Champneys Health Resort & Spa. 140
Chewton Glen Hotel, Health & Country Club. 142
Forest Mere Health Farm. 144

Mandarin Otiental Hotel, Hyde Park 146
Thermae Bath Spa 148
Scotland
The Sheraton Grand Hotel and Spa. 150
Westin Turnberry Resort and Spa. 152
Wales
The Celtic Manor Resort—Forum Health Club
   and Spa 154

INDIA/AFRICA

INDIA
Rajvilas 158

SOUTH AFRICA
Western Cape Hotel & Spa: Acquabella
   Wellness Center 160

TUNISIA
The Residence—Phytomer Spa 162

MIDDLE EAST

ISRAEL
Carmel Forest Spa Resort 166
The Dead Sea: Spa Town 168
Herods Vitalis 170

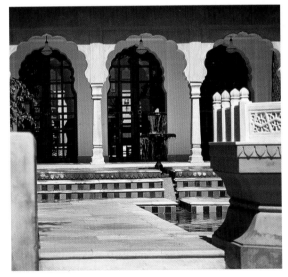

PACIFIC RIM

INDONESIA
Four Seasons Resort Bali at Jimbaran Bay 174
Le Meridien Nirwana Golf & Spa Resort 176

JAPAN
Inn Seiryuso 178

MALAYSIA
The Datai—Mandara Spa 180

REPUBLIC OF MALDIVES
Banyan Tree Maldives 182

THAILAND
Banyan Tree Phuket 184
Chiva-Som International Health Resort 186
The Oriental Hotel Bangkok—The Oriental Spa 188
The Regent Resort Chiang Mai—Lanna Spa 190

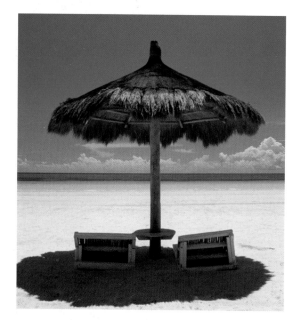

CARIBBEAN ISLANDS & THE BAHAMAS

ANGUILLA
CuisinArt Resort & Spa 194

THE BAHAMAS
Mandara Spa at the Ocean Club 196

BARBADOS
Sandy Lane Hotel 198

JAMAICA
Grand Lido Sans Souci Resort—Charlie's Spa 200

PUERTO RICO
The Golden Door at Las Casitas Village: Wyndham
    El Conquistador Resort & Country Club 202

SAINT LUCIA
The Body Holiday at LeSPORT 204

SOUTH AMERICA

BRAZIL
Kurotel 208

URUGUAY
Four Seasons Resort Carmelo 210

SPAS AT SEA

Judith Jackson's SeaSpa—Radisson *Seven Seas*
    Mariner 213
Spa du Soleil—Holland America MS *Prinsendam* . . . 214
Steiner Spa—Cunard *Queen Elizabeth 2* 215
WindSpa—Windstar's *Wind Surf* 216

Glossary 217
About the Authors 219

The prices and rates listed in this guidebook were confirmed at press time but under no circumstances are they guaranteed. We recommend that you call establishments before traveling to obtain current information. For international travel, check with the State Department on current travel conditions prior to your departure (www.travel.state.gov/travel_warnings.html).

INTRODUCTION

Defining the Spa Experience

The mystique of spas is as ancient as the Roman baths, and yet spas are on the cutting edge of the way we vacation in the twenty-first century. Still, the spa experience is a very personal one. Whether you want to be pampered on an exotic island, learn the latest techniques for stress management, or simply seek a relaxing retreat, you have more choices than ever.

Each spa visit becomes an adventure, sensory and physical, that helps you learn how to cope with the stress of your personal and professional life. But expectations don't always match the experience. Increasingly there is confusion about terminology—what's a "full-service" spa?—and professional standards for staffing and operating. Throughout this book you will learn not only the best places to spa, but also how to get the best values in services, treatments, and accommodations.

The New Spa

During our journeys (which span forty years) as travel and spa journalists, we have seen the evolution of a new breed of health resort—one that provides a variety of options in wellness and well-being along with spa services. Ancient traditions of natural healing such as ayurvedic medicine and yoga are meeting high-tech methods for the prevention of illness. Indeed, spas these days must do more than offer massages or trendy treatments to be ranked as world class. The most basic ingredients of the spa experience are being redefined. You can expect cutting-edge developments in:

Design: As old distinctions make way for new approaches to total wellness, spa designers are creating environments where you feel comfortable, safe, and well cared for. For example, in the beautiful Laurel Highlands of western Pennsylvania, the distinguished interior design consultant Clodagh used natural elements of water and light, wood and stone to create spaces that

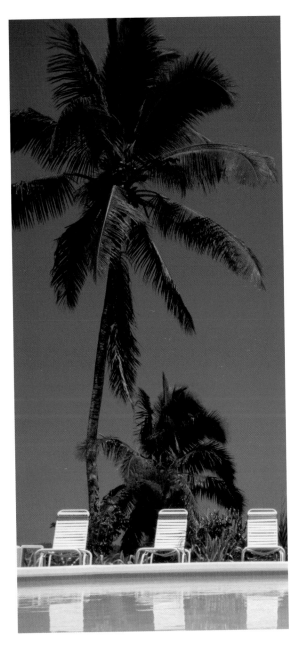

inspire a surge of energy along with your workout at Nemacolin Woodlands Resort & Spa. At her New York design studio, Clodagh speaks of her inspirations, from Zen Buddhism to feng shui, the Chinese art of placement, as well as astrology and channeling: "I just channel some kind of energy." Blending Asian and Western sensibilities, she adds, is not a logical process, but the result is a total design that creates an experience.

The Seven Kinds of Spas

Not all spas are created equal. The seven categories described by the International Spa Association (ISPA) can help you choose the best experience for you:

1. **Club spa:** Primarily a fitness facility, with services offered on a day-use basis.
2. **Cruise ship spa:** Aboard a cruise ship, professional treatments, personal training, and salon services are offered on an a la carte basis.
3. **Day spa:** Professionally administered services offered on a day-use basis.
4. **Destination spa:** Focused on lifestyle improvement and health enhancement through professionally administered services, physical fitness, educational programs, and on-site accommodations.
5. **Medispa:** Individuals, solo practices, groups, and institutions composed of medical and spa professionals whose primary purpose is to provide comprehensive medical and wellness care in an environment that integrates spa services with conventional and complementary therapies and treatments.
6. **Mineral springs spa:** Hydrotherapy treatments that use natural mineral or thermal waters, or seawater, from an on-site source.
7. **Resort hotel spa:** Located within a resort or hotel, professionally administered spa services, fitness and wellness components, and spa cuisine menu choices that are available on a daily or multiday basis.

Fitness and exercise: Whether it's aerobics, walking, or jogging—on a treadmill or a mountain trail—fitness and exercise are the basics of a wellness program. Each workout at a spa gives you new perspectives on your personal progress—and nowadays there may be new equipment with lots of bells and whistles to try. At Canyon Ranch, Champneys in Great Britain, and Rancho La Puerto in Mexico, as many as five classes each hour (all rated according to fitness level) are yours to choose from. The camaraderie of group exercise and sessions with a personal trainer will help you learn what works and add value to your daily regime at home.

Cuisines: Eating healthy is another part of the spa experience that's getting a new look. Tofu and veggie burgers, once staples of spa cuisine, now share the menu with meat, fish, and pasta. According to trends forecaster David Pursglove, some spas are now serving wine as well as waters.

The Spa Criteria

From London to Singapore, Malaysia, Thailand, Italy, and the American Southwest, at the pioneering Canyon Ranch in Arizona and its sibling SpaClub at the Venetian Resort in Las Vegas, the new health resorts offer something for everybody. Still, some of our favorite places to relax and be pampered are at hot

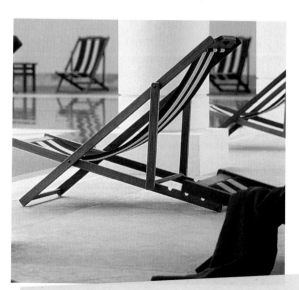

springs in historic towns that haven't changed much since our first visits. Bringing all of these experiences together for the first time into this book has been a voyage of discovery that encompasses some of the oldest and newest places to rejuvenate. Ultimately, all of these one hundred spas are the best of their type, be it a destination spa or resort spa, day spa, or mineral springs spa. What distinguishes them might be the program, the location, the design—or that indefinable look of happiness on people's faces as they leave.

Packing for Your Spa Vacation

Visiting a spa presents a packing dilemma: What to bring? You'll be changing clothes often for hiking, exercise classes, evening programs, and special events. Should you bring hiking boots, socks, warm-ups, comfortable jeans, a bathing suit, all-weather jackets? Assembling your wardrobe and compressing it into one easy, compact suitcase can be a challenge. But a little planning can solve the problem. Take easy-care but rugged fabrics woven from microfiber; you can wad them up in your suitcase and just shake them out later. They are entirely presentable. *TravelSmith*, a company that specializes in travel clothing and accessories, suggests that travelers pack such items as Supplex shirts, Coolmax T-shirts, explorer's shorts, Coolmax socks, trekking boots, a hat that offers sun protection, a travel twill shirt, a Great Escape shirt, a warm-up suit, and a bathing suit. To prevent spills, pack a leakproof bottle set (with screw-on tops for each container). You can consult with a TravelSmith outfitter who can send you free packing lists and reports on your destination. Call TravelSmith for a catalog at (800) 950–1600 or check out their Web site at www.travelsmith. com. New products are fun and functional, including the portable plug-in air purifiers.

Here's what we looked for:

1. *The design:* Does the physical setting have trend-setting infrastructure?
2. *The experience:* Does it live up to reputation, advertisements, and hype?
3. *The treatments:* Is the range of treatments indicative of current advances?
4. *The products:* Are product lines tested and reputable?
5. *The sense of place:* How does the program complement the location?
6. *The staffing:* Do therapists and aestheticians enjoy thorough education and in-service training?
7. *The cuisine:* Rather than spa cuisine, think healthy cuisine. Does the food have eye appeal and taste as well as low-fat nutritional value?
8. *The cleanliness:* How are housekeeping standards maintained?
9. *The facilities:* Regardless of size, does the combination of treatment areas, outdoor recreation, fitness equipment, and staff provide complete satisfaction?
10. *The journey:* Would you go out of your way to experience this spa?

Price guidelines used in this book are based on a typical package or one-week program:

$$$$ Ultraluxurious . . $7,000 and up per person.
$$$ Luxurious . . . . . . $5,000 and up per person.
$$ Superior . . . . $3,500 and up per person.
$ Value . . . . Less than $3,500 per person.

All prices are given in U.S. dollars and have been rounded to even dollar amounts.

The Spa Journey

What you need from your own spa experience can't always be measured. Each experience is unique—there's really no such thing as "the best." With this book you will discover multiple subtle and not-so-subtle variables that can make each spa visit an experience that enhances your life. The choices are yours to enjoy.

The merger of traditional medicine with the spirit of spa therapy defines our selection of the one hundred best spas of the world. The union will bring life to our years and years to our lives.

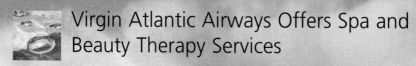

Virgin Atlantic Airways Offers Spa and Beauty Therapy Services

If ever there was a solution to challenging jet lag and looking terrific at the same time, Virgin Atlantic Airways has made it happen. A pioneer in taking the spa experience to the highest heights ever, the airline has brought new meaning to the oft-used phrase "a heavenly spa experience."

It all starts even before take off, should you be in London and should you be holding a ticket in upper class. Credit goes to Jane Breeden, who heads up Virgin's team of in-flight beauty therapists. In 1989 she proposed the innovative idea to the airline's founder, Richard Branson: Why not offer passengers something special when crossing the Atlantic, such as a massage?

The rest is history. Today there are 200 in-flight beauty therapists plus nine hairdressers and eighteen therapists based at the Virgin Clubhouse at London's Heathrow International Airport. The service boils down to complimentary preflight grooming services. Just as at any day or destination spa, choices range from massage to facial and beauty treatments, such as a pressure point massage to a rejuvenating foot spa. Specialty treatments reflect Virgin's pioneering spirit, such as the Ready for Takeoff, a facial designed to eliminate dead cells, hydrate for a fresh complexion, and provide a protective moisturizer.

Arriving at London Heathrow, upper-class passengers are encouraged to visit Revivals in Terminal 3. This is the first spa of its kind exclusively for upper class. The transition from air to land is dealt with sensibly here.

A high-power luxury shower with a choice of radio stations helps passengers adjust to their time zone. While you shower, a personal valet service takes care of shirt pressing and suit steaming. A choice of breakfast foods, from smoked salmon to scrambled eggs, kicks off a new day.

In addition Virgin offers special assistance to all passengers with restricted mobility, such as providing onboard wheelchairs. Sight-restricted passengers are provided with briefing cards in braille. Virgin Atlantic is a "green" airline that never gets the blues when it comes to recycling. Even printer toner cartridges are collected and donated to the Roy Castle Lung Cancer Appeal for recycling. Onboard, economy amenity kits are collected by recycling agents and sorted out for future use. Virgin Atlantic has taken initiatives in many ways, from spa services to socially responsive flight management.

Serving many of the one hundred best spas of the world, Virgin Atlantic operates flights between New York, Miami, Boston, Los Angeles, and San Francisco and Heathrow/London, and between Las Vegas, Orlando, and Miami and Gatwick International. From London's Heathrow there is service to Tokyo, Shanghai, Delhi, and Hong Kong.

For further information call (800) 862–8621, or visit www.virgin.com/atlantic.

HOW TO SPA

Knowing what to expect before you go will enhance both the spa experience and the value of your vacation. Talk to the spa director by telephone or e-mail to learn about services and treatments offered. If you've never been to a spa, discuss your goals with a qualified professional, and consult your personal physician to set guidelines. Study the daily routine of scheduled group exercise and personal time to select a balanced program that suits your needs and fitness level. Hardline, fixed programs are a thing of the past; today the key word is *revitalize*. Become an empowered spagoer with these ten questions:

What's included in my spa package?
Ask about seasonal specials, as well as the best combinations of services and treatments offered in daily and multiday programs. Get a description of each treatment and its therapeutic value.

How much does it cost?
All-inclusive programs are typical at destination spas, which offer fixed packages that include accommodations, meals, treatments, and exercise/fitness training. Seasonal specials include mother-daughter weeks and bring-a-friend-for-free weeks. Resort and cruise ship spas offer more options and flexible pricing. At historic spa towns, such as Palm Springs, California, and Budapest, Hungary, you will find a wide range of accommodations at all price levels.

Are tips included?
Although some resorts include gratuities for therapists as well as staff in the restaurant and hotel, the policy varies, especially in Asia and Europe. Ask at the reception desk. Spa tipping is actually similar to salon and restaurant tipping: 15 to 20 percent, depending on how satisfied you are with the service. Take small envelopes to reward special people with extra cash.

What do I wear?
Modesty is never compromised. Most often robes are supplied. Under the robe? It's up to you. If water therapy is involved, a swimsuit may be appropriate. Bring exercise clothing and shoes, but ask what the spa provides, like jogging suits, slippers, and rain gear. Basics may be fine for dinner, or you might enjoy changing into something more dressy.

Are there special health considerations?
Before strenuous exercise or thermal treatments, a physical evaluation or fitness screening is recommended. European spa doctors require a checkup (usually a separate fee) as the basis for scheduling services. If you have a particular injury or physical condition, explain it to the therapists and instructors. They can suggest appropriate adjustments or enhancements.

Can I request a male or female therapist?
Usually, yes, but some spas have only female therapists. And most spas are coed but offer separate facilities for men and women.

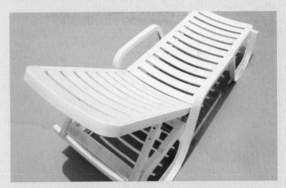

What is the size of the group during a typical week?
Get a profile of the typical guest as well as typical activities. You may prefer destination spas with fixed programs and a small band of fellow spa-goers. Sharing experiences builds camaraderie.

Can I bring my family?
Resort spas cater to all ages, and some have special programs for children. Destination spas usually have a minimum age limit of sixteen or eighteen.

What else should I bring?
Sunscreen, alarm clock, gym bag or fanny pack, lots of socks, well-worn aerobics shoes, and hiking gear. Don't forget business cards—spas have become networking hot spots.

And leave behind?
Don't bring jewelry, alcohol, office work, or food. Distance yourself from the people, problems, and responsibilities of your real life.

ACKNOWLEDGMENTS

Countless experiences and conversations with spa professionals went into the preparation of this book. We were inspired by Deborah Szekely, cofounder of the Golden Door and Rancho La Puerta, as well as her son Alex. The leadership of Canyon Ranch cofounder Mel Zuckerman and his associates can be found at three resorts featured in the book. Sharing insights from world travels, Jenni Lipa of Spa Trek Travel and Susie Ellis of Spa Finder in New York opened doors for us. And then there's Sheila Cluff, who shared Pamela's vision of spas from the beginning, as well as Sharon Norling, M.D.

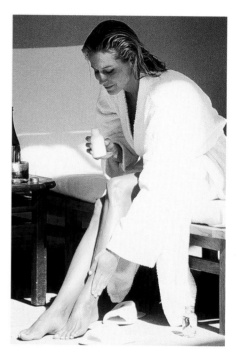

Special thanks to Mary Tabacchi, Ph.D., School of Hotel Administration at Cornell University, who is a dedicated educator in spa management. The archival collection of spa materials covering two decades (1976–1996) contributed by Pamela Price is now housed at Cornell. We are also indebted to the publisher of *Spa Management Journal*, Guy Jonkman, and to Vincenzo Marra, CEO of Italian Beauty Innovations, for continuing support of industrywide education programs. For technical advice, Dr. Reinhard R. Bergel of H.E.A.T., Inc., in California and Dr. Jonathan de Vierville at the Alamo Plaza Spa in San Antonio, Texas, were invaluable. European colleagues guided our selection of new destinations: Josef Bartholemy, former Kurhouse director in Baden-Baden, Germany, who now writes and lectures on spas worldwide; Dr. Susan Horsewood-Lee in London; and Jane Crebbin-Bailey of HCB Associates, vice president of the ISPA European Chapter. In Asia we had input from longtime residents Kim and Cary Collier, founders of Jamu; Darryll Leiman and Donna Wells at Mandara Spas; and Diana Moody of Sheila Donnelly & Associates. Jean Kolb at the Kohler Water Spa in Wisconsin provided much useful information.

Family support was indispensable. Tony Lechtman, in New York, and Arthur Lechtman, Washington, D.C.–based attorney, shared their mother's enthusiasm for spas. Jeffrey A. Burt keeps tabs on his uncle. And our extended family includes the founders of ISPA who have made this book possible. Thanks also to Robert Mishkin, The RobeWorks, Jennifer Kottom, Joey English, Jackie Olden, David Goss, Autumn Bates, and to Jamie Lee Pricer for her editorial assistance.

To our editors at The Globe Pequot Press, Laura Strom and Mimi Egan, and to Jane Reilly, senior publicist, deep appreciation for believing in this book.

Bernard Burt   Pamela Price
Washington, D.C.   Palm Springs, California

NORTH AMERICA

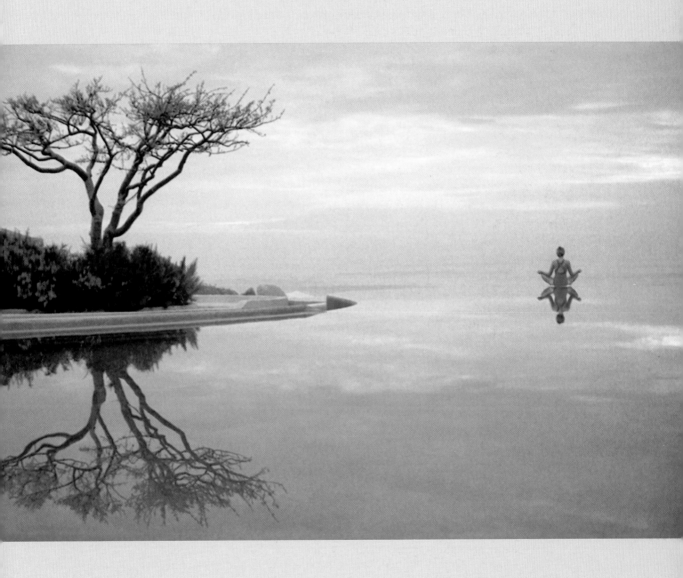

CANYON RANCH
Tucson, Arizona

Established in 1979, this year-round, award-winning destination spa accommodates up to 240 guests in single-story, adobe-style cottages on seventy acres in the foothills of the Santa Catalina Mountains. Canyon Ranch was voted "Best Spa" by *Condé Nast Traveler* magazine in 1990, 1992, and 1997 and is an internationally recognized pioneer in preventive health programs for every stage of life and every fitness level.

The staff at Canyon Ranch is composed of physicians, nurses, psychologists, fitness instructors, bodywork therapists, art and music therapists, hiking guides, and nutritionists. The staff-to-guest ratio is nearly three to one. It requires a seventy-page guide to describe the activities and services, and it will take you at least a week to benefit from the range of offerings, from classes focused on spiritual awareness to behavioral health.

The health resort's ambience is created by natural desert vegetation highlighted by tropical trees, streams, pools, fountains, original sculpture, and cactus gardens. It takes about a day to become oriented with the comprehensive facilities, including the 64,000-square-foot spa complex honeycombed with treatment rooms for massages and facials, whirlpools, sunbathing areas, and herbal wrap and hydromassage rooms. There are seven gyms, seven lighted tennis courts, a yoga/meditation dome, a large Pilates studio, and men's and women's locker rooms complete with sauna, steam, and inhalation rooms. New at the spa is the aquatic center with three Watsu pools, an exercise pool, two aqua-therapy pools, and a whirlpool. The golf school, staffed by PGA professionals, is another impressive addition.

The daily program is exciting, with guided walks

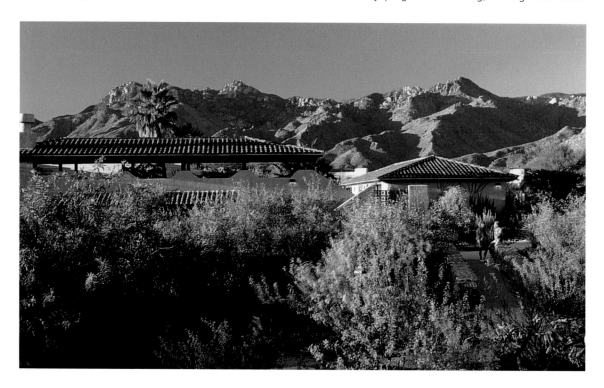

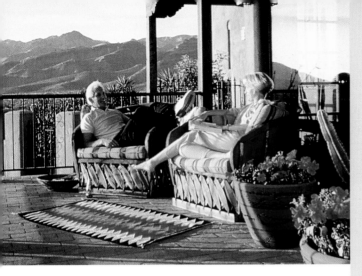

starting as early as 6:30 A.M., and there are lots of choices. For example, at 10:00 A.M. you may select from seven classes, such as H_2O Power Hour in the pool or a cardio circuit. After lunch, there are lectures, such as "Is It My Hormones?" or "The Skinny on Fat." The upbeat attitude of the staff and guests is motivating, and the ambience is casual and unpretentious. In the evening, there are concerts, watercolor classes, and a variety of presentations, from travelogues to health lectures.

Leading the way to quality aging, the Life Enhancement Program has its own spa and health center designed to serve small groups in a supportive environment. Group members share common life-improvement goals, ranging from controlling cardio-vascular disease, diabetes, stress, or weight to smoking cessation and healthy aging issues. Group members participate in a structured week-long program.

Everything at Canyon Ranch is touched by the spirit of health, including Lunch & Learn. This special cafe is devoted to those who want to learn how to prepare Canyon Ranch cuisine at home. There is a demonstration kitchen, and guests are seated at tables for four to watch as a full lunch is prepared from scratch. The "show" might include such healthy choices as tomato soup, ahi tuna with salsa, and dessert, which could be chocolate chip cookies, blueberry cobbler, or fudge brownies—low in fat and calories, of course.

Canyon Ranch is definitely the vacation you take home with you!

Taking Control of Your Health and Well-Being

Canyon Ranch
8600 East Rockcliff Road
Tucson, AZ 85750
Phone: (520) 749–9000
Fax: (520) 749–7755
Web site: www.canyonranch.com
Season: Year-round
General Manager: Karen Ramirez
Spa Director: Sharon Stricker
Fitness Director: Eduardo Perez
Reservations: (520) 749–9000 or (800) 742–9000
Accommodations: 175 rooms; variety of room styles and sizes, accommodating 240 guests.
Meals: The Spanish-Colonial clubhouse hosts the spacious dining room. Canyon Ranch offers healthy menus that include gourmet favorites.
Facilities: The grounds include cactus gardens, streams, pools, and fountains; the clubhouse holds the dining room, registration, guest services, meeting rooms, and boutique. The demonstration kitchen and creative arts center are adjacent to the clubhouse. The spa has skin care and beauty salons, as well as massage and hydrotherapy rooms. Medical clinic. Coed gym with full cardio and strength-training equipment; aquatic center, golf school.
Services & Special Programs: Lunch & Learn cooking classes; Life Enhancement Program; medical assessments; golf school; daily guided biking and hiking programs.
Rates: $$$
Best Spa Package: Between September and June, seven nights in a standard accommodation, double occupancy, is $4,376 per person, which includes tax and service charges. The week's stay covers three meals daily; use of spa facilities; fitness classes; hiking; biking; a health and fitness assessment; a selection of spa, sports, and health and healing services. Also offers fifteen minutes with an exercise physiologist and group presentations. Service charges cover round-trip transfers from the airport, gratuities, and unlimited local phone calls.
Credit Cards: Most major
Getting There: Airport transfers are provided for guests from Tucson International Airport, 21 miles from the ranch.
What's Nearby: Sabino Canyon Recreation Area; all Tucson area shops, restaurants, and attractions; Nogales, Mexico; the Arizona-Sonora Desert Museum.

MII'AMO

Sedona, Arizona

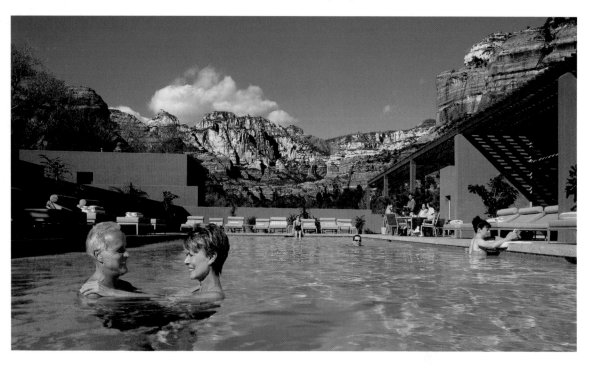

Opened in January 2001, this stunning 24,000-square-foot spa housed in a two-level building with twenty-four treatment rooms captures the spirit of Sedona's Boynton Canyon in more ways than one. Sedona has been called a "New Age Mecca," and justifiably so with the opening of this charismatic spa. Generations of Hopi and Apache found the rock cliffs in the area sacred because of their healing power. Today's spa seekers choose to stay here because they seek a life-enhancing experience. There does seem to be a mystical aspect to this extraordinary location.

Mii' Amo is in a secluded location on the property of the Enchantment Resort, and spa guests stay in one of sixteen comfortable casitas adjacent to the "organic" spa structure. The design is an authentic reflection of Native American pueblos and is a first for an American destination spa. Glowing reviews of Mii'

Amo in magazines ranging from *Arizona Food & Lifestyles* to *Departures* emphasize the architecture as well as the treatments, which offer a fascinating escape from reality.

The Enchantment Resort has been ranked among the top one hundred resort hotels of the world. The addition of this spa, which was built to be totally separate from the main hotel, confirms the fine reputation that Enchantment has earned over the years.

The simple, yet energy-charged ambience of the spa is reinforced by a world-class program that covers every aspect of the wellness experience—from an 8:30 A.M. Hiking Powerstart to a ninety-minute Sedona Clay Wrap. Then there are the signature treatments, such as the Mii' Amo Crystal Bath and the Blue Corn Body Polish and Massage, which gets down to basics and uses ground blue corn with mineral salt crystals to cleanse and purify the skin.

Waking up to a Mii' Amo morning, surrounded by the subtle red rocks of Boyton Canyon, is a natural energizer. The spa restaurant, with indoor-outdoor seating, specializes in contemporary, eclectic spa cuisine—a nutritious range of fresh fruits and vegetables prepared with a flourish of color and fresh herbs, but barely any fat. Yet a glass of wine is permissible. The food philosophy here is simple: "Have it, metabolize it, and move on!"

The spa is organized for contemplation and reflection. The intense feeling of spiritual connection to Native American culture is nearly instant, especially at the spa's inimitable Crystal Grotto, a place of meditation. When you feel it is time to slip away from a world of stress, techno-overload, and Palm Pilots, Mii' Amo is the spa journey for you.

Tea for Tired Skin

Pat Riley, CEO and founder of Clientele, specializing in skincare, says radiant skin begins with the right nutrition. Tomislav Podreka, author of *Serendipitea: A Guide to the Varieties, Origins and Rituals of Tea,* agrees. They both recommend a cup of green tea.

You'll find green tea for sipping between spa treatments in the relaxation areas of many spas. Vitamins, minerals, and antioxidants can nourish and protect the skin from the inside; the result is younger-looking skin throughout your life. Riley and Podreka recommend a cup of green tea daily. This provides a rich source of natural antioxidants and also helps protect the skin from sun damage. A daily multivitamin also contributes to radiant skin.

Selecting a green tea is like a journey. One exotic choice is Ti Kuan Yin (Iron Goddess of Mercy), an oolong tea from Fujian provence in China. The tea tastes tender and peachy on the palate. Healthy, tantalizing green tea is a tradition that is enjoying rediscovery in the spa world.

A Spa Journey with Native American Spirit

Mii' Amo
525 Boynton Canyon Road
Sedona, AZ 86336
Phone: (928) 203–8500
Fax: (928) 203–8599
E-mail: info@miiamo.com
Web site: www.miiamo.com
Season: Year-round
General Manager: Annika Chane
Director of Spa Operations: Dorah Waldvogel
Reservations: (888) 749–2137. Enchantment Resort is a member of the Leading Hotels of the World and the Small Luxury Hotels of the World.
Spa Appointments: (928) 203–8599
Accommodations: Fourteen spa guest rooms and two deluxe spa suites, housed in six traditional adobe-style casitas, each with private patio, beehive fireplace, and spa-inspired bathrooms with deep tubs.
Meals: Mii' Amo Cafe accommodates eighty for breakfast, lunch, and dinner. A group table near the open kitchen is ideal for guests who prefer not to dine alone.
Facilities: The 24,000-square-foot, two-level spa is nestled in the slope of a canyon wall with spa pool, lap pool.
Services & Special Programs: Guests can use facilities at Enchantment Resort, including concierge services.
Rates: $$$
Best Spa Package: The seven-night package starts at $2,800 per person (November–February) with a Sunday arrival staying in a Spa Casita. All packages include three Mii' Amo Cafe meals daily, use of fitness facilities, scheduled fitness classes, lectures, and cooking demonstrations. A visitor day package, such as Mii' Amo Magic (custom massage, facial, manicure), is $265 if reserved in advance.
Credit Cards: Most major
Getting There: From Phoenix, travel time is approximately two-and-a-half hours.
What's Nearby: Numerous art galleries and boutiques in Sedona, red rock Jeep tours. Hikes to Deer Bear Mountain and Grasshopper Point and horseback riding can be arranged through the concierge.

MIRAVAL
Catalina, Arizona

A recent guest appropriately nicknamed this spa "Miracle." At Miraval guests discover a carefully planned strategy focused on a "single belief that each of us has the innate capacity to live a more fulfilling life." It is no wonder that Miraval has been cited as the number-one spa in the world by *Condé Nast Traveler* Readers' Choice Awards and was rated in the top one-third of all travel destinations in the world by the same publication.

When experts gathered to create a new educational vacation alternative at Miraval, the bottom line became "balance of life." And that goal is embraced in every aspect of the program, from the self-discovery and stress management work-shops to the spa's Conscious Cuisine (the use of foods that are appealing, satisfying, and healthy) developed by Chef Cary E. Neff. The experts also made another precise decision to categorize Miraval as a "health leisure resort" rather than as a spa.

Miraval literally means "view of the valley," which it indeed grants in its setting on 135 acres at the foot of the Santa Catalina Mountains. Resembling a dude ranch with adobe-style build-ings, Miraval is worthy of its four-star resort status.

One glance through the fifteen-page Personal Services Guide will give you an under-standing of the structure and depth of this program, which covers every aspect of body

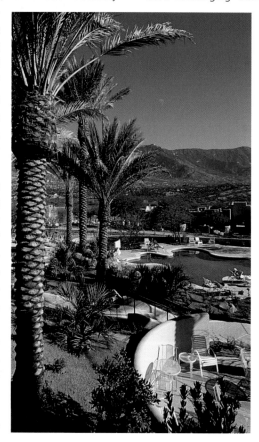

care, from a self-heating mud and massage treatment to nine kinds of facials. If your goal is to jump-start your life, this is the place to make it happen. Miraval has expanded on the usual spa offerings to include such unique programs as the Equine Experience. Self-awareness is increased through greater "communication" with your horse, including increased awareness while cleaning the horse's shoes and hooves. Other self-challenging activ-ities include mountain biking, meditation, yoga, and specialized body work ranging from craniosacral to ayurvedic body treatments. For the intrepid there are extra-challenging activities, such as wall climbing, night climbing, and desert and mountain hiking. For the imaginative there are classes in the sacred art of sand painting and an introduction to journal writing. In fact, there is almost everything under the Arizona sun to stimulate your creativ-ity. You may do as little or as much as you choose, but, if you want to do it all, plan to stay about a week.

At Miraval there are no required classes or rules against drinking alcohol or wine, which are available in the dining room and bar. Abstinence and deprivation are not part of the well-planned agenda. This fact sets Miraval apart from the many spas that eschew alcohol, sweets, and other decadences. If ever there was a feel-good resort, this is it! The key here is to make

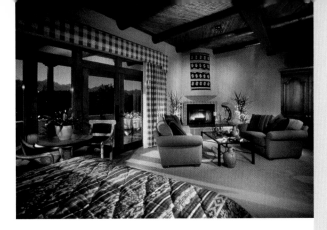

Miraval
5000 East Via Estancia Miraval
Catalina, AZ 85739
Phone: (520) 825–4000
Fax: (520) 825–5163
E-mail: miravalaz@aol.com
Web site: www.miravalresort.com

Season: Year-round

General Manager: Jack O'Donnell

Spa Director: Amy McDonald

Fitness Director: Nordine Zouareg

Reservations: (800) 232–3969

Spa Appointments: (800) 363–0819

Accommodations: 106 casita-style rooms (most with private patios), two luxury suites, four king rooms with fireplaces. All have cotton velour bathrobes, minibar, two-line telephones, morning newspaper.

Meals: The Cactus Flower (breakfast, lunch, and dinner); the Palm Court (continental breakfasts, gourmet sandwiches, snacks); the Brave Bull (4:00–10:00 P.M.; wine, alcoholic drinks, light snacks).

Facilities: Three swimming pool areas; fitness center; conference rooms; horseback riding; tennis courts; volleyball; croquet; hiking and mountain biking trails; Zen and desert gardens; nearby golf; climbing wall; personalized spa treatments; facials and salon services.

Services & Special Programs: Flexible, personalized programs, classes, and services, including self-discovery, lifestyle management, recreation/fitness.

Rates: $$–$$$

Best Spa Package: Miraval's Life in Balance Deluxe Package is the only option. It includes casita-style accommodations; three gourmet meals daily; all nonalcoholic beverages; access to group programs and activities; one personal spa service or one one-on-one consultation or round of golf per night of stay; use of facility; round-trip Tucson International Airport transfers. Low season (June–September): $420 per person per night, double occupancy; high season (October–mid-June): $445; with 7.5% tax and 17.5% service charge.

Credit Cards: Most major

Getting There: Miraval is located 20 miles outside of Tucson, between Tucson and Phoenix, near the small community of Catalina. Guests most conveniently fly into Tucson International Airport.

What's Nearby: Biosphere; two golf courses; a multitude of attractions in Phoenix and Tucson.

choices that work for you, based on "mindfulness." Mindfulness simply means that there is something for everyone at Miraval. The positive environment that surrounds the guest at this spa nurtures sensible choices—from fitness to food—that lead to a life in balance.

Weight Control through Mindfulness

Weight loss without dieting is possible according to Lisa O'Donnell, registered dietitian at Miraval. She recommends you get in touch with your own body by paying attention to how food affects your energy level and your general health (for example, noting if eating dairy products causes stomachaches). She also suggests you notice how emotions affect your food choices. The idea is to slow down and focus your attention on eating: Scrutinize the junk food in your diet, and take a look at your family's medical history. O'Donnell advises her clients to always eat breakfast and to include protein in it (a few almonds, natural peanut butter, or cottage cheese will do), to eat frequently to keep blood sugar stabilized, and to balance carbohydrates and proteins. She also suggests you take at least twenty minutes a day away from your workplace for lunch and also plan a healthy afternoon snack. "There is no such thing as a good or bad food," she stresses. "It's a matter of how much you eat and how often."

SCOTTSDALE: SPA TOWN
Scottsdale, Arizona

Called the "rising star of the spa world" by *USA Today*, Scottsdale's positive energy has given birth to an impressive number of spas, each presenting its own concept of therapeutic healing treatments, nutritional dining, and fitness choices. Thriving in this desert community, each has a distinctive personality while sharing similar goals for healing and wellness. The common bond of Scotts- dale's spas is their orientation to the mountains and focus on treatments reflecting a high level of individuality. Concentrating on Native American modalities and natural products, each spa offers a dramatic range of skin care treatments, massages, and wraps, combined with fitness opportunities, which echo the relaxed lifestyle of this vacation paradise.

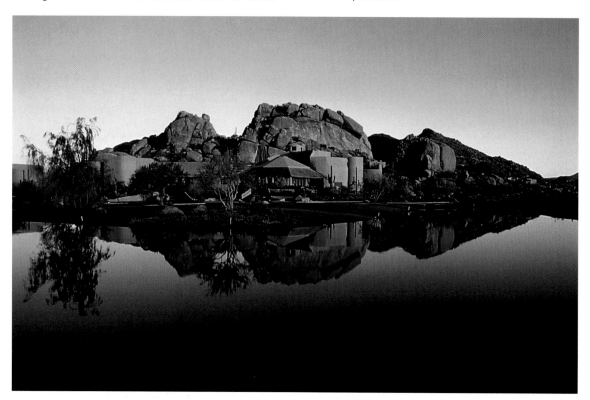

The Boulders Resort and Golden Door Spa
34631 North Tom Darlington Drive
Carefree, AZ 85377
Phone: (480) 488–9009 or (800) 553–1717
Fax: (480) 488–4118
Web site: www.wyndham.com/luxury
Spa director: Lorraine Park

Boulders is known as the ultimate desert hideaway, and the impressive addition of the spacious Golden Door Spa, in a freestanding 33,000-square-foot shrine to healthy living, has burnished its reputation. There are many Golden Door touches here, including the Labyrinth (a path to tranquility), the Japanese Gardens, and a spa cafe serving recipes made legendary by

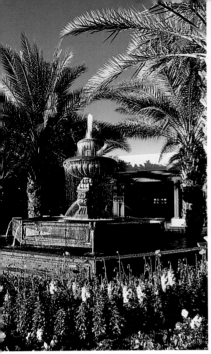
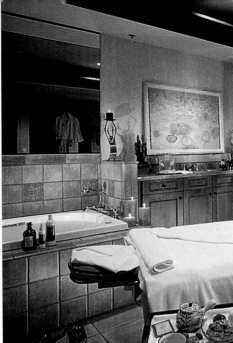
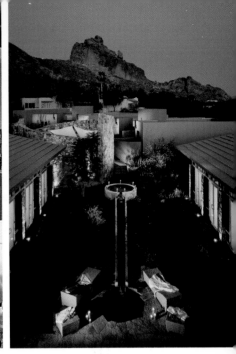

Executive Chef Michel Stroot at the original Golden Door in Escondido, California. The spa building, looking like a surrealistic sand sculpture, wraps around the north side of the base of the resort's signature boulder monument. An ambitious range of fitness classes and Native American-inspired treatments, such as a turquoise wrap and Native grain exfoliation, impart an authentic feeling of traditional culture. The wide-open spaces, 1,300 acres in the Sonoran Desert, ensure maximum privacy. There are 160 casitas and fifty one-, two-, and three-bedroom villas, many on the golf course.

Four Seasons Resort Scottsdale at Troon North
10600 East Crescent Moon Drive
Scottsdale, AZ 85262
Phone: (480) 515–7000 or (800) 332–3442
Fax: (480) 515–5599
Web site: www.fourseasons.com/scottsdale
Spa Director: Karen Steidl

It's easy to see why guests are high on spas at this tranquil resort. Not only are you at an altitude of 2,651 feet, but the air is clean and crisp, and clusters of casitas are removed from annoying traffic. In other words, this is the right choice for those who want to get away from the madding crowds. Opened in 1999, this contemporary 210-room resort on forty acres houses guests in spacious one- and two-story Southwestern casitas, all with spectacular desert views. The heart of this resort for many is the intimate 12,000-square-foot spa with an impressive menu of skin and body treatments. The most outstanding is the 110-minute Pinnacle, which is certain to put the most stressed urban dweller into a state of nirvana. It begins with a gentle exfoliation, followed by lavender oil, then a Sonoran honey dip to warm hands and feet; the finale is a champagne and caviar collagen facial. All spa suites have a sauna and steam/shower combination unit and a specialty jet bath.

Marriott's Camelback Inn Resort
The Spa at Camelback Inn
5402 East Lincoln Drive
Scottsdale, AZ 85253
Phone: (480) 948–1700 or (800) 24–CAMEL
Fax: (480) 951–5452 (reservations)
Web site: www.camelbackinn.com
Spa Director: Kelli Royer-Ziegler

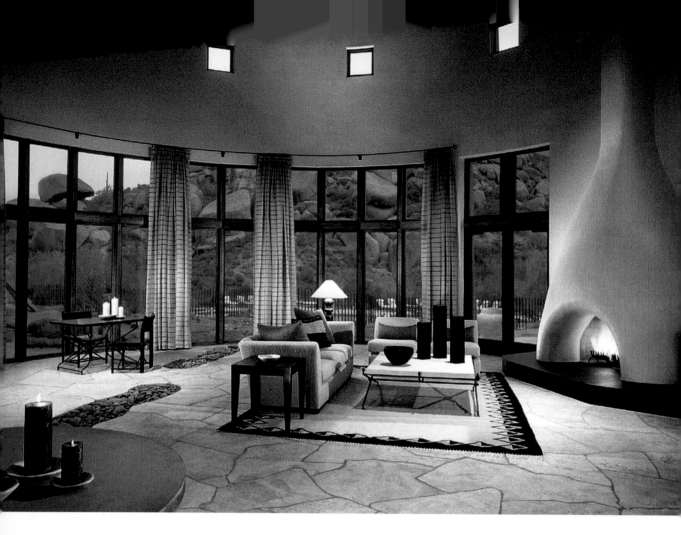

This 31,000-square-foot spa opened in 1981 in a historic 453-room 1936 resort. It covers 125 acres overlooking Camelback Mountain and was one of the first spas in the United States to offer what we now recognize as a harmonious blend of the most serious spa components: diagnostic testing, nutrition counseling, education, individualized spa treatments, and lifestyle-enhancing wellness programs. From hot stone massage to healthy back stretch classes, this unpretentious spa opened the eyes of the spa world with a simple yet successful program that draws crowds from dawn to dusk. Their recipe for success has a proven track record. Their signature treatments feature vitamin E and blends of citrus and fruits. The experienced staff runs the spa like clockwork, with twenty-seven treatment rooms, sunbathing terraces, hot tubs, cold plunge pools, Finnish saunas, and Sprouts, a signature restaurant with a heart-healthy menu.

Willow Stream—
The Spa at the Fairmont Scottsdale Princess
7575 East Princess Drive
Scottsdale, AZ 85255
Spa Phone: (480) 585–2732 or (800) 908–9540
Web site: www.fairmont.com
Spa Director: Jill Eisenhut

A serious freestanding spa (44,000 square feet) inspired by Havasu Falls, a hidden oasis in Arizona's

Grand Canyon, sets this stunning spa apart from other hotel spas. The Scottsdale Princess is a popular convention hotel that now has a world-class spa impressive enough to attract those seeking a destination experience. You can reserve a package for two to seven days. The resort, opened in 1987, has 650 guest rooms and is set against the backdrop of the McDowell Mountains. The architecture reflects the Spanish colonial style with wide, open spaces. The spa's logo—air, fire, water, and earth—sets the stage for signature experiences, such as the ninety-minute Willow Stream Body Experience and the Willow Stream Relaxation Massage. The spa serves freshly baked muffins and other refreshments throughout the day. A spa representative greets guests. A plus here is the Lifestyle Cuisine menu created by Executive Chef Reed Groban and his team. Guests make their own informed choices.

The Sanctuary on Camelback Mountain

5700 East McDonald Drive
Paradise Valley, AZ 85253
Phone: (480) 948–2100 or (800) 245–2051
Fax: (480) 483–3386
Web site: www.sanctuaryaz.com
Spa director: Jennifer Braddock

Here is a spa that captures the essence of the mountains, sunsets, and desert tranquility. The 12,000-square-foot spa perches high on the north slope of Camelback Mountain, with eleven treatment rooms located around a Zen meditation garden. The courtyard is the spa's interactive area near the gym. Spa enthusiasts should reserve accommodations in one of the twenty-four new luxury spa casitas surrounding the pool. Each has an outdoor steeping tub, which is best enjoyed at sunset. Unique to the Sanctuary is the Sanctum, a circular treatment suite for two with a 16-foot yin/yang wall, vitality pool, deluge shower, misting system, and fire pit, which brings the desert spa experience to a new level for those seeking the ultimate in private rejuvenation.

Getting There: Phoenix Sky Harbor International Airport is the gateway to Scottsdale. Currently served by Aero California, Alaska Airlines, America West Airlines, American Airlines, American Trans Air, British Airways, Continental Airlines, Delta Airlines, Frontier, KLM, Northwest, Southwest Airlines, United Airlines, and US Airways.

What's nearby: For information, contact the Scottsdale Convention and Visitor's Bureau, 7343 Scottsdale Mall, Scottsdale, AZ 85251; Phone: (480) 945–8481; Fax: (480) 947–4523 or (800) 805–0471. Consult "Discover Scottsdale," the visitor bureau's official destination guide for the latest on art galleries, dining, and outdoor activities. Cosanti, home of Paolo Soleri bells, and Taliesin West are two major attractions. The three main museums are Fleischer Museum, Phoenix Art Museum, and the Scottsdale Museum of Contemporary Art. Golfers flock to the more than 175 courses in the area.

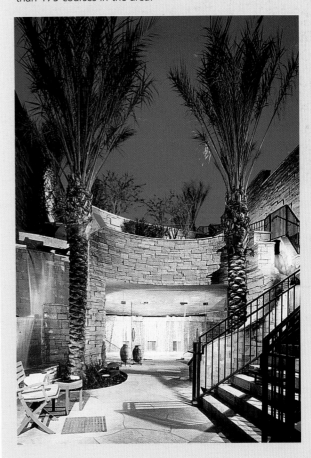

CAL-A-VIE
Vista, California

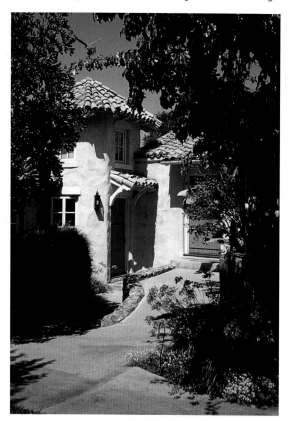

Leave the city stress behind once you arrive at Cal-a-Vie, a destination spa in a garden setting 40 miles north of San Diego. Opened in 1986, this oasis of serenity has attracted considerable media attention thanks to dozens of celebrities who have "spa-ed" here. No more than twenty-four guests at a time attend this posh hideaway sequestered on 150 acres. Cal-a-Vie demands that you invest 100 percent of yourself; chores are left to an attentive staff of seventy. During the year, there are coed weeks as well as exclusive women's weeks. The standard program runs Sunday to Sunday.

Guests stay in European-inspired cottages furnished with a country French decor. The huge armoire could go empty because fitness attire is provided—right down to jacket and sweatpants—fresh daily. The ambience is egalitarian; you can even wear your sweats to dinner and feel comfortable. The king-size bed is turned down each evening, but don't expect a chocolate truffle on your pillow! The calorie count, presided over by Chef Steven Pernetti, is 1,200, but it can be adjusted to fit individual requirements.

The day begins at 6:15 A.M. with a before-breakfast hike that revs up the system for what is ahead. To soften the "boot camp" agenda, there is a break at 10:50 A.M. when a tray with beautifully arranged fruit and glass mugs filled with vegetable broth is delivered to the lounge. By 1:00 P.M. guests have challenged their heart rate with aerobic circuit training, sports training, and a killer abdominals class, as well as water volleyball when the sun is shining (about 320 days a year!). And before you can say "aromatherapy," the day has slipped away and it is time for dinner at 7:00 P.M.

Everyone starts their spa journey with a fitness assessment, so this is the time to set your goal, whether the focus is weight loss, inch loss, or—the best goal of all—to attain a healthier lifestyle. Cal-a-Vie offers a concentrated spa program designed to produce results. Fitness is enhanced by daily spa treatments ranging from two-hour European hydrotherapy treatments and body scrubs to daily massages and a series of three facials. The beauty salon offers the finishing touches, from hand and foot treatments to scalp treatments. Special women's weeks (approximately sixteen per year) have a sorority-house feel, but without the agonizing over finals!

Three evenings a week feature lectures on nutrition, stress, and current health topics. On Friday nights Chef Pernetti shares spa secrets on how to prepare the recipes used throughout the week. A typical menu might include vine-ripened tomato salad with fresh mozzarella and basil, asparagus-stuffed chicken breast,

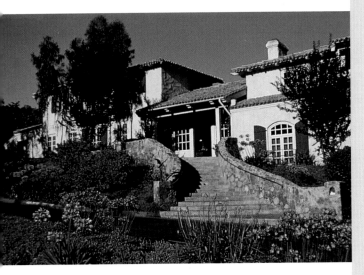

roasted red peppers, grilled zucchini, and potatoes with roasted garlic sauce. Desserts are consistently beguiling—the chocolate mousse made with tofu and maple syrup is a perfect example.

If you can splurge on one spa experience this year, Cal-a-Vie would be the place to consider for a concentrated one-week program.

Breathe to Destress

Many spas offer guests strategies for stress management, because stress is considered the disease of our time by many health and fitness professionals. One recommendation for coping with stress is through proper breathing. We should all learn to breathe deeply. When under stress, oxygen requirements increase. Breathing abdominally is energizing, yet will calm the mind and body. Breathe in to a comfortable count, such as six or twelve, and hold for the same length if possible or to a natural point. Then exhale to the same count. This method of "cycle breathing" is effective in maximizing oxygen intake and carbon waste removal. This psycho-physio therapy is one way of dealing with stress.

Oasis of Serenity and Service

Cal-a-Vie
2249 Somerset Road
Vista, CA 92084
Phone: (760) 945–2055
Fax: (760) 630–0074
E-mail: info@cal-a-vie.com
Web site: www.cal-a-vie.com
Season: Year-round
Owners: John and Terri Havens
General Manager: Deborah Zie
Spa Director: Deborah Zie
Fitness Director: Judy Wood
Reservations: (760) 945–2055
Spa Appointments: (760) 945–2055
Accommodations: Twenty-four guest cottages, individually decorated in the style of a European country villa with hand-carved furniture and pastel floral chintz fabrics; private terraces.
Meals: Carefully prepared spa cuisine with low calorie count built around herbs, fruits, and vegetables from the spa's own gardens; flavors are Provençal and Mediterranean style.
Facilities: Gym with state-of-the-art equipment; tennis courts; adjacent private golf club; swimming pool; hydrotherapy pool.
Services & Special Programs: Cooking classes; individualized fitness courses; morning and afternoon hikes; massages; aromatherapy; seaweed wraps; skin, hair, hand, and foot treatments; evening lectures on various healthy living topics; hydrotherapy; reflexology.
Rates: $$$
Best Spa Package: The three-night La Petite Week, at $2,495 with Sunday arrival and Wednesday departure, includes three meals a day, accommodations, fitness classes, two massages, one reflexology, one hydrotherapy, one facial, and one hair and scalp. The seven-night California Plan is $4,995.
Credit Cards: American Express, MasterCard, VISA
Getting There: The spa is 40 miles from San Diego International Airport; complimentary transfers provided on Sunday.
What's Nearby: This 150-acre site is in a secluded valley north of San Diego, yet close to all the San Diego area attractions, shopping, and beach.

THE CENTURY PLAZA HOTEL AND SPA
Los Angeles, California

Whether you arrive at the hotel's 35,000 square-foot Spa Mystique via the VIP entrance on Constellation Boulevard or simply pick up the phone in a chic, sleek guestroom to make an appointment, you will be made to feel welcome at this serene spa. Whether you are a weary traveler arriving from a long-haul flight or a member of a wedding party spending the day, you will find this heart-of-the-city oasis to be a serious spa. The two-story structure, which looks like an office building from the outside, was once a popular Japanese restaurant. Today, thanks to a complete overhaul, it has emerged as the city's largest hotel-based spa staffed by professionals who can personally create programs for individuals and groups.

The building's design has brought together the elements of water, fire, metal, and earth with the goal of symbolizing harmony. Feng shui played a vital role in the design, according to Sylvia Sepielli, a world-class design consultant. The impact of such a soothing environment, enhanced by quiet music, is immediate. For those needing some positive energy after the demands of travel have taken their toll, this is the spa where you can pull yourself back together with treatments such as Mystique Yang facial, designed especially for men, or a Twin Tigers massage performed by two therapists.

As you leave the hectic traffic of overurbanized LA to experience the spa menu, whether it be a single treatment or a full day, the feeling of peace and calm is nearly overwhelming. First, check in at the small desk. After wrapping up in a kimono-style bathrobe, experience the Japanese tea ceremony and then relax in a traditional *furo* pool (which is deep and designed for quiet bathing). Bathing at Spa Mystique is an art form, with four varieties of experiences, including a Vichy shower. Imported from France, it provides a mild shower of water with alternating temperature and pressure and is the ideal way to prepare for more intensive massages, such as shiatsu, Thai, and aro-

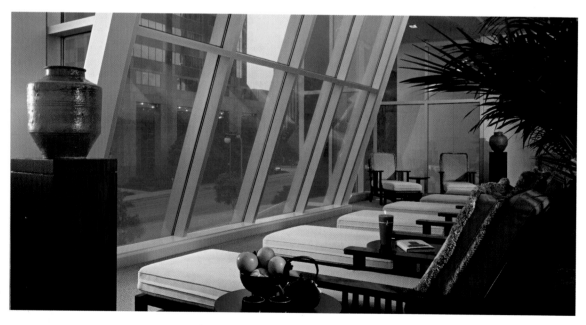

matherapy. A feeling of calm permeates the spa and, without exception, is echoed throughout the building. In the lounge, with views of the city, one still feels enveloped in a protective cocoon.

Having the convenience of a serious hotel linked to a spa with services to satisfy the business and pleasure traveler is a challenge. The Century Plaza Hotel & Spa has set an example by combining spa treatments, a 4,500-square-foot gym with cardiovascular equipment and weight-training machines, private fitness counseling, and a delightful spa cafe with reasonable prices. Travelers contemplating a stopover in Los Angeles will find this approach to wellness a worthwhile experience, from the first sip of Japanese tea to the warm towels waiting for them after their Akasuri scrub.

Traveling Tooth Tips

Travelers should change their toothbrush monthly and when traveling should keep it in a separate container to fend off bacteria, according to Diane McLaughlin, a Palm Springs dental hygienist.

"Never leave your toothbrush out on the bathroom counter," McLaughlin advises, because the cleaning staff might spray the brush head with chemicals. Portable battery-operated toothbrushes are ideal to pack, especially when traveling internationally.

McLaughlin advises gently massaging gums and methodically brushing teeth in the morning and before bed. It's not easy to find a dentist in the Seychelles Islands or the Great Barrier Reef at a moment's notice! Dental care is important, and you should pack an ample supply of toothpaste, a nonalcohol mouthwash, dental floss, and other favorite implements with you in a separate plastic case. Be wary of purchasing toothpaste and other dental products in a foreign country unless you are certain the ingredients will not harm your veneers, crowns, or implants.

Serenity in Glamour Central

Century Plaza Hotel and Spa
2025 Avenue of the Stars-Century City
Los Angeles, CA 90067
Phone: (310) 277–2000
Fax: (310) 551–3355
Season: Year-round
General Manager: William A. Hall
Spa Manager: Diego Heredia
Reservations: (800) 937–8461; spa direct (877) 544–2256 or (310) 556–2256.
Accommodations: 724 renovated rooms make this a stylish urban resort. With its new image as a full-service resort in the heart of LA's west side, all rooms feature double and king-size Heavenly Beds, which invite guests to curl up and relax; three telephones; comfortable robes; deluxe bath amenities; individual climate control; and a private bar.
Meals: The Spa Cafe, open for breakfast and lunch, has an excellent variety of specialty salads, wraps, and desserts. There are healthy beverages, including teas and fruit juices. The hotel's only restaurant, Breeze, seats 250 and focuses on fresh, seasonal cuisine with a California grill menu.
Facilities: Located on seven exquisitely landscaped acres with a swimming pool, lounge areas, and the new 35,000-square-foot Spa Mystique. There is a 4,500-square-foot fully equipped gym with cardiovascular equipment, personal training services, and fitness classes.
Services & Special Programs: The full-service spa has twenty-seven treatment rooms and four outdoor treatment cabanas. Of special note is a private entrance on Constellation Boulevard, much appreciated by celebrities, and a secluded "west wing," ideal for day-spa guests, groups, and those hosting a special event, such as a spa day for wedding parties, birthdays, and business gatherings. The Yamaguchi Salon offers hair styling, makeup, manicure, and pedicure services.
Rates: $$$
Best Spa Package: Executive Escape is five to six hours and includes a signature Akasuri scrub, Sleeping Tiger Massage, Mystique yin/yang facial, lunch at Cafe Mystique, and a Hayaku manicure and pedicure for $295. There are no packages that include room stays.
Credit cards: Most major
Getting There: Twenty-five minutes from the Los Angeles International Airport
What's nearby: Century City Shopping Center and Marketplace, five minutes from Beverly Hills, ten minutes from West Hollywood. Easy access to the Getty Center and Museum, the Museum of Tolerance, the Armand Hammer Museum, the Santa Monica Pier, Universal Studios/City Walk and downtown, and the Museum of Contemporary Art.

THE GOLDEN DOOR
Escondido, California

The Golden Door, the stellar spa that set the stage for the others, has retained its crown by keeping pace with the times, from the personalized spa day to cuisine that thwarts pounds while satisfying even the fussiest guest. Awards are too numerous to list. The highest accolades range from its being rated the number one spa in the *Robb Report*'s 1998 "Best of the Best" to its coveted rating as the number one spa in America by *Zagat's U.S. Hotel, Resort and Spa Guide* every year since that survey began in 1988.

The Golden Door opened in 1958 and from the beginning has added programs that reflect the changing needs of men and women: fitness classes, creative

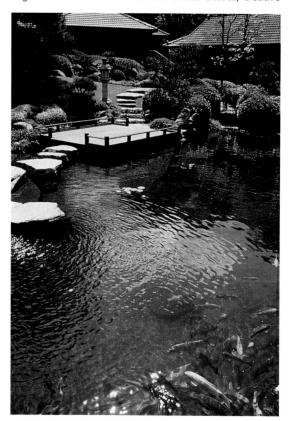

spa cuisine for specific dietary requirements, and perfectly maintained accommodations. The spa accepts only thirty-nine guests on a seven-day program that begins each Sunday. There are more than four staff members per guest, including twenty-two instructors in the fitness department, each with a university degree. You'll get a perfect night's rest after putting yourself through a plethora of classes, ranging from sunrise hiking to tap or jazz dancing, from weight training and water volleyball to strength and flexibility classes. The day is a harmonious schedule of upbeat fitness in the morning tempered by a generous array of passive activities later in the day.

In addition to a conventional daily massage, you can choose from aromatherapy, seaweed thalassotherapy, moortherapy, and deep-cleansing facials that combine mineral masques with chamomile. A personal exercise therapist is assigned to each guest for the entire week with the goal of overseeing the schedule and charting daily progress.

The weather is year-round perfect in this 377-acre rural corner of San Diego County, 30 miles north of San Diego and 8 miles north of Escondido. Sunny days here number 341, making it one of the most geographically desirable spots in the United States. In this utopian setting, the Golden Door unfolds its serene Japanese theme, reflected in the bell courtyard, sand garden, and architecture. Each guest is given a Japanese *yukata* (cotton robe) along with warm-up clothing, T-shirts, and shorts. The "uniform" is a great equalizer and takes the competitive edge off dressing up (or down, as the case may be).

The spa's inclusive gourmet menus, prepared by noted spa cuisine chef and author Michel Stroot, feature healthful, natural foods—many from on-site organic vegetable gardens and fruit orchards. The evenings are reserved for guest lecturers. The informative topics range from cooking demonstrations and

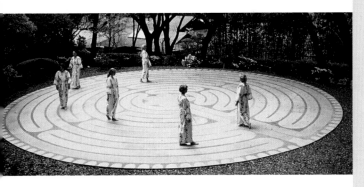

lifestyle programs to stress management and dried flower arranging.

Deborah Szekely, founder of Rancho La Puerta in 1940, created the Golden Door's programs, the first destination spa recognized for lavish personalized service in a stunning Asian ambience. With dedication and ability to change with the times, the Golden Door legend continues to flourish and recharge the lives of those who participate in its time-tested program.

Tips to Improve Your Body Image

You don't have to change your appearance to improve the way you feel about your body. Find ways to regularly give your self-esteem a boost: Stop reinforcing the negative. Every time you say to yourself, "I hate my flabby thighs," you reinforce exactly what you don't want. Focus on your attributes. Make a list of the things about your appearance that you like. If you don't like something about your body that you can't change, make peace with it. Replace judgments about your body with real knowledge and understanding of how your body works. Focus more on health and energy than on appearance. Increase your awareness of your physical self. Monitor your body for areas of stress or tension (relax your shoulders, etc., at least once an hour). Before you eat, calm yourself and check in with your body to see if food is really what you need at that time.

The Golden Door
P.O. Box 463077
Escondido, CA 92046-3077
Phone: (760) 744–5777
Fax: (760) 471–2393
Web site: www.goldendoor.com

Season: Year-round

General Manager: Rachel Caldwell

Spa Director: Judy Bird

Fitness Director: Judy Bird

Reservations: (760) 744–5777 or (800) 424-0777

Accommodations: Thirty-nine private guest rooms, with shoji screens, black jalousie windows, CD players, outdoor decks, and private gardens.

Meals: All meals and snacks are included in the stay. Pre-hike, midmorning, and late afternoon snacks are provided. Hors d'oeuvres are served in the early evening; dinner is in the dining room.

Facilities: This is a self-contained destination spa whose 377 acres are filled with hiking trails, gardens, groves, a lake, and two swimming pools. The 45,000-square-foot facility contains a boutique, beauty court, three lounges, dining room, two gyms, and a bathhouse.

Services & Special Programs: Private lessons and consultations; archery and fencing; evening lectures and demonstrations; all clothing provided; special dietary needs; weekly cooking class; library; personal laundry service; safety deposit boxes. Men's weeks are scheduled five times yearly in March, June, September, November, and December. Coed weeks are four times yearly in March, June, September, and December. Otherwise all women.

Rates: $$$

Best Spa Package: There are summer and special rates, such as coed weeks. The regular week includes meals, accommodations, all fitness classes, and six body treatments for one weekly fee of $5,975, plus room tax.

Credit Cards: American Express, MasterCard, VISA

Getting There: Limousine pickup and return Sundays is complimentary from the San Diego International Airport (forty-five-minute drive). By car: from Orange County's John Wayne Airport (ninety minutes) and from Los Angeles International Airport (three hours).

What's Nearby: All San Diego area attractions: Old Globe Theatre, Old Town, Tijuana, SeaWorld, Wild Animal Park, La Jolla.

THE OAKS AT OJAI

Ojai, California

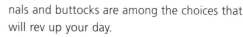

Just being in the lively art community of Ojai melts away stress. The Oaks opened in this small town in Ventura County—ninety minutes from Los Angeles—in 1977. It inhabited a former country inn that had held landmark status since the 1920s. Since its inception, the spa has hosted nearly 50,000 health seekers who have reveled in the Oaks program created by Sheila Cluff. Cluff, a former professional figure skater and physical education teacher, has devoted her energy over the last forty-plus years to spreading the fitness gospel.

The Oaks keeps the cost of this spa experience at an affordable level without sacrificing a quality fitness, nutrition, skin-care, and wellness program. From the moment you enter the intimate inn, you will be surrounded by a beehive of activity. Announcements remind guests of evening lectures, menu choices, and special events. There is hardly an idle moment.

The majority of the spa's guests are executive women who enjoy a nonstop schedule that starts at 6:30 A.M. with a mountain hike and ends with a stimulating evening program, covering anything from Ukrainian egg decorating to lectures by well-known authors.

Fifteen optional fitness classes daily provide ample opportunity for those who are serious about shaping up. Low-impact aerobics, aqua-toning, yoga, and classes geared toward shaping up the abdominals and buttocks are among the choices that will rev up your day.

Three gourmet, low-calorie meals are served daily. There is a broth break at 10:45 A.M. and a happy hour, featuring juice cocktails, at 5:15 P.M. The basic 1,000-calories-a-day menu designed by Chef David Dal Nagro is imaginative and nutritious. Alternative menus, such as those for high-fiber, high-protein, athletic, or vegetarian diets, may be ordered.

The Spa Sanctuary has a eucalyptus steam room, redwood sauna, indoor whirlpool, and locker room. The adjacent gym has Lifecycles, StairMasters, treadmills, and Paramount equipment. A facial and massage department features aromatherapy, body scrubs, reflexology, a full-service beauty salon, a nail salon, and a well-stocked boutique in case you lose so many pounds and inches you need to freshen up your wardrobe.

The staff-to-guest ratio is one to three, which means everyone receives ample personal attention in this casual and informal setting. Personal trainers are available for yoga, weight training, and even ballroom dancing.

The Oaks is situated in the heart of downtown Ojai, surrounded by boutiques, antiques shops, and a noticeable absence of fast-food outlets. Guests have ample opportunity to explore the area. Pack only the essentials—a warm-up suit, fitness wear, and hiking/ biking shoes—to blend into this unpretentious environment.

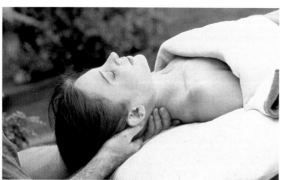

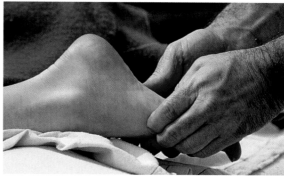

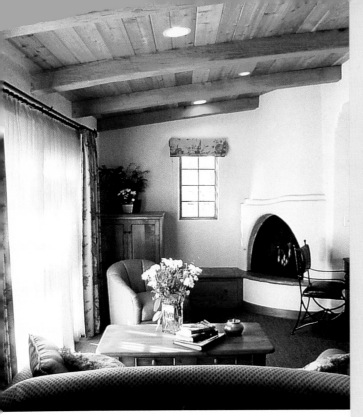

The Oaks at Ojai
122 East Ojai Avenue
Ojai, CA 93023
Phone: (805) 646–5573
Fax: (805) 640–1504
E-mail: info@oaksspa.com
Web site: www.oaksspa.com

Season: Year-round

Owners: Sheila and Don Cluff

General Manager: Dietrich Pahnke

Activities Director: Elizabeth Horton

Reservations: (800) 753–6257

Spa Appointments: (805) 646–5573 (for day use)

Accommodations: Forty-six guest rooms, including private rooms, double lodge rooms, double cottage rooms, and three new spacious suites with fireplaces.

Meals: Three meals a day with menus based on 1,000 calories per day; alternative menus and additional dishes offered. Meals are served in the dining room and poolside.

Facilities: Swimming pool, whirlpools, saunas, Lifecycles, StairMasters, treadmills; hiking and biking; special area for women includes a locker room, eucalyptus steam room, redwood sauna, indoor whirlpool, and washrooms/showers. Handicap accessible.

Services & Special Programs: Full range of fitness classes; treatments a la carte: reflexology, aromatherapy, massages, facials, body scrubs, paraffin treatments, manicures/pedicures; hair salon, acupuncture, body analysis, private fitness consultation. Special weekend and weekday programs on such topics as spa cuisine, yoga, and feng shui. Theme weeks (water aerobics, hiking, and biking) with guest instructors.

Rates: $

Best Spa Package: The seven-night package, which includes accommodations in a standard double room, three meals daily, activities, and two complimentary treatments. The base price is $1,085 per person.

Credit Cards: Most major

Getting There: The spa is located in northern Ventura County, two hours from the Los Angeles International Airport and forty-five minutes from Santa Barbara. Inquire about shuttle services when making your reservation. Rental cars are also an option.

What's Nearby: The Ojai Music Festival at the Libby Bowl, for four nights in May and June, is an annual event.

Exercise "For the Road"

Sheila Cluff, founder of this popular health spa, was so sure that a mere five minutes of daily exercise could be beneficial she implemented a study on the concept at Cornell University. Ultimately, along with Toni McBride and Mary Tabacchi, she authored a book about her revolutionary findings. The book, *Take 5,* outlines an exercise program that even travels well, according to Cluff. Cluff recommends assembling an exercise kit that includes exercise clothing appropriate for your destination, proper footwear, a tape player and extra batteries, a variety of tapes that include some for unwinding following busy days on the road, a few exercise videos in case your hotel room has a VCR, and your favorite bath products (aromatherapy essential oils and lotions are a good choice) to help you relax before you retire for the night.

OJAI VALLEY INN & SPA

Ojai, California

Just getting to Ojai will raise your spirits. And by the time you reach the narrow country road that leads you to the historic Ojai Valley Inn & Spa, you'll understand why filmmaker Frank Capra chose this valley to depict Shangri-la in his 1937 classic movie, *Lost Horizon*. Surrounded by the Topa Topa Mountains, this 206-room inn, set on 220 scenic acres and designed in the Andalusian Spanish architectural style, conveys casual elegance.

The spa portion of the Mediterranean-style village creates a self-contained cocoon where guests leave the world of cellular phones, computers, deadlines, and stress behind. The spa consists of twenty-eight treatment rooms and the 1,600-square-foot mind/body center with a fully equipped exercise room, a cardiovascular workout area, and a studio for yoga, Spinning, meditation, and tai chi.

The centerpiece of the spa experience is the Kuyam, a fifty-minute purifying session that in Native American Chumash culture means a "place to rest together." This communal experience starts with a self-application of cleansing clay, followed by guided meditation. Herb-infused steam softens the mud (and you!) before you walk through a Swiss shower. After the shower, lotion is gently applied, and you are rewrapped in warm linen and led to the outdoor loggia to rest. If the treatment sounds tempting, consider the Ojai honey body masque, the elderberry herbal wrap, and the orange blossom facial as well.

Enhancing the spa treatment program is a schedule of mind/body classes that begin daily

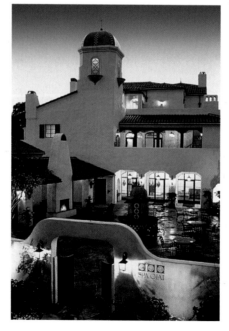

with morning walks, yoga, and hikes. The last classes of the day begin at 5:00 P.M. and include guided meditation, healing bowls, and Spinning. Because Ojai stands as an internationally known art community, the spa, not surprisingly, offers a comprehensive list of enrichment/art programs from basic watercolor to landscape painting.

The newest program at the spa is a health assessment developed by Florence Comite, M.D., which includes a complete physical examination, nutritional evaluation, and lab tests.

Cuisine stresses the use of local ingredients, ranging from seafood to produce. Maravilla is the signature restaurant of the resort. Other dining spots offer casual outdoor dining and spa cuisine.

This is no ordinary spa, and neither is the inn's 3,500-square-foot ultraluxurious penthouse with private elevator, treatment room, sauna, indoor and outdoor fireplaces, and whirlpools. The terrace of the indulgent retreat provides an ideal spot to view Ojai's legendary "pink moment"— when sunsets and the sky reveal a marvelous panoply of pink.

The resort's 6,235-yard, par-70 golf course has hosted seven Senior PGA Tour events and the EMC Golf Skills Challenge televised by NBC Sports. If golf isn't your game, visit the inn's 800-acre ranch and stables with horseback riding for all levels. The Ojai Valley Inn & Spa is one of those rare destinations offering something for everyone, including Camp Ojai—a children's program operating year-round.

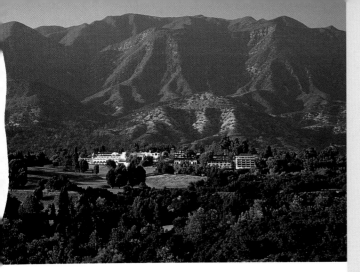

A Creative Spa Experience in a Village Hideaway

Ojai Valley Inn & Spa
Country Club Road
Ojai, CA 93023
Phone: (805) 646–5511
Fax: (805) 640–0305
Web site: www.ojairesort.com or www.spaojai.com

Season: Year-round
Managing Director: Thad Hyland
General Manager: Anna Olson
Spa Director: Suzy Bordeau-Johlfs
Mind/Body Manager: Kent Burden
Reservations: (805) 646–5511 or (800) 422–6524
Spa Appointments: (805) 640–2000 or (888) SPA–OJAI
Accommodations: Deluxe guest rooms and suites, many with private balconies or patios, all with king-size or double-queen beds, minibars, hair dryers, personal amenities.
Meals: Maravilla for Pacific Provincial cooking and panoramic mountain views; the Oak Grill & Terrace for casual lunches and dinners; the Club Bar for light fare, wine, and cocktails. Light fare lunches, drinks, and snacks served poolside. Room service available.
Facilities: Championship golf course; weight room, workout area; horseback riding; spa with treatment rooms, whirlpools, steam rooms, sunbathing loggias, hair and nail salon, lap/exercise pool; meditation garden; four tennis courts (four lighted); meeting center; two heated swimming pools; jogging and bicycling trails.
Services & Special Programs: Camp Ojai children's program for ages three to twelve; bird-watching; wine tours; shopping; jeep tours; health assessment program; gardening and art classes.
Rates: $$
Best Spa Package: The Spa Ojai Discovery Package includes a luxurious guest room, welcome gift, unlimited use of spa facilities and mind/body center, and two spa treatments per person, per night; rates start at $318 per person, per night, double occupancy. A two-night stay is required. Tax and gratuities not included.
Credit Cards: Most major
Getting There: The resort is 73 miles northwest of Los Angeles, 35 miles southeast of Santa Barbara, and 14 miles from the Pacific Ocean. Airport transfers can be arranged through the concierge desk.
What's Nearby: Lake Casitas, with boating, kayaking, and fishing; the town of Ojai, with art galleries, boutiques, cafes; Santa Barbara and Ventura attractions.

Signature Blends for the Perfect Massage

The spa at Ojai Valley Inn has blended eight specialty massage oils and a massage lotion that guests may choose from when experiencing their massages. The specialty blends are attributed to certain massage goals—you choose your goal and enjoy!

Creative Energies: grapefruit, lemon, bergamot, and jasmine

Ojai Elements: French lavender, sage, and bitter orange

Health Potential: vanilla, sandalwood, sweet orange, and ylang-ylang

Vital Energy: lavender and rosemary

Protection: eucalyptus, rosemary, peppermint, and spearmint

Ojai Dreams (to promote tranquility): lavender, geranium, ylang ylang, and tangerine

Citrus Grove (to promote healthy circulation and relieve tension): tangerine, lemon, orange, and grapefruit

Pink Moments (to relieve muscle and joint discomfort): juniper, cypress, pine, rosemary, grapefruit, lime, and lemongrass

Indian Summer (stimulates circulation to promote detixification): lemongrass and ginger

PALM SPRINGS DESERT RESORTS: SPA TOWN

Palm Springs, California

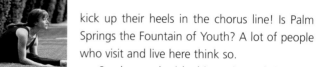

Palm Springs has been blessed with more than enough spas to keep visitors rejuvenated—all year round. Nestled between the San Jacinto and Santa Rosa Mountains, the area affords views of peaks glistening with snow in the desert sunshine. The Agua Caliente Indians flocked here in centuries past, and their sacred healing waters have evolved into the essence of the spa experience here today.

Discovered in the 1930s by the movie industry, Palm Spring's prominence accelerated during World War II when General George S. Patton chose the area to train more than a million troops just east of Palm Springs. In addition, the U.S. Army established an air base and a general hospital.

The movie stars who flocked to the area left legendary marks and hideaway homes that still attract sight-seers. Today many celebrities retire here, often taking up second careers. At the Fabulous Palm Springs Follies, long-legged lovelies (as producer Rif Markowitz refers to them) must be fifty years or older in order to kick up their heels in the chorus line! Is Palm Springs the Fountain of Youth? A lot of people who visit and live here think so.

Spa-lovers cherish this oasis, and day spas continue to proliferate along El Paseo, the resort area's legendary shopping avenue that features a tree-lined promenade accentuated by contemporary outdoor sculpture. The El Paseo directory lists more than 150 expert aestheticians, manicurists, and hairstylists, who staff more than fifty spas and beauty salons along this chic avenue. It is obvious that the healthy, wealthy, and wise are serious about looking good for the charity events and the society pages. This social whirl monopolizes the season (November through April) with nonstop golf and tennis tournaments and the endless array of parties for charitable causes.

This environment is paradise for spa-lovers. The Palm Springs Desert Resorts Convention and Visitors Bureau lists twenty-two spas in the immediate area, and there are dozens more in nearby Desert Hot Springs, where

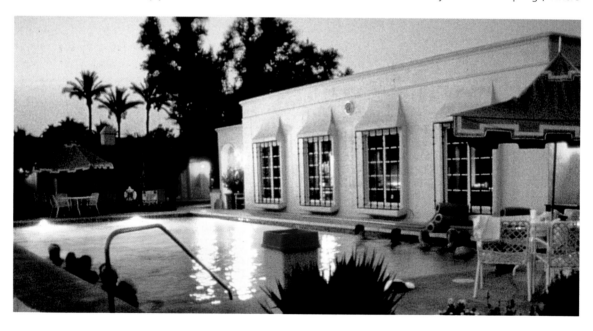

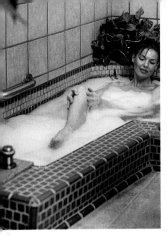
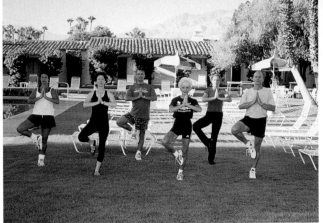
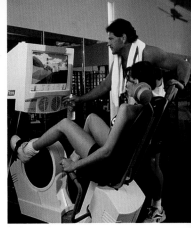

smaller spas beckon with healing waters.

Here is our list of the best spa resorts offering a complete range of spa programs, from one-day packages to a full week of fitness, spa dining, and treatments.

Marriott's Desert Springs Resort & Spa

74855 Country Club Drive
Palm Desert, CA 92260
Phone: (760) 341–1865 or (800) 255–0848
Fax: (760) 341–1846

Although the resort is a magnet for conferences, the full-service spa is off on its own, creating a more private feel within this immense resort property.

Rancho Las Palmas Marriott Resort & Spa

41000 Bob Hope Drive
Rancho Mirage, CA 92270
Phone: (760) 568–2727
Spa reservations: (800) 228–9290
Fax: (760) 568–5845

Two-level spa with twenty-six treatment rooms features spa cuisine at Fresca's.

The Palms at Palm Springs

572 North Indian Canyon Way
Palm Springs, CA 92262
Phone: (760) 325–1111
Spa reservations: (800) 753–7256
Fax: (760) 327–0867

This is a serious spa resort, housed in a historic structure; the ambience is hospitable and friendly. Under the guidance of Sheila Cluff, one of the world's leading health and fitness experts, the well-qualified staff shepherds guests through a comprehensive health and fitness experience. Marilu Rogers, general manager, directs hikes beginning at 6:00 A.M.; sixteen classes for all fitness levels, from walks to water classes, fill the remainder of the day. The all-inclusive rate is one of the desert's best spa values.

Hyatt Grand Champions Resort and Spa

44-600 Indian Wells Lane
Indian Wells, CA 92210
Phone: (760) 341–1000 or (800) 223–1234
Fax: (760) 674–4382

This 30,000 square foot spa, with an emphasis on anti-aging, is the newest spa in the desert. Its spa menu is diverse. Guests will find accommodations at the resort luxurious. The resort has access to excellent golf and tennis, as well.

La Quinta Resort & Club

49-499 Eisenhower Drive
La Quinta, CA 92253
Phone: (760) 564–4111 or (800) 598–3828
Fax: (760) 564–5723

This resort marks the debut of the WellMax Clinic, which, under the supervision of Dan Cosgrove M.D., provides a detailed medical history and analysis of those seeking more than a routine physical. This evaluation may be linked to determining your spa services and exercise program at Spa La Quinta.

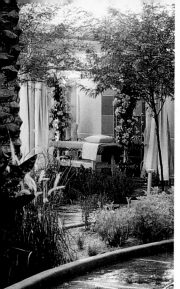
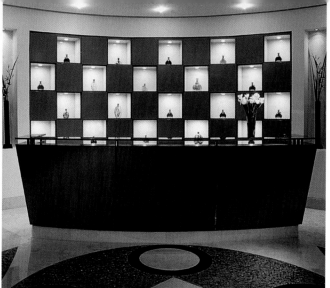
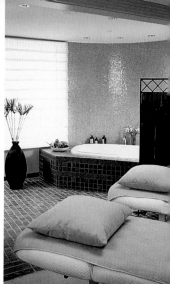

Estrella

415 South Belardo Rd.
Palm Springs, CA 92262
Phone: (760) 320–4117 or (800) 237–3687
Fax: (760) 323–3303

An ultra-private five-acre retreat built in the 1920s and exquisitely renovated to reflect today's hip spa culture. From outdoor tsunami showers to couple's treatments, this vintage resort represents glamour "under the sun."

Spa Esmeralda: Renaissance Esmeralda Resort and Spa

44-000 Indian Wells Lane
Indian Wells, California
Phone: (760) 773–4444

An oasis of absolute tranquility and beauty, the 13,000-square-foot Spa Esmeralda features nineteen indoor and outdoor treatments rooms and lush gardens with waterfalls. A wide variety of personal treatments, including massage and facial therapies and skin and body care, are offered. Facial therapies feature freshly made skincare products from the Body Deli. The men's and women's areas, furnished in elegant woods and granite, have private relaxation lounges where complimentary ayurvedic teas, coffee, and flavored waters are served.

The Spa Hotel & Casino

100 North Indian Avenue
Palm Springs, CA 92262
Phone: (760) 325–1461
Reservations: (800) 854–1279
Fax: (760) 778–1519

The building is classic 1960s-style architecture. The spa's traditional treatments, such as massage and facials, feature the legendary mineral water that helped put Palm Springs on the map. The spa boasts two outdoor mineral pools. The Spa Experience is a forty-five-minute treatment that includes steam, sauna, eucalyptus inhalation, mineral bath, and a relaxation room. This is a popular choice for those casino-goers wanting a quick rejuvenation. The spa is best considered for day use.

Two Bunch Palms Resort and Spa

67-425 Two Bunch Palms Trail
Desert Hot Springs, CA 92240-6034
Phone: (760) 329–8791 or (800) 472–4334

Two Bunch Palms, one of the most interesting resorts in Southern California and the world, caters to the elite of the entertainment and corporate worlds. It is an oasis of elegant informality in splendid isolation. The spa's natural mineral water is enriched with green clay noted for its healing qualities. The secret plan of Two Bunch Palms is absolutely no plan at all. There are no structured exercise programs, no regimented schedules, and no calorie-restricted diets. Resort facilities include forty-four guest casitas and villas, a restaurant and spa, several hot mineral water pools, a man-made lake, two lighted tennis courts, a grotto swimming pool, mud-bath treatment rooms, outdoor salt rooms with steam baths, and sun deck.

Swiss Health Resort

66-729 Eighth Street
Desert Hot Springs, CA 92240
Phone: (760) 329–6912
Fax: (760) 329–5641

Relief from stress and arthritis to stiffness and pain in bones and joints is found in the hot mineral waters at Swiss Health Spa. The specialty is Swiss water massage—massage while you float in the pool. This desert retreat's program also includes a standard massage that is a combination of Swedish, deep tissue, trigger points, stretching, joint mobilization, and reflexology. A popular specialty is the spa's Swiss-style breakfast buffet featuring meusli.

An Apple a Day

If there is one recipe that can start your day on a healthy note, Bircher Meusli is it. Prepared from scratch every morning at the Swiss Health Resort in Desert Hot Springs, California, owner Ursula Furer says "Meusli aids in digestion," because it is preservative free and calls for fresh ingredients.

This traditional recipe proves that "an apple a day" can keep the doctor at bay (serves 4).

Bircher Meusli
    1 oz. oatmeal flakes, freshly rolled
    1 oz. wheat flakes, from the whole grain
    1 cup plain yogurt
    2 oz. grated nuts (filberts, almonds)
    4 large apples, unpeeled and grated

Soak the flakes overnight in a little water; mix with yogurt, nuts, and apples. Serve fresh.

Stellar Spas in the Desert Sun

Palm Springs Desert Resorts

Getting There: The Palm Springs International Airport is three minutes from downtown Palm Springs and is served by the following airlines: Alaska Airlines, American Airlines, American Eagle, American West Express, United Airlines, USAir Express/Northwest Airlines, and Canadian Airlines.

What's Nearby: For information contact the Palm Springs Desert Resorts Convention and Visitors Authority, 69–030 Highway 111, Suite 201, Rancho Mirage, CA 92277; Phone: (760) 770–9000; (800) 42–RELAX (reservations in the United States and Canada); Fax: (760) 770–9001; Web site: palmspringsusa.com. The bureau covers the desert resort communities of Palm Springs, Palm Desert, Cathedral City, Indian Wells, Indio, Rancho Mirage, and Desert Hot Springs.

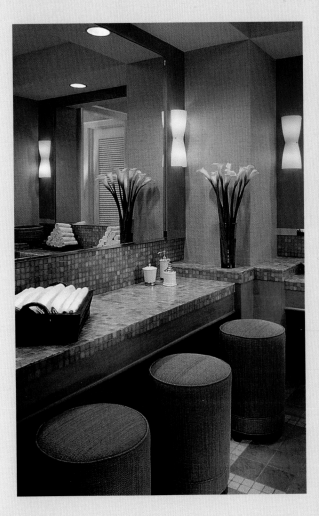

THE POST RANCH INN
Big Sur, California

Stunning and dramatic from the moment you veer off California State Highway 1, the Post Ranch Inn has a sense of place and spirit attracting those who want to strike out on their own when it comes to a free-form spa experience.

Symbolizing the independent, spiritual side of the spa experience, with more emphasis on individual needs rather than a structured program, the Post Ranch Inn, rich in history but avant garde in design, beckons those who are receptive to the essence of the spa experience without the benefit of a state-of-the-art megagym or a ready staff to serve every need. This spa reflects nonconformity, and it works harmoniously with those who march to a different drummer.

When you check in, you leave your television, car, and cell phone behind. Your car is whisked away upon arrival, and after a few days you may never want to see it again. Replace all that civilization has wrought with the dramatic majesty of the Big Sur's rugged coastline, studded with redwood trees and framed by mountains.

Put yourself in this picture, and you are at the threshold of one of North America's stellar resort destinations,

a totally controlled environment where you can contemplate, meditate, and challenge yourself, spiritually and physically, in the lap of luxury.

This is definitely a no-stress zone, and those who want to be alone with their thoughts or their partner will find the ambience made to order. Designed to take advantage of views that overwhelm and ultimately calm, the infinite boundary of the Pacific Ocean sets the stage for spa treatments that transcend the ordinary. South on Highway 1 about twenty minutes from the Post Ranch Inn is the Esalen Insititute, a retreat center known for its educational offerings on personal growth. The Post Ranch Inn has therapists schooled there who are on the cutting edge of bodywork and massage. All of this positive energy has led the Post Ranch Inn to offer two-night theme programs throughout the year, such as the Outdoor Inspiration, and to implement more New Age treatments, such as spa-tested crystal and gemstone therapy designed by Patricia Edge.

The goal of this 90-minute treatment is to clear blocked energy; the therapist uses smooth Big Sur jade and other carefully selected gemstones that are

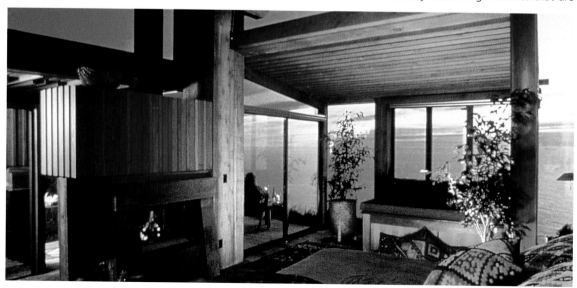

positioned on the seven chakras. For those who are intrepid and who are willing to go beyond chocolate scrubs and blueberry facials, there are specialized therapies: craniosacral, reiki, reflexology, and Thai massage.

Post Ranch Inn treatments, including some facials, can be done in guest rooms, even if it means bringing it all to a tree house! Cuisine, though not specifically conforming to strict guidelines, is inventive and fresh, and Executive Chef Craig von Foerster and his staff handle special requests gracefully.

Some call the Post Ranch Inn nirvana. It's a protective perch jutting above the Pacific Ocean, where a fortunate few enjoy their days and evenings with their heart's desires: a quiet hike, steeping in the basking pool, or simply chilling out. And the day doesn't end with a magical sunset. Enhancing this romantic spa rendezvous is nightly stargazing with the resort's amateur astronomer.

Best Foot Forward

If you plan to wear sandals or slippers during your spa vacation, take a good look at your feet before your heels and toes sabotage you. There's no excuse for dry patches or swollen or rough cracked heels. Get into the habit of preventing this unsightly situation by taking your feet in hand!

Check out the spa boutique. You'll probably find a selection of foot-care products. The ingredients are designed to alleviate foot discomfort from long airline flights, hiking, and biking.

CCS foot-care cream has as its most important ingredient urea, which aids in softening skin. Masada's mineral foot scrub with peppermint and thyme softens skin while removing rough, dry patches. At the Mandara spas, feet are transformed with shea butter and essential oils of rosemary, cypress, and eucalyptus. Sundance starts treatments with a relaxing fifteen-minute footbath. Why not pamper your feet every day? You will see and feel the difference.

The Post Ranch Inn
Highway One, P.O. Box 219
Big Sur, CA 93920
Phone: (831) 667–2200
Fax: (831) 667–2824
E-mail: info@postranchinn.com
Web site: www.postranchinn.com
Season: Year-round
General Manager: Dan Priano
Spa Director: Monica Jalovec
Reservations: (800) 527–2200
Spa Reservations: (831) 667–2887
Accommodations: Thirty luxurious rooms, all with views. All accommodations reflect high environmental standards. All rooms have a digital music system, king-size bed, wood-burning fireplace, indoor spa tub, in-room massage table, wet bar and complimentary minibar, terry cloth robes, hair dryer, and walking sticks.
Meals: Breakfast is included. The Sierra Mar, with a bar and deck, overlooks the Pacific and serves internationally influenced California cuisine.
Facilities: Lap pool, basking pool, spa with three treatment rooms, a yurt near the pool for yoga and other classes, gift shop, library.
Services & Special Programs: Exploring Big Sur is a must-do hiking experience for guests. Hikes to Pfeiffer Big Sur State Park, Julie Pfeiffer Burns State Park Beach, Molera State Park, Mount Manuel, and a drive and bike tour on the Old Coast Road. At Pfeiffer Beach nude sunbathing is allowed in one out-of-the way section.
Rates: $$$$
Best Spa Package: Guests can select their treatments from the spa menu and combine these with hiking, biking, and complimentary classes. Complimentary guest activities are offered daily with no pressure to participate. Rates are based on single or double occupancy and range from $485 to $935 per room. There is a two-night minimum stay on weekdays and weekends. Treatments range from $115 for a one-hour Post Ranch massage to a two-hour Wild Flower facial ($215). There are two-night/three-day theme weekends.
Credit Cards: All major
Getting There: From the Monterey Airport, forty-five minutes to an hour by car; from San Francisco International Airport, three to three-and-a-half hours by car; and from Los Angeles, seven to eight hours by car.
What's Nearby: Hiking, biking, horseback riding.

WYNDHAM PEAKS RESORT & GOLDEN DOOR SPA

Telluride, Colorado

Up, up, and away if you choose to take the 9,500-foot uphill tram to this spa hideaway in the San Juan Mountain Range, about a ten-minute car trip from Telluride Mountain Village. Within the handsome 174-room Wyndham Hotel is a full-service, 42,000-square-foot spa spread over four levels and honeycombed with forty-four treatment rooms. Many of Golden Door's signature massage techniques and body treatments are offered here. The Southwestern motif throughout the hotel reflects Telluride's colorful history. Not only is this town the site of one of America's most complete spas, it was also the site of Butch Cassidy's first bank robbery in the late nineteenth century.

Considered one of the nation's best ski mountains and rated by readers of *Snow Country* magazine as the most scenic resort in America, the mountain is known for vertical drops of more than 3,000 feet and for some of the most challenging ski trails on the continent.

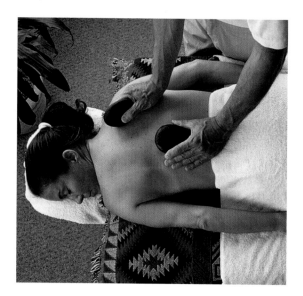

What better place is there to relax after a day on the slopes than at the Golden Door, ranked second among the top five spa resorts in the world by the *Condé Nast Traveler* magazine? And during the summer, hiking and biking opportunities test fitness levels with a challenging terrain.

Here, under one roof, is a spa that has it all, including a Cybex weight room, cardiovascular deck, squash and racquetball courts, an indoor climbing wall, saunas, steam rooms, Jacuzzi, and a water slide that invites swimmers to plunge from an indoor lap pool to a lower-level indoor/outdoor pool. Exercise classes are scheduled throughout the day and can be combined with the latest spa therapy. Reflexology, bindi balancing, reiki, shiatsu, targeted massage with fango, and facials for any skin type are among the offerings from which to choose. It is essential to speak with a spa concierge first to personalize your program.

Accommodations at the resort are spacious, with luxury-sized rooms (400 square feet) overlooking Telluride village. Rooms are equipped with either a king-size bed or two full-size beds, and children sixteen and younger are free. The KidSpa offers day care and scheduled adventure-oriented activities, making this a family destination. A separate enclave of thirteen guest rooms offer twenty-four-hour spa access with one-on-one attention provided by a spa concierge. This spa-within-a-spa is the first of its kind in the United States.

Golden Door cuisine, which is light and healthy, is served in both the Legends and Appaloosa restaurants. Colorado ingredients are used and incorporated into flavors from all over the world.

Cradled on three sides by the majestic peaks of the San Juan Mountain Range, this first-class resort and spa has become the standard by which other North American mountain resorts are measured.

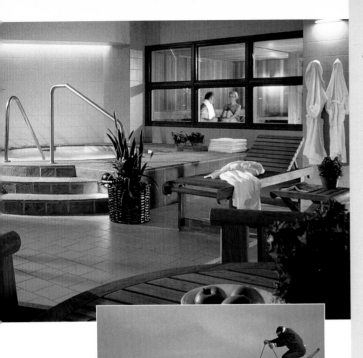

A Mountaintop Golden Door

Wyndham Peaks Resort & Golden Door Spa
136 Country Club Drive
PO Box 2702
Telluride, CO 81435
Phone: (970) 728–6800
Fax: (970) 728–6175 (resort); (970) 728–2525 (spa)
Web site: www.wyndham.com, www.thepeaksresort.com

Season: Closes four to five weeks in the spring and fall

General Manager: John Paul Olivier

Spa Director: Carla Stoehr

Reservations: (800) 789–2220

Spa Appointments: (970) 728–6800 or (888) 772–4584

Accommodations: The 174 guest rooms, including twenty-eight suites, one- to four-bedroom condominiums, and penthouses; minibars, cable TV, VCRs, CD players.

Meals: Legends and Appaloosa restaurants offer healthy cuisine with an emphasis on local ingredients and flavors of the world, as well as Golden Door spa cuisine.

Facilities: Forty-four treatment rooms, saunas, steam rooms, Jacuzzis, Cybex weight room, cardiovascular deck, squash and racquetball courts, indoor climbing wall; full-service salon, men's and women's kivas; ski rental and retail shops; adjacent Telluride Ski and Golf Company with 18-hole championship course; five outdoor tennis courts; conference and banquet facilities.

Services & Special Programs: Customized spa programs; ski-in/ski-out access to ski area; complimentary ski valet; group and private tennis instruction; jeep tours; hiking and mountain sports available; KidSpa program.

Rates: $$$

Best Spa Package: The Ski & Spa Five-Night Package offers upgraded accommodations, four lift tickets per person, four fifty-minute spa treatments per person, breakfast daily. Rates are seasonal and range from $2,460 to $3,237 per person double occupancy.

Credit Cards: Most major

Getting There: The resort is a ten-minute drive from the Telluride Regional Airport and a one-and-a-quarter-hour drive from Montrose Airport. It is two-and-one-half hours to airports in Grand Junction, Durango, and Gunnison.

What's Nearby: The historic town of Telluride; skiing and all mountain sports; Durango and Grand Junction; Mesa Verde National Park, famous for Anasazi cliff dwellings.

Spa 101

For those of you who are new to spa-going, Wyndham Peak's Golden Door publishes a handy "guide for the uninitiated" titled "How to Spa Like a Pro." The pamphlet includes information on types of spas, the spa experience, planning a spa vacation, and spa etiquette. And it lists a glossary of spa terms. Have you wondered if you should wear makeup? What should you avoid if you are claustrophobic? How to tip? Their glossary clears up the meaning of *phytotherapy, fango,* and *lomi lomi.* Even if this is your first spa experience, a quick brushup with this brochure will make you a spa scholar. Best yet, study time won't exceed fifteen minutes; you'll have plenty left over for a Vichy shower!

MANDARIN ORIENTAL HOTEL, MIAMI

Miami, Florida

Asian accents and state-of-the art technology combine at Mandarin Oriental, Miami. Built into Biscayne Bay, the fan-shaped $100 million, twenty-story hotel is as sleek as can be. Enjoy a luxuriously funky retreat and total serenity.

The Spa, managed by London-based ESPA, blends Eastern and Western philosophies. Think candles, pottery, bamboo flooring, Zen-like lounges. Hotel guests have direct access to a movement studio for group sessions of yoga and Pilates, to a workout room with Cybex equipment, and to the outdoor lap pool. Individual treatments or holistic rituals are scheduled in private suites; there are seventeen rooms for massage and skin care.

Start your daily program as a two-hour ritual based on Asian cultures. Therapists can be Bangkok-trained or Latino. You are welcomed with traditional washing of feet, then relax as warm aromatherapy oil is massaged on reflex zones. Treatments suited to your dosha or body type aid in purification. Bliss comes after an aromatherapy bath when herbal tea is served.

The treatments elevate your senses: try a salt and oil scrub, spearmint body polish, and hot herbal linen wrap. Other options include hot stone massage, Indian scalp massage, or shirodhara, where warm oil is dropped soothingly on your forehead. The six spa suites have whirlpool tubs, showers, floor-to-ceiling windows, and water views.

Surrounded by water, the hotel feels like a cruise ship. Vaulted ceilings and enormous windows enhance the lobby's bay view. Terraces curve from restaurants to swimming pool at spa level. Jog along Brickell Key seawall, or cross the causeway to Miami's financial district.

For sophisticated dining, the hotel's Azul Restaurant features the cuisine of Chef Michelle Bernstein. Seafood is the specialty. Dine alfresco all day at casual Cafe Sambal on the waterfront; two can share appetizers of stone crab and sushi.

Guest rooms are done in a tranquil palette of beige

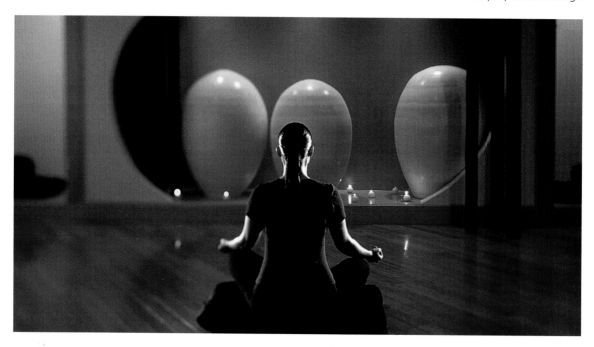

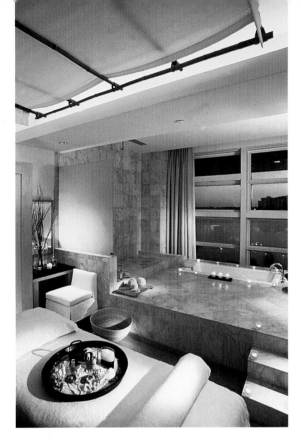

Mandarin Oriental Hotel, Miami
500 Brickell Key Drive
Miami, FL 33131
Phone: (305) 913–8288
Fax: (305) 913–8300
E-mail: miamispa@mohg.com
Web site: www.mandarinoriental.com
Season: Year-round
General Manager: Jorge Gonzalez
Spa Director: Tracey Chappell
Reservations: (866) 888–6780 or (305) 913–8288
Accommodations: 329 rooms, including thirty-one suites, with balcony and marble bathroom. Suites tucked into corners have bamboo-like floors; entertainment center with DVD, CD, and TV and a bathroom divided by walk-in shower, with a deep bathtub. Amenities include robes, Moulton Brown toiletries, hair dryer, and magnified mirror.
Meals: Waterfront dining at Azul blends Latin flavors with Asian, Caribbean, and French influences. Dinner can be braised Florida snapper, Caribbean bouillabaisse, seared tuna, churrasco steak, or chèvre-stuffed free-range chicken with couscous. Vegetarian selections include truffled risotto with grilled shiitake mushrooms, miso-glazed tofu with Thai curry, and Asian vegetables. Cafe Sambal serves breakfast through evening light fare with wok specialties. Spa cuisine lunch is served poolside.
Facilities: Seventeen treatment rooms, plus six suites; Cybex cardiovascular and strength-training equipment; studio for group exercise, meditation; hydrotherapy bath with color therapy lighting; changing rooms with relaxation lounge, sauna, steam room. Outdoor heated pool and whirlpool, jogging track.
Services & Special Programs: Wide range of body care and massage with ESPA aromatherapy oils, organic lotions, muds, and seaweed. Rituals (two hours) combine treatments for holistic effect. Aesthetic services include hair and nail care and waxing.
Rates: $$$
Best Spa Package: Two-night Spa Exclusive package for two persons sharing room, with breakfast daily, one spa lunch poolside, two-hour ritual per person: $1,350 for two, including tax.
Credit Cards: All major
Getting There: From Miami International Airport, take I–395 to downtown Miami, Brickell Avenue exit to Highway 1, causeway at Brickell Key (twenty minutes).
What's Nearby: Port of Miami, Vizcaya Museum & Gardens, Miami Beach, Key Biscayne State Park (aquarium, beach, golf, water sports).

and white, with dark wood furnishings and Spanish marble bath tiles. Suites are enhanced by bamboo hardwood floors and a double balcony. And Biscayne Bay adds ocean colors as well as sea air.

Beyond Beach and Bay: The Golf Alternative

Combine golf, tennis, and spa at Turnberry Isle Resort & Club in Aventura, about forty minutes from downtown Miami. Arrangements must be made in advance by the concierge at Mandarin Oriental to use facilities at its sister resort. Guests enjoy access to a lavish new spa, two golf courses, and a private beach club. Chef Todd Weisz creates contemporary Floridean cuisine at the Veranda restaurant, which overlooks the hotel's tropical garden. Shop at Aventura Mall's designer boutiques and department stores.

MARRIOTT'S HARBOR BEACH RESORT & SPA

Fort Lauderdale, Florida

Marriott's Harbor Beach Resort & Spa in Fort Lauderdale is located on a quiet, clean beach; the resort caters to families as well as adults—upscale but affordable—and recently added an oceanfront spa. Fresh from a $36 million renovation, public areas gleam with tropical Art Deco lounges and restaurants. Join the crowd for Sunday brunch on the beach terrace, swim amid tropical gardens, hike the broad beach and dunes bordered by Australian pines, and work out in the spa.

Staffed by professionals, the 24,000-square-foot spa is an oasis of relaxation for adults only. Swimmers have a heated outdoor lap pool, and there's a co-ed whirlpool on the outside deck. There are separate locker facilities for men and women, each equipped with saunas, steam rooms, and a whirlpool. There is a tiny cafe serving spa cuisine, and meals there are included in full-day or half-day packages. Recognizing that today's spa visitors no longer seek the "fat farm" and fitness "boot camp" experiences of yesteryear, Marriott designed the facility

to mirror contemporary vacationers' visions of tranquility, wellness, and rejuvenation. "It's about living a healthier life," says George Lopez, executive spa director.

Imaginative, indulgent services and amenities set the mood: chamomile-infused iced towels at the sauna; Tara neck pillows during treatments; complimentary bowls of fruit and herbal tea; grooming products and stacks of big towels in the locker rooms. The boutique encourages you to take home spa accessories and gifts.

Thai massage is the specialty of lead therapist Ted Kaminski, a veteran of PGA National Resort and Canyon Ranch SpaClub. Working on a floor mat, Ted integrates traditional rocking and stretching techniques with his stimulating Thai massage. Reflexology in the hands of therapist Deborah Jones becomes a rejuvenating experience. In the nail salon, the pedicures are pure pleasure.

The eighteen treatment rooms connect to an oceanview lounge and gym. Join sessions of yoga,

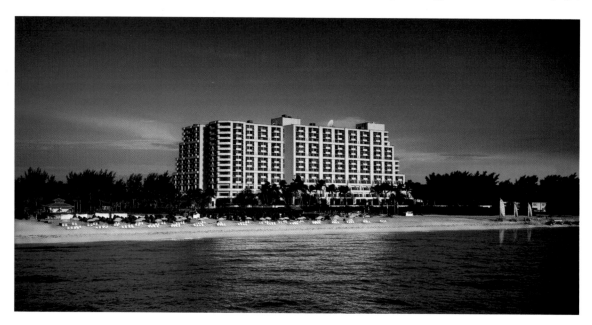

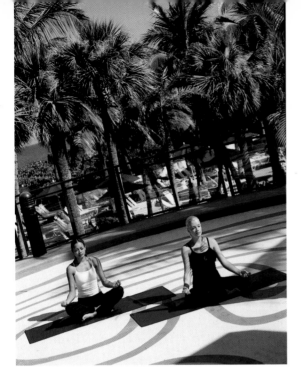

Pilates, and Spinning in the movement studio. Workouts on LifeFitness strength-training units, Softrac cardio equipment, and Johnny G. Spinning bikes require a $25 daily facility fee, but when you book spa services, you have free access to the fitness center. Personal trainers are on staff, helping you plan a serious shape-up. And all the attractions of Fort Lauderdale are minutes away.

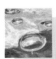

Labyrinth Walk Aids Healing

Known since ancient times as sacred spaces, labyrinths are the latest aid to stress management.

Moving through the spiral is said to change perceptions connecting your inner and outer self. The spiral pattern created for the Spa at Marriott's Harbor Beach follows classical lines. Start your walking meditation by simply placing one foot in front of the other; find your way to the center, then follow the path back out. At the full moon, join a meditation circle and experience yoga in tropical gardens.

Beach Resort Bliss

Marriott's Harbor Beach Resort & Spa
3030 Holiday Drive
Fort Lauderdale, FL 33316
Phone: (954) 525–4000
Fax: (954) 766–6101
E-mail: george.lopez@marriott.com
Web site: www.marriottharborbeach.com
Season: Year-round
General Manager: John Hearns
Spa Executive Director: George Lopez
Program Director: Tanya Lee
Reservations: (800) 222–6543
Spa Appointments: (866) 303–0772
Accommodations: 632 spacious rooms, all with balcony, ocean view, or vista of Intracoastal Waterway. Tropical colors and floral prints decorate rooms furnished in traditional Florida style. Amenities include coffeemaker, daily newspaper delivery, standard telephone, TV, air-conditioning.
Meals: Casual bistro fare at 3030 Ocean Restaurant features seared Chilean sea bass, seafood pasta, tuna tartare stack, herb-crusted sea bass, lobster, stone crab. Breakfast buffet includes tropical fruit, yogurt, cereals, egg-white omelet. Spa Cafe offers salads, sandwiches.
Facilities: Resort hotel with family recreation, extensive gardens, and swimming pools adjoining wide, sandy beach on the Atlantic Ocean. Spa complex entered from hotel lobby, open daily, has indoor and outdoor whirlpools, heated lap pool, private treatment rooms, fitness center with full line of cardiovascular and strength-training equipment, personal trainers, scheduled group exercise. Nail salon and makeup consultation. Locker rooms with sauna, steam rooms.
Services & Special Programs: Massage, facials, body wraps. Children's massage and nail treatments with adult supervision.
Rates: $$
Best Spa Package: AquaVie, $500. Signature treatments in this package include an eighty-minute facial, a fifty-minute massage, an eighty-minute body wrap, a manicure, a pedicure, and one spa cuisine lunch.
Credit Cards: American Express, MasterCard, VISA
Getting There: Located twenty minutes from Fort Lauderdale/Hollywood International Airport, the resort is reached from Highway A1A.
What's Nearby: Golf; major league sports venues, including baseball spring training; Everglades National Park; Bahia Mar Marina (charter and excursion boats); Broward Center for Performing Arts; Bonnet House Museum (Florida history); Fort Lauderdale Museum of Art; Port Everglades (cruise ships); Intracoastal Waterway (boat shuttle to downtown).

PGA NATIONAL RESORT & SPA

Palm Beach Gardens, Florida

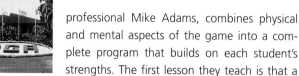

Get into championship shape at the home of the Professional Golfers Association of America. Five golf courses, a nineteen-court tennis club, racquetball courts, and a croquet lawn give the PGA resort a winning combination of sports and spa.

Like a cool oasis, the spa at PGA provides a refreshing change of pace. Here you are in the hands of professionals who know how to make you look and feel your best. You can set up a personalized regimen that includes workouts with a trainer at the fitness center, salon services for hair and nails, and nutrition-balanced meals in the resort's theme restaurants.

Drenched with light, the Mediterranean-style spa building is surrounded by subtropical gardens and bubbling fountains. Soak in pools infused with mineral salts from springs in Europe and Israel, or try Watsu, a water-borne massage therapy for total relaxation. The spa has a full complement of hydrotherapy tubs, mud and algae wraps, and Swiss showers to relieve muscular aches and pains.

Sports massage, neuromuscular and craniosacral therapy, and skin care to repair sun damage help keep you in shape. The spa aestheticians are schooled in the latest European face and body treatments. Aromatherapies, detoxifying seaweed body masques, remineralizing gel treatments, and oxygenating facials are among the one hundred services offered. Spa services and treatments are available a la carte. Or choose from among several packages, including half-day getaways and four-night escapes.

From the reception area in the spacious, glass-walled lobby, which overlooks palm-lined fairways, to the guest rooms furnished in tropical tones, this is a country club with world-class credentials. Day-spa packages come with workout clothing and poolside lunch at the signature Waters of the World garden. Sport-specific exercise gets you in shape for the main game: golf. The Academy of Golf, directed by PGA professional Mike Adams, combines physical and mental aspects of the game into a complete program that builds on each student's strengths. The first lesson they teach is that a perfect swing is not based on one-size-fits-all form. In the hands of these seasoned instructors, you learn how to maximize your body type to deliver the club on the most direct route to the ball. The three-day golf school, as well as the three-times-daily clinics, are for acers and duffers of all ages.

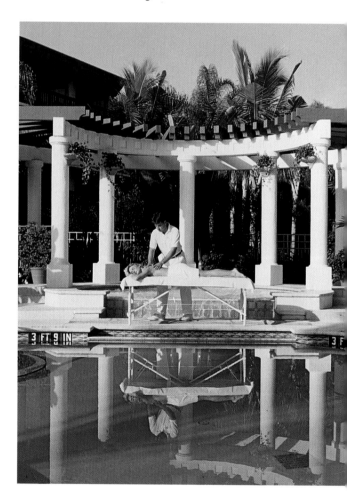

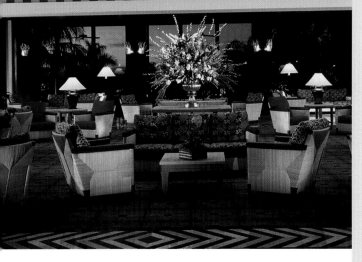

Dining at the resort's eight restaurants means everything from Italian cuisine at Arezzo to spa cuisine. A fusion of Floridian and Asian flavors, the spa cuisine menu is available for breakfast and lunch at the Citrus Tree, an informal cafe and outdoor terrace, as well as poolside at the spa. Dinner menus highlight heart-healthy versions of classic dishes created by Executive Chef Michael Vlasich. Selections from the sports nutrition plan provide a diet high in complex carbohydrates but low in fat.

Designed to complement an active lifestyle, the resort is a two-hour drive from Disney World and twenty minutes from West Palm Beach. Making you feel like a champion is what PGA does best.

One Side at a Time

Isolateral conditioning strengthens muscles on each side of the body. At the PGA health club, Fitness Director Randy Myers recommends using light dumbbells and free weights for optimal benefits. Stretching between sets assists in muscle development, endurance, and functioning. After age thirty-five, adults lose approximately 2 percent of their muscle mass per year. Weight training offsets this loss.

PGA National Resort & Spa
400 Avenue of the Champions
Palm Beach Gardens, FL 33418
Phone: (561) 627–2000
Fax: (561) 622–0261
E-mail: marketing@pga-resorts.com
Web site: www.pga-resorts.com
Season: Year-round
General Manager: Ronald Vuy
Spa Director: Margaret Byrnes
Fitness Director: Randy Myers
Reservations: (800) 633–9150
Spa Appointments: (800) 843–7725
Accommodations: 339 rooms and suites in main hotel; sixty-five golf course cottage villas with two-bedroom suites.
Meals: Spa Plan breakfast and lunch includes spa cuisine of the world. Dinner a la carte at eight restaurants, including Shula's Steak House and Italian-themed Arezzo.
Facilities: Hydrotherapy rooms equipped with tubs, Vichy shower, nine swimming pools, lap pool; salon for hair/nails and makeup consultation; golf on five 18-hole courses; Health & Racquet Club with cardiovascular/strength-building equipment by Cybex, Trotter, Nautilus; nineteen tennis courts (twelve lighted), two racquetball courts (air-conditioned); croquet complex.
Services & Special Programs: Full-service menu of massages and skin care. Fitness evaluation, personal trainers, golf clinics, golf school, tennis clinics, tennis camp, croquet instruction, concierge, laundry, dry cleaning, Budget Rent-A-Car.
Rates: $$
Best Spa Package: Two-night Ultimate Getaway with daily golf, spa treatments, breakfast and lunch. Single, $568–$1,120; double, $498–$815.
Credit Cards: American Express, Diners, Discover, MasterCard, VISA
Getting There: From Palm Beach International Airport, transfers by limousine, van. By car from West Palm Beach: I–95 to exit 57, PGA Boulevard west to resort entrance; Florida Turnpike to exit 44.
What's Nearby: Palm Beach has Worth Avenue shops, Flagler Museum; West Palm Beach for Clematis Street arts district, CityPlace, Kravis Center for the Performing Arts, Norton Museum of Art, the Gardens Mall, Palm Beach Polo Club. Day trips to Kennedy Space Center, Walt Disney World, Orlando, Delray Beach, Morikami Museum & Japanese Gardens, the Everglades.

GRAND WAILEA RESORT HOTEL & SPA

Wailea, Maui, Hawaii

What would Hawaii be without volcanoes, beaches, hula skirts, and a world-class spa? Welcome to the Grand Wailea Resort Hotel & Spa. This 780-room hotel, on the southwestern shore of Maui, opened its 50,000-square-foot Spa Grande in 1989. The spa has become known for its blending of Hawaiian and ancient Eastern healing and relaxation techniques with European rejuvenation therapies. The signature Terme Wailea Hydrotherapy Circuit—a selection of international water therapies—forms the basis of all the treatments here. The circuit begins with a brief shower, followed by a soak in the Roman tub. Then guests are invited to use the steam, sauna, and cold plunge pool. A loofah scrub is next, followed by a cascading waterfall shower. Then come the specialty baths, with a choice of moor mud, aromatherapy, tropical enzyme, limu (seaweed), or mineral salt. The final step is the Swiss jet shower. If you arrived feeling jet-lagged, this water treatment is a perfect antidote.

The spa facilities are divided into the wet and dry areas, and both are accentuated with inlaid Italian marble, original artwork, Venetian chandeliers, and mahogany millwork. The spa's interiors harmonize beautifully with the resort's $30 million art collection, which includes original works by Pablo Picasso and Andy Warhol.

Thirteen types of massage are offered, so if you don't want to try the Lomi Pohaku (a thermal massage using smooth steamed lava stones to massage avocado and olive oil into your skin), there is always the Hawaiian Lomi Lomi Wela Pohaku, a total body massage that incorporates heated lava pebbles in a small denim bag. The less adventurous can choose from ten varieties of Swedish massage and aromatherapy facials.

For those who overdose on the irresistible Maui sun, the spa offers an aloe mud wrap, using a blend of natural aloe vera gel and herbal mud to cool the skin. The spa's color light therapy is a combination of colored light, warmth, music, and natural aromatherapy to soothe the body and mind. Couples will enjoy the abhyanga-pizichili, a two-step treatment that includes a massage by two therapists and a moisturizing warm oil treatment. It is advisable to make spa appointments in advance.

Pampering aside, there are squash and racquetball courts and cardiovascular and strength-training facilities. Fitness services include one-on-one instruction. And if you aren't interested in a conventional stretch class or boxercise, try the hula class for an overall workout!

The spa's juice bar offers smoothies and energy drinks. Spa cuisine is served in the Bistro Molokini, an open-air cafe.

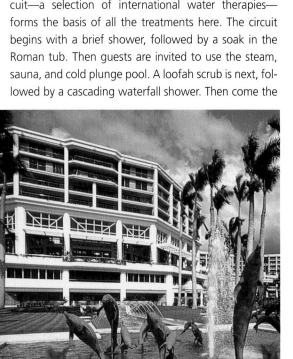

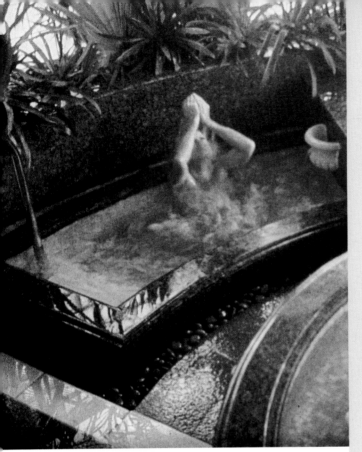

Grand Wailea Resort Hotel & Spa
3850 Wailea Alanui Drive
Wailea, Maui, HI 96753
Phone: (808) 875–1234
Fax: (808) 874–2411
E-mail: spa@grandwailea.com or info@grandwailea.com
Web site: www.grandwailea.com
Season: Year-round
General Manager: Johnny So
Spa Director: Lucia Rodriguez
Reservations: (808) 875–1234 or (800) 888–6100
Spa Appointments: (800) SPA–1933
Accommodations: 780 guest rooms, including sixty suites. Napua Tower is a one-hundred-room exclusive small hotel within the resort. Accommodations are spacious, surrounded by six gardens with sculptures and tropical flowers.
Meals: At the Humu Humu restaurant, a cluster of thatched-roof Polynesian huts, guests are able to "catch" their own lobster; Kincha is a creative Japanese restaurant; the Grand Dining Room serves a breakfast buffet and a la carte; Bistro Molokini is an open-air cafe with an exhibition kitchen; Cafe Kula offers casual terrace dining.
Facilities: Tsunami, a high-tech nightclub; Camp Grande for children; seaside chapel for weddings; the Canyon Activity Pool (nine separate pools, a baby beach, waterslides, waterfalls, caves, rapids, and grottoes); three 18-hole golf courses; an eleven-court tennis complex; meeting facilities; shops.
Services & Special Programs: Scuba diving lessons; business center; wedding services and packages; cruises on the resort's 60-foot catamaran for picnics, snorkeling. Winter whale-watching cruises.
Rates: $$$
Best Spa Package: The best room and spa package starts at $468 per night, double occupancy, and includes accommodations, two massage treatments, and the hydrotherapy circuit.
Credit Cards: Most major
Getting There: Twenty-minute drive from Kahului Airport; Maui is a twenty-minute flight from Honolulu.
What's Nearby: Wailea Beach; Lahaina; all island attractions.

This resort attracts major conferences and is a popular venue for weddings and romantic getaways. Guests can also stay at the Napua Tower, a small hotel within the resort that offers exclusive access to a private lounge serving complimentary continental breakfasts and evening hors d'oeuvres and cocktails. Children aged five to twelve can enjoy the resort's Camp Grande.

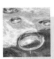

A Tropical Bath to Go

The tropical enzyme bath, which accompanies the Terme Wailea Hydrotherapy Circuit, uses a secret recipe mixed right on the property. Key ingredients include Japanese bath crystals and dried papaya enzyme. In addition to enjoying the special blend at the spa, guests may take home or mail order the private-label product.

MAUNA LANI SPA AT MAUNA LANI RESORT

Kohala Coast, Hawaii

This is one of those rare island spas one fondly remembers, and for reasons that extend beyond a creatively charged spa menu. The Flowering Chakra session or Seaside Massages can predictably erase the trauma and drama of everyday life, but this is just part of staying in this 3,200-acre sanctuary.

The Hawaiian-inspired treatments combined with fitness classes, swaying palm trees, and a caring staff make this the leading spa on the Island of Hawaii. It's obvious why this 25,000-square-foot spa, with another 15,000 square feet of outdoor treatment space, has set a new spa standard in the state. Their theme as a Fire and Ice Spa was carefully planned to integrate native healing practices with local products, a rare commodity in the hotel industry. This has resulted in treatments reflecting the culture and traditions of old Hawaii.

At check-in, you are presented with a sarong with the Mauna Lani Spa logo and a pair of brown sandals. Throughout your spa appointments the staff looks after you—you will not get lost in the crowd.

The genuine aloha attitude of the staff is evident, from the treatments to the serene resonance in the Hale Nahenahe (house of gentle sounds). Here charms frozen in an ice bell slowly drop into a metal plate as the sculpture slowly melts. The result is a mesmerizing tone. There's no Kenny G. music or anything intrusive to break the spell at this pristine hideaway.

Just finding your way to the Mauna Lani Resort is a trip in itself. An old-fashioned highway takes you along lava-strewn terrain. This truly magical journey is fully realized when you arrive at the resort's new spa. Designed by Sylvia Sepielli, it reflects the ambience of an old Hawaiian Village. From the healing garden (lapa'au) to nine authentic thatched huts (hales), it is the closest you can come to a Hawaiian experience in all the Hawaiian Islands. Surrounded by an abundance of lush tropical flowers, from ginger and gardenia to pikake and pakalana, all five senses are touched here; taste, sound, smell, sight, and touch.

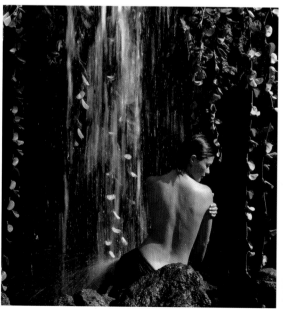

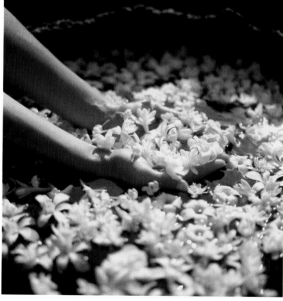

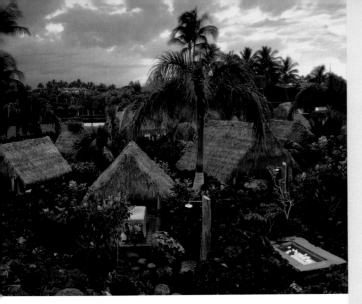

Sound Sense

Music is a vital part of the spa experience. When we embark on a detoxifying seaweed wrap or a fountain of youth facial, our sense of sound is attuned to quieting music. Intrusive music is the last thing we want to hear. Spa music should not overpower but add dimension to a treatment. Selecting the correct music to enhance the spa experience has become an art. New age or soft music creates an ambience of calm and tranquility.

Aeoliah, a composer of music designed to "enhance the total health experience," feels that music can enhance one's sense of well-being and rejuvenation. His music has been clinically tested and proven to be stress reducing and calming while balancing the mind, body, and emotions. Aeoliah's music is smooth as silk, with titles such as "The Healing Heart," "Angel's Touch," "Angel Feather," and "Phoenix Rising."

Some spas offer a choice of music. Depending on the sound system, you might want to bring your favorite music to your spa treatment and ask for it to be played. Aeoliah (www.aeoliah.com) blends various sounds and themes that soothe the senses. The harmonious blend of music and massage is sure to put you in a better frame of mind.

Vintage Hawaii

Mauna Lani Spa at the Mauna Lani Resort
68-1400 Mauna Lani Drive
Kohala Coast, HI 96743-9796
Phone: (808) 881–7922
Fax: (808) 885–6375
Web site: www.maunalani.com
Season: Year-round
General Manager: Roy Honjo
Spa Director: Crystal Poe-Cabatbat
Spa Reservations: (808) 881–7922 or (888) 977–2139
Reservations: (800) 367–2323
Accommodations: 350 guestrooms and suites; five bungalows with private swimming pools and views of the Pacific Ocean or Mauna Kea.
Meals: Five restaurants include alfresco Bay Terrace for American cuisines; poolside Ocean Grill; the resort's signature restaurant, the Canoe House, with Pacific Asian cuisine, and casual dining at Beach Club and Gallery Restaurant.
Facilities: The Mauna Lani Spa, with the Fire and Ice theme, reflects geographical wonders of the Big Island, from flowing lava of Kilauea Crater to snowy peaks of Mauna Kea, two 18-hole golf courses carved from ancient lava fields, and the Racquet Club.
Services & Special Programs: Daily aerobics classes, aquatoning, hula lessons.
Rates: $$$
Best Spa Package: The Mauna Lani Hawaiian Experience, seven to eight hours, should be reserved in advance. It includes the Pu'olo Pa'aki (using Hawaiian rock salt) and pohau (stones) used to sooth tight muscles, a lava sauna, hula facial, Cocanilla (fresh coconut pulp) manicure and pedicure ($638).
Credit Cards: All major
Getting There: Aloha Airlines operates daily flights to the Kona Airport. By taxi, rental car, or hotel car to the resort.
What's Nearby: Parker Ranch in Waimea with a Visitor Center and the John Palmer Parker Museum, historic downtown Hilo, Hawaii Volcanos National Park, and the state's number-one visitor attraction: Kiluea.

CANYON RANCH IN THE BERKSHIRES
Lenox, Massachusetts

If improving your lifestyle is your objective, the New England version of Tucson's Canyon Ranch has the solution. This state-of-the-art destination spa is a beautiful sprawling complex, and one of the main buildings here is an 1897 mansion, known as Bellefontaine, designed to echo Louis XV's Petit Trianon at Versailles. Nowadays guests wearing warm-up suits and leotards walk briskly through the lobby, symbolizing a new life for this vintage landmark.

Opened in 1989, Canyon Ranch offers an ambitious program of fitness, therapeutic bodywork, lifestyle management, sports activities, wellness consultations, and nutrition that has set the standard for the spa industry. This spa holds the distinction of being a five-time winner in the Best Spa award given by *Condé Nast Traveler* magazine.

The daily program is similar to a camp for adults on a grand, luxurious scale. The 100,000-square-foot spa is connected to the guest rooms by a glass-enclosed walkway. Women predominate during the week, and men arriving for the weekend balance out the gender ratio.

The approach to wellness spans mind, body, and spirit. You will learn new ways to walk, breathe, exercise, and eat. You won't want to skip exercise class or anything else on your schedule, because it is fun to be here and participate without having to worry about being graded. There are three indoor tennis courts, three outdoor courts, an indoor track, and two racquetball courts. Other outdoor options include canoeing, hiking, biking, and kayaking. Forget television and videos; excellent evening programs cover a multitude of topics, from time management to tarot cards.

Fitness, the nerve center of Canyon Ranch, is considered a reward here, not a punishment. And you do see a lot of happy faces. As the week progresses, those who once led a sedentary lifestyle acquire a glow. The

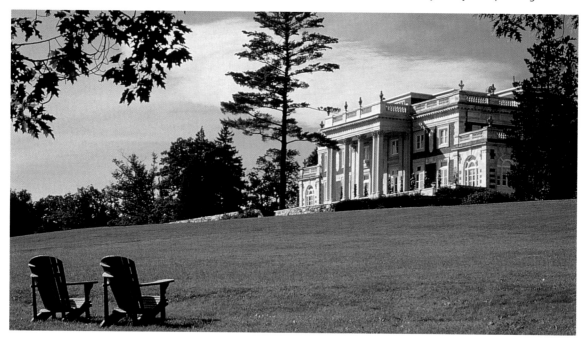

goal is to keep the glow going once you check out.

Chefs produce healthy, great-tasting cuisine. Fitness takes the lead over weight loss, and it is the guests who decide how much to eat. There is no incentive to smuggle in pizza and soda because the menu is diverse, with entrees ranging from ahi tuna dressed with fresh salsa and risotto to Santa Fe–style chicken. Cooking demonstrations show you how to prepare it all at home. The salad and pasta bar are popular with buffet enthusiasts, and there is always plenty of iced tea and water to keep you properly hydrated.

Stress and tension get attention here, with information and ideas that can transform your life. Fending off heart disease is taken seriously at the Ranch, and if you want to confront this issue, this is the spa where you can make it happen. Canyon Ranch helps you acquire the skills to make health choices that will add years to your life and life to your years!

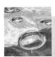

Living Longer

The *Canyon Ranch Guide to Living Younger Longer* reveals the top "secrets" of people who live to be one hundred or more.

- Work hard throughout your life, and never functionally retire.
- Exercise for fun and pleasure—keep "playing."
- Make and maintain social connections.
- Be a contributing member of one or more close-knit social systems.
- Stay curious, explore, learn—and keep laughing.
- Follow a disciplined, regular daily schedule; live efficiently.
- Cherish and preserve your independence.
- Eat and drink in moderation.
- Lighten your emotional load.
- Accept what cannot be changed.
- Find meaning and purpose in living.
- Believe in something bigger and better than yourself.
- Stay in contact with the young, and share your wisdom.

Wellness and Lifestyle Management

Canyon Ranch in the Berkshires
165 Kemble Street
Lenox, MA 01240
Phone: (413) 637–4100
Fax: (413) 637–0057
Web site: www.canyonranch.com

Season: Year-round
General Manager: Carl Pratt
Spa Director: Simon Marxer
Fitness Director: Michelle Adams
Reservations: (413) 637–4100 or (800) 742–9000
Spa Appointments: (413) 637–4100 or (800) 726–9900
Accommodations: The 120 guest rooms are located in a modern New England–style inn that connects via glass-enclosed walkway to either the spa or the mansion.
Meals: Healthy, imaginative cuisine with a high degree of customer service and satisfaction served in the mansion. New spa cafe serving light bistro fare; open noon to 2:30 P.M.
Facilities: 120 woodland acres, with the turn-of-the-twentieth-century mansion as its centerpiece, containing the dining room, restored library, and Health & Healing Center. The two other structures are the spa complex and the inn. All three buildings are connected by climate-controlled, glass-enclosed walkways. Indoor and outdoor tennis courts; racquetball; squash; indoor and outdoor pools; indoor running track; salon facilities.
Services & Special Programs: Hiking, bicycling, canoeing, kayaking, cross-country skiing, snowshoeing, downhill skiing. Wellness consultations, workshops, and cooking demonstrations are offered year-round.
Rates: $$$
Best Spa Package: December to March, the seven-night package, double occupancy, in deluxe accommodations is $3,700. The all-inclusive package covers accommodations, meals, hiking and biking programs, selection of spa services, health and fitness assessment, and health and healing services.
Credit Cards: Most major
Getting There: Arrive via Albany International Airport (New York) with a one-hour drive to the resort or via Bradley International Airport (Hartford, Connecticut/Springfield, Massachussetts), a one-and-one-half-hour drive away. Transfers are available.
What's Nearby: Skiing; fall colors; Williamstown Theater Festival; Jacob's Pillow Dance Festival; Tanglewood Festival.

CRANWELL RESORT, SPA & GOLF CLUB
Lenox, Massachusetts

Edith Wharton would have loved the new spa at Cranwell Resort, just a few miles from the famed novelist's summer home in the Berkshire Mountains. Built in the style of grand mansions at the turn of the twentieth century, the resort and spa are complemented by spacious grounds, a championship golf course, and some of America's leading cultural centers.

Opened in March 2002, The Spa at Cranwell is a 35,000-square-foot full-service resort spa, the largest of its type in the Northeast. Choose from dozens of treatments, and enjoy the comprehensive fitness facilities, including the 5,000-square-foot cardiovascular fitness center and the 60-foot indoor lap pool. The Spa affords every opportunity to keep up a fitness regimen, destress, or relax after playing the championship golf course.

Glass walkways connect the spa to the four main guest-room buildings. Once inside the dramatic light-filled structure, visitors find a glass-enclosed atrium showcasing a 60-by-30-foot heated indoor pool, a lounging patio, and scenic views of the Berkshires.

Highlights of the Cranwell Resort include: a comprehensive menu of massages, facials, body treatments, and signature therapies, including wraps, aromatherapy, and Swedish, stone, clay, and reflexology massages. There are luxuriously appointed men's and women's spas, each with a fireplace, sauna, steam room, whirlpool, and locker area. The Image Center, offering cosmetics and the latest nail, hair, and scalp treatments. The Spa Shop carries imported products for skin and hair, along with wellness books and tapes. The fitness center has a complete line of cardiovascular equipment, strength-training equipment, and specially designed aerobic and yoga rooms with spring-loaded floors. The

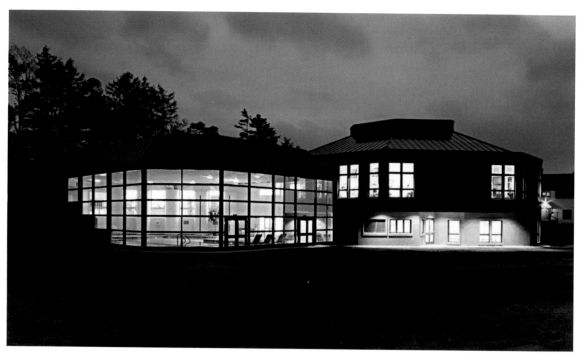

outdoor adventure fitness program offers a seasonal variety of activities led by skilled guides. The Spa Cafe serves spa luncheon cuisine created by the resort's award-winning culinary team under the direction of Executive Chef Carl DeLuce.

Built during the Gilded Age of the 1890s, the Tudor-style country manor remains the centerpiece of today's 380-acre resort. Renowned nineteenth-century landscape architect Frederick Law Olmstead designed the original grounds, and the picturesque Berkshires can be viewed from the manor's hilltop dining rooms. The baronial mansion boasts a richly decorated great hall and guest rooms furnished in the nineteenth-century Arts and Crafts style.

Located two hours from both Boston and New York, the area is a center for the arts as well as recreation. It is minutes from Tanglewood, summer home of the Boston Symphony Orchestra. Just down the road are antiques shops and crafts boutiques in Stockbridge, and masterpieces of French Impressionism at the Clark Institute of Art in Williamstown.

Devoted to enjoying the good life, Cranwell, a Historic Hotel of America, preserves the best of past and present.

Good Enough to Eat

Warm plum tonic, summer tomato cream, peach masque, carrot vitamin masque . . . it sounds as if we just went to the supermarket to create a skin-care line. That's the direction many skin-care experts are moving toward, with ingredients that are fresh and fragrant. These moisture-rich products for dry skin and other customized lotions for specific problems, from couperose and rosacea to acne and sun damage, are making news in the spa world. Eminence handmade organic skin-care products (www. eminenceorganics.com), based on old-world knowledge of herbs and fruits, are designed to treat these problems.

Cranwell Resort, Spa & Golf Club
55 Lee Road
Lenox, MA 01240
Phone: (413) 637–1364
Fax: (413) 637–4364
E-mail: info@cranwell.com
Web site: www.cranwell.com
Season: Year-round
General Manager: Lew Kiesler
Spa Director: Helen Pierce
Reservations: (800) 572–6935; Historic Hotels of America (800) 678–8946
Spa Appointments: (800) 572–8938, ext. 674
Accommodations: 107 deluxe rooms with private bath, all air-conditioned. Original manor rooms have high ceilings, period furniture. Contemporary rooms are in new lodges connected by a glass-enclosed walkway to the manor house. All have TV, telephones, data port, and minibar.
Meals: Spa Cafe serves lunch daily. Three resort dining rooms offer spa cuisine options. Complimentary tea, coffee, and fruit are offered throughout the day.
Facilities: Full-service spa with indoor swimming pool, hydrotherapy, private treatment rooms linked to men's and women's lounges, saunas and steam rooms. Movement studio with spring-loaded floor for aerobics, yoga. Fitness center with cardiovascular and strength-training equipment. Salon for hair, nail, and skin care. Golf, tennis, cross-country skiing, mountain biking.
Services & Special Programs: Massage, hydrotherapy, facials, manicure and pedicure, hair and scalp treatments. Fitness evaluation and personal trainers.
Rates: $$
Best Spa Package: The Two-Night Weekend Spa Stay includes overnight resort room accommodations for two nights, one fifty-minute service (Swedish massage or classic facial), one floral scrub, two fitness classes, one spa cuisine lunch, and use of the spa, fitness center, and indoor pool. Package prices change by season and range from $365 to $525 per person, double occupancy. Rates do not include taxes, gratuities, or service charges.
Credit Cards: Most major
Getting There: By car from New York, Taconic Parkway, to Massasschussettes Route 7; from Boston by I-90 (Massachusetts Turnpike) to Route 7.
What's Nearby: Tanglewood summer festival (Berkshire Music Center), Jacob's Pillow (Dance), MassMoCa (North Adams arts center), Appalachian Trail, Hancock Shaker Village, Clark Art Institute, Norman Rockwell Museum.

CANYON RANCH SPACLUB AT THE VENETIAN

Las Vegas, Nevada

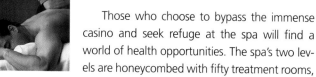

You can spend your time exercising at a one-armed bandit or you can make a more sensible choice and check into the Venetian's 65,000-square-foot Canyon Ranch SpaClub and really be a winner.

Just being at this $1.2 billion, 3,036-suite megaresort is a trip in itself. Imagine yourself in Venice, recreated in all its charm right down to a gondola ride through an elaborate Grand Canal and a Rialto Bridge. Everything is on a grand scale here, from stunning 700-square-foot guest rooms replete with private bed chambers draped in canopies to a 500,000-square-foot themed indoor retail mall with its own St. Mark's Square.

Those who choose to bypass the immense casino and seek refuge at the spa will find a world of health opportunities. The spa's two levels are honeycombed with fifty treatment rooms, offering 120 spa services. Spa-goers enjoy dozens of treatment options with enticing names, such as Euphoria and Royal King's Bath. Ten different facials await.

Fitness reaches a new level with fifty pieces of cardio equipment, thirty Spinning bikes, and classes such as boxercise, qigong, yoga, and strength training. A staff of nutritionists, exercise physiologists, health educators, and physical therapists use an integrated approach that combines Western and alternative health practices. There is a daily fee ($30) for hotel guests to use the facilities.

If you have decided to trim down and get fit (a healthy anticasino move), the SpaClub has the cure, with nutritionists and exercise physiologists to design weight-loss programs. The Canyon Ranch Cafe (note the absence of burgers and fries) presents daily menu selections such as egg-white omelettes, wraps, pancakes, fresh fish dishes, and unforgettable desserts.

The goal of the SpaClub is to provide sanctuary from the nonstop, frenetic ambience of the Las Vegas Strip, with its smoke-filled casinos, rich food, and surging traffic. And, amazingly, it does.

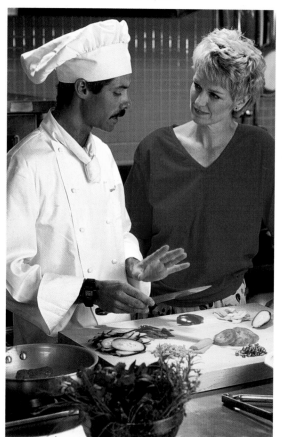

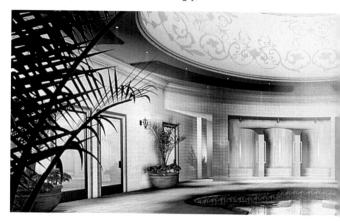

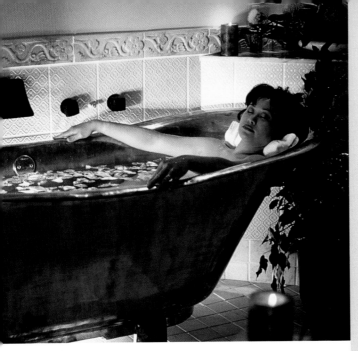

Canyon Ranch SpaClub at the Venetian
3355 Las Vegas Boulevard South
Las Vegas, NV 89109
Phone: (702) 414–3600 or (877) 220–2688
Fax: (702) 414–1100
Web site: www.canyonranch.com

Season: Year-round

General Manager: Blake Feeney

Spa Director: Michael Leboeuf

Wellness Manager: Laura Shmiel

Reservations: (877) 220–2688

Spa Appointments: (877) 220–2688

Accommodations: The Venetian, the world's largest all-suite hotel/resort, shopping, casino, and convention complex, offers 3,036 suites featuring 130-square-foot bathrooms finished in Italian marble, a sunken living room, minibar, fax machine/copier; telephones with dual lines and dataport, color TVs, and a living room entertainment center.

Meals: Upscale dining in more than a dozen restaurants, including Wolfgang Puck's Postrio and the Canyon Ranch Cafe, serving world-famous spa cuisine.

Facilities: 65,000-square-foot SpaClub with beauty salon, fitness center, fifty treatment rooms, three aerobics studios, and 40-foot indoor rock-climbing wall.

Services & Special Programs: Several spa packages, including massage, fitness, and sport and beauty consultations.

Rates: $$$

Best Spa Package: The Personal Creation III enables you to design your own package. Selecting three services from twelve possibilities is an exciting prospect. Some of the services included in the $395 fee are a fifty-minute Swedish massage, a European facial, a fifty-minute rock-climbing session, an Essential Signature Pedicure, or a Canyon Ranch Body Cocoon. There is a separate charge for accommodations.

Credit Cards: Most major

Getting There: The resort is a short drive from the McCarran International Airport.

What's Nearby: All Las Vegas Strip attractions, Valley of Fire National Park, Red Rock Canyon, Lake Mead.

Eyes, Thighs, and Sighs!

Health food stores hold a world of remedies for spa-goers. Here are three products you should consider adding to your home spa. Herbal chamomile is available as an eye stick that soothes while firming and can reduce the appearance of puffiness and dark circles under the eyes. Thigh cream has been getting a lot of press. Results have been noticed by those who report it helps smooth out the appearance of spongy tissue (cellulite) from the thighs and buttocks. And finally, consider skin formulas containing alpha hydroxy acids. These are natural biological substances found in fruits. They have several beneficial effects on the outer and deeper layers of the skin. Similar to Retin-A, they slow down the aging process, which is accelerated by stress and UV exposure. Unlike Retin-A, they are safe and gentle and do not cause photosensitivity, excess redness, or excessive skin peeling. When these products are used in conjunction with a sensible nutrition and fitness program, you may see results.

ELEMIS SPA AT THE ALADDIN HOTEL

Las Vegas, Nevada

Morocco meets Las Vegas at the heart-stopping 32,000-square-foot Elemis Spa at the Aladdin Hotel. Call it a sensory haven, a magical temple, or just one of the most exquisite spas in Las Vegas. What wondrous sights lie behind the exotic facade of this megahotel designed by Stephen John Ltd., a British firm whose credits include Crystal Cruises, Norwegian Cruise Lines, and P & O Princess Cruises. Attention to detail at this opulent spa is to be credited to John O. Picken, who handpicked many of the Moroccan antiques displayed throughout this luxurious hideaway. You leave the Las Vegas glitz behind as you cross over the threshold, where traditional fragrant herbal tea is served. It's the spa therapy menu that sets this spa apart from all others in Las Vegas, which has more megaspas per square foot than any other stretch of real estate in North America.

The objective of the spa is to "seduce the six senses," starting with sound (the music is ethereal, the tinkling fountains enchanting), smell (Elemis aromatherapy products are used in treatments and sold in the boutique), taste (fresh fruit and cool tea are served in the lounge area), touch (experienced therapists for body, hand, foot, and chakra-balancing massages), and most of all, sight, as you view the magnificent works of Moroccan art displayed throughout. Treatments are enhanced by Elemis products, which are noted for their range of medicinal and active therapeutic plant extracts. These are best exemplified in five facials that focus on protection, cleans-

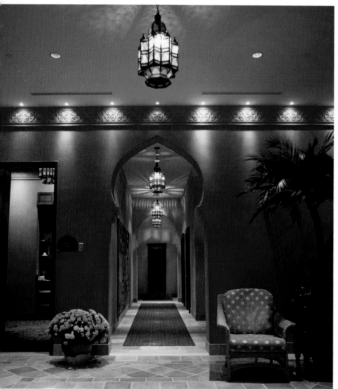

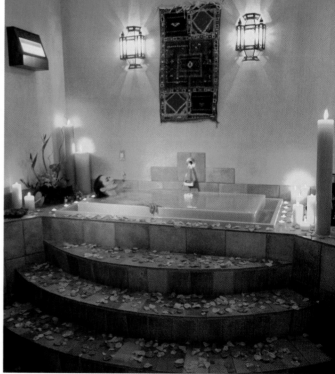

ing, and oxygenating the skin. Specialized treatments include the Japanese Silk Eye Zone Therapy, designed to minimize that look of bags under the eyes, and the Hawaiian Wave Four-Hand Massage, with two therapists working simultaneously to create "a mystical experience of the sublime."

Spa guests may lose their way in the maze of treatment rooms—there are twenty-nine—relaxation areas, and therapy pools. But getting lost in this Moroccan paradise is more delightful than daunting, as every turn reveals the fascinating world of spa life in an exotic culture that's been transplanted to Las Vegas. Just imagine finding yourself in a softly lit inner sanctum soaking in a pool of water infused with essential oils, strewn with rose petals, and surrounded by candles of various heights. What you'll find here is a tranquil haven that makes you forget that the cacophony of nonstop gambling is just footsteps away.

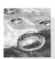

Guaranteed Winners

If you want to explore spas in Las Vegas, access *The Spa Guide* **at www.lasvegas24hours.com, call (702) 892–0711, or fax (702) 892–2824 for information about the bursting spa world in Las Vegas. Spas off the Strip are getting into the act, with the opening of the Palms on West Flamingo Road. Their new 20,000-square-foot spa has hosted botox (wrinkle therapy) cocktail hours on Saturday nights, with a Beverly Hills plastic surgeon on call.**

If you can't get an appointment for a Nectarine-Basil Body Scrub or a Japanese Silk Booster Facial in Las Vegas proper, you can head out of town and visit the JW Marriott two-level superspa in Summerlin, about a twenty-minute ride from the the Strip. With thirty-six treatment rooms in a more suburban setting, this spa has an equally diverse menu. Soak in a European-inspired hydrocircuit exercise pool as strategically placed jets soothe and relax your body from head to toes.

Elemis Spa at the Aladdin Hotel
3667 Las Vegas Boulevard South
Las Vegas, NV 80191
Phone: (702) 785–5555 or (877) 333–9474
Fax: (702) 785–5558
Web site: www.aladdincasino.com
Season: Year–round
VP Hotel Operations: Frank Vignola
Spa Director: Darryll Leiman
Reservations: (702) 785–5772 or (866) 935–3647
Accommodations: 2,567 guest rooms
Meals: The Aladdin has Elements for fresh seafood and pasta, and the Spice Market Buffet and the Zanzibar Cafe for breakfast, lunch, and dinner.
Facilities: The spa has a fully equipped gym.
Services & Special Program: There is a fennel-cleansing and Ionithermie Detox program.
Rates: $$$
Best Spa Package: Suggested is the Absolute Spa Ceremony for $345, which includes a Japanese Silk Booster Facial; Well-Being Massage; shampoo, set, and blow dry; and Sole Delight. Or try the Elemis Health and Well-Being package for $385. The Elemis does not yet offer spa packages that include accommodations.
Credit Cards: Most major
Getting There: About thirty-minutes by car from the Las Vegas International Airport.
What's Nearby: Badlands 18-hole golf course; Angel Park; and Red Rock Recreation Area for hiking and mountain biking (recently designated a vortex by Nevada state officials).

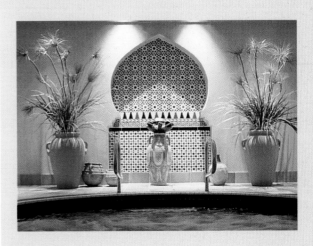

THE GROVE PARK INN

Asheville, North Carolina

Opened in 2000, The Spa at The Grove Park Inn capped the hotel's transformation from southern inn to world-class resort. Owner Elaine D. Sammons committed to building the finest spa in North America on this historic property.

With the goal of bringing the Blue Ridge Mountains indoors, the designers have combined elements of earth, water, and light to create a new American spa. Ancient granite boulders arch over the pools and reception area, creating the feeling that you are deep inside a grotto devoted to health and fitness. Waterfalls and soaring glass skylights frame indoor and outdoor swimming pools. Designed by award-winning Canadian architect Robert LeBlond of Calgary, Alberta, the 40,000-square-foot spa is spread out among hillside gardens. With an expanded sports complex and outdoor pool terrace, the new spa complex integrates the U-shaped hotel, yet retains a sense of refuge and sanctuary.

Beyond the reception desk, the spa is divided into men's and women's lounges, each with locker rooms, showers, and shaving/makeup areas. Fireplaces warm the lounges, and there is a view of the pools below. Skylit steps lead to the indoor swimming pool, sauna, inhalation room, hot tubs, and cool plunge pool. A lap pool and two therapeutic waterfall pools face a wall of windows with stunning views of the city and valley below.

Staying here is like returning to another era. The hotel was first opened in 1913 to offer sophisticated travelers an exclusive retreat in the Blue Ridge Mountains of North Carolina. The resort is on the National Register of Historic Places. It currently houses the world's largest collection of Arts and Crafts antiques and lighting fixtures. Just across town is the Biltmore Estate, George Vanderbilt's 250-room mansion, which awes visitors with its French chateau grandeur and 250-acre gardens designed by Frederick Law Olmsted in 1895. For collectors of Americana, the area remains a source of inspiration and discovery.

Emerging from a $36 million makeover in 2000, the Grove Park Inn preserves its period grandeur with touches of modern comfort. In the great hall lobby, guests encounter two massive fireplaces, which flank a hall full of antique furnishings, and a stenciled ceiling with hand-hammered copper chandeliers that give off a warm glow. Original guest rooms at the main inn have new wall, window, and floor treatments, new armoires and stereos, and updated bathrooms. Two wings of contemporary rooms boast mountain and garden views.

Downtown Asheville, only five minutes away, has become a thriving center for the arts. Situated at an elevation of 2,500 feet in the spectacular Blue Ridge Mountains of western North Carolina, the area is blessed with four distinct seasons. Yet the mild climate permits golf year-round on the resort's par-70 Donald Ross–designed golf course. Tennis fans can choose from three hard-surface outdoor courts and three indoor courts. The spa has a complete menu of services and total fitness equipment.

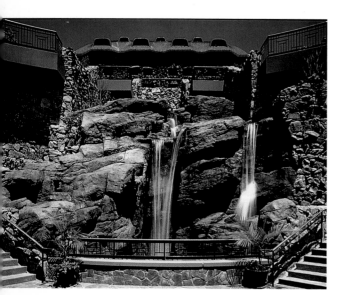

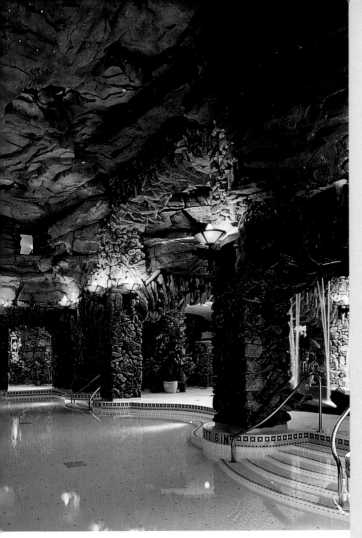

Going to the Mountain, Southern Style

The Grove Park Inn
290 Macon Avenue
Asheville, NC 28804
Phone: (828) 252–2711
Fax: (800) 374–7432 or (828) 253–7053
E-mail: dtomsky@groveparkinn.com
Web site: www.groveparkinn.com

Season: Year-round

General Manager: Craig Madison

Spa Director: Ellen McGinnis

Reservations: (800) 438–5800

Spa Appointments: (800) 438–0050 (Call in advance.)

Accommodations: 510 rooms, including suites, featuring Arts and Crafts movement furniture and decorative objects from the early 1900s. Newly renovated and updated rooms and bathrooms. Completely air-conditioned, all with TV. Deluxe rooms enjoy best views; value rooms in main inn are small, have one bed, and no view. The club floor has twenty-eight oversized guest rooms with Jacuzzi tub.

Meals: A la carte menus in two restaurants: Sunset Terrace, newly covered and heated, features broiled steak, lamb, and pork chops; grilled tuna; pan-seared salmon. Horizons has classic cuisine; no spa menu available. The spa has a juice bar and light snacks.

Facilities: Hydrotherapy underwater massage tubs, couples treatment room, waterfall pools, swimming pool, lap pool. Fitness center with exercise equipment. Sports include golf, tennis, racquetball. Rocking chairs on the terrace and in great hall are traditional. Inhalation steam and sauna.

Services & Special Programs: Massage, aromatherapy, exfoliation, bath, spirulina wrap, moor mud bath, lymphatic drainage, facials.

Rates: $$

Best Spa Package: Spa Sampler for two people includes overnight accommodations, breakfast, and choice of two treatments (massage, facial, or body wrap). Package price includes tax and 20 percent gratuity and ranges from $465 to $605 weekdays, $490 to $645 weekends in season.

Credit Cards: Most major

Getting There: From Atlanta, by car I-40 (204 miles). By air, Continental Express, USAir, or ASA to Asheville Regional Airport.

What's Nearby: Biltmore Estate, Blue Ridge Parkway, Charlotte, Southern Highlands Folk Art Center, Mount Pisgah, Chimney Rock Park (hiking trails).

Sanctuary of the Senses

The signature treatment at Grove Park is much more than a facial. Using sounds, smells, and sensations associated with the Blue Ridge Mountains, as well as light, water, and rock, it transports you to a place of complete relaxation. A massage therapist moves to the gentle sounds of water and ends by applying a skin-rejuvenating refining cream scented with mountain herbs. A final touch: honey body paint and cold stone facial.

NEMACOLIN WOODLANDS RESORT & SPA

Farmington, Pennsylvania

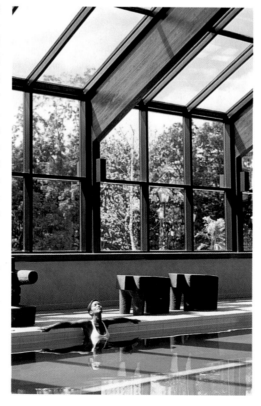

Sprawling over 1,500 acres of the Laurel Highlands mountains in southwestern Pennsylvania, this is one of the most original resorts in America. Nemacolin's two PGA-rated championship golf courses wrap around a French Renaissance–style chateau and English lodge. The resort's centerpiece is the Woodlands Spa. Energized by natural light, water, wood, and native stone, and designed according to feng shui principles, it is a place that sends spirits soaring.

Framed by trees, boulders, and a reflecting pool, the Woodlands Spa harmonizes natural elements inside with the mountains and meadows surrounding the resort. Designed by environmental architect Clodagh, the three-story spa building was transformed in 1999 by Nemacolin's owners to serve the diverse interests of families and fitness buffs, as well as sophisticated spagoers. Spaces for aerobics and swimming enjoy woodland views, and treatment rooms are secluded, with nature-inspired furnishings, crystals, and wall coverings in soothing tones. And the menu at Seasons, the Woodland Spa's restaurant, satisfies hearty appetites while meeting the nutritional needs of active or weight-conscious guests.

Scents of the forest and a cascading waterfall set the scene as you enter from an arched bridge over the reflecting pool. The garden-terrace restaurant is open to all guests, breakfast through dinner. Group activities include fitness walks, water aerobics, and hikes, plus trail rides, ski lessons, and golf instruction. Or simply relax at the outdoor pool, complete with swim-up bar.

Services range from eight types of massage and nine body therapies to a variety of facials and hydrotherapy baths. Special treatments include a vitamin facial by Dermalogica, which repairs the skin's elasticity and tone by combining vitamin-infused cream cleansing and hydroxy acid exfoliation. Body kurs by Kerstin Florian utilize European moor mud, marine algae, and thermal water salts. Treatments can be reserved individually or as part of a value-added package. The daily facility fee of $20 is waived when you book treatments.

Family-oriented programs let parents share spa experiences with kids. In the beauty salon, teenagers can have a manicure or facial. The Kidz Klub has supervised activity for children ages four to twelve, full or half-day. Saddle up for a trail ride at the Equestrian Center, which has ponies for youngsters; practice target shooting with an instructor (minimum age sixteen) at the Shooting Academy; go to golf school or schedule private lessons at the Golf Academy for adults and juniors (sixteen and younger). There are two golf courses, which are open to the public. Nemacolin guests get reduced greens fees of $125 at the top-rated Mystic Rock course; the fee for eighteen holes at the Links course is $79 for guests. (Fees

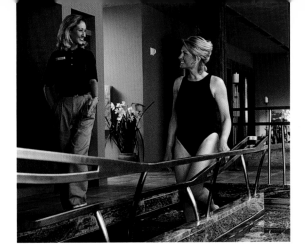

are lower after 3:30 P.M.) Winter adds a different outdoor dimension to the activities: downhill and cross-country skiing at Mystic Mountain, tubing, and snowboarding on a half-pipe. Lessons are available.

Accommodations are equally varied. Families can occupy an entire townhouse or get additional bedrooms in the main lodges for 50 percent off the applicable rate. Rooms at both Chateau Lafayette and the mountain lodge are spacious, tastefully furnished, and have all the usual amenities. Some come with whirlpool bathtub, balcony, and suites.

Whether taking tea or indulging in gourmet dining or luxury pampering, you are king of this mountain.

Water Walk
Stimulates Circulation

Adapting a European thermal therapy, the Woodlands Spa has the first American water path. Designed to stimulate circulation and improve immune functions, the experience consists of a guided walk through shallow pools of water, alternately warm and cold, followed by a relaxing soak in a pool infused with salts from European hot springs. Similar to treatments in Kneipp spas in Bad Woerishofen, the water path is a sure way to enhance your energy and a feeling of well-being. Available by reservation; $65 per session.

Mountain Retreat for Families and Sports and Fitness Buffs

Nemacolin Woodlands Resort & Spa
1001 Lafayette Drive
Farmington, PA 15437-9901
Phone: (724) 329–6922
Fax: (724) 329–6385
E-mail: spa@nwir.com
Web site: www.nemacolin.com

Season: Year-round

General Manager: Ron Cadrette

Spa Director: Kaite Hurley Laguna

Reservations: (800) 422–2736

Spa Appointments: (800) 422–2736

Accommodations: Chateau Lafayette has 124 oversized rooms, including twenty-five suites. The Lodge offers ninety-eight inn-style rooms. Both buildings are linked to the Woodlands Spa via walkway. Townhouses also available.

Meals: Seasons restaurant serves organic food. The Caddy Shack, country club fare; the Golden Trout, regional specialties; Lautrec, contemporary French cuisine.

Facilities: Twenty-eight private treatment rooms. Fitness center with full line of equipment; indoor swimming pool, therapy pool, and whirlpools for men and women. Swimming pools, fly-fishing, volleyball, croquet, bocce ball, skiing, polo field, sleigh and surrey rides.

Services & Special Programs: Hydrotherapy, bodywork, krauter baths, massages, wraps, facials, hair and nail care. Fitness instruction. Full salon services. Registered dietitian available.

Rates: $$–$$$

Best Spa Package: The Laurel Relaxer half-day package for $190 includes a facial or Swedish massage, body scrub or reflexology, and spa cuisine lunch. Full use of the Woodlands Spa swimming pools, fitness equipment, scheduled group exercise and walks, plus a spa gift.

Credit Cards: Most major

Getting There: Located 61 miles southeast of Pittsburgh International Airport, the resort offers transfers (fee) by limousine. By car, on scenic I-70 west to I-68, exit 14 to Route 40 west; from I-70 east, Route 43 south to Route 40 east.

What's Nearby: Frank Lloyd Wright's Fallingwater and Kentuck Knob; Youghiogheny River whitewater rafting; kayaking; Fort Necessity (French and Indian War).

GREEN VALLEY SPA & TENNIS RESORT

St. George, Utah

From the decor to the lay of the land to the services, Green Valley Spa & Tennis Resort is an authentic slice of the Southwest. Set amid the red rock canyons of Utah, the spa draws inspiration and products from the desert. Combined with an active hiking program, this is one of the best destination spa programs in America.

Rugged terrain changes to rolling high desert hills as you approach St. George. Following trails set by Mormon pioneers, hikers head into wilderness areas and the breathtaking heights of Zion National Park. Each day brings a new challenge, and knowledgeable staffers encourage you to go the extra mile.

Vistas of mountains against blue sky and a multi-hued desert surround the resort complex. Located within an affluent community of ranch-style homes set on immaculate lawns, Green Valley is an upscale version of the Old West. Spa guests are housed in deluxe suites at Coyote Inn. Spread among cactus gardens and tennis courts, the Coyote suites are the best of the west. A sunny swimming pool is steps from your private patio, and a communal pantry is stocked with refreshments. These secluded suites perfectly complement an active, outdoor-oriented program, pampering the inner person with freshly ground Starbucks coffee beans (regular and decaf), feather beds in front of real fireplaces, TVs, and microwave ovens for food cravings.

Hiking is the main event; groups often depart before sunup, avoiding the midday heat. Winter schedules allow more time for breakfast, although the weather in southern Utah can be surprisingly warm in January and February. St. George's quiet western lifestyle is an attractive alternative to Las Vegas, 120 miles to the south. Gateway to the largest concentration of national parks and monuments in America, the town also hosts the World Senior Games every year in mid-October.

Scampering over rocks and ravines, hikers are awed by the contrasting hues and textures of the red sandstone rocks. Bathed in the warm, hazy light of morning sun, Snow Canyon State Park is a place of stunning views. Native American pictographs invite exploration. Longer hikes in Bryce Canyon National Park, as well as Zion, include transportation to trailheads. Water canteens and lunch packs are supplied, and there are warm-up stretches before and after the hike.

Tennis camp is an alternative to hikes. With indoor and outdoor courts, and a team of teaching professionals at the Vic Braden Tennis College, the spa offers choices between pampering and playing. Also available are an indoor golf learning center and two racquetball courts. A fully equipped gymnasium is open day and night for shape-ups.

Reward yourself with a deep-tissue massage and soothing soaks scented with desert sage and lavender. Treatments can be scheduled outdoors in warm weather; baths are color coded for energy and relaxation and feature Green Valley's personalized Good

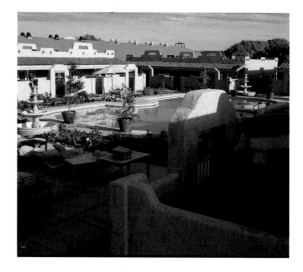

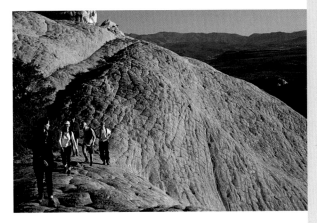

Medicine products. Join scheduled sessions of aquacise, step class, stretch, or meditation. Evening programs in the spa's auditorium include an introduction to Native American healing. And there is line dancing in the gym. Bring your boots and jeans for a vacation that combines New Age holistic healing with New West fun and adventure.

The Body Code

How does your body shape affect your weight and well-being? Green Valley teamed up with Jay Cooper, author of *The Body Code,* to develop a weight management program. After a physical evaluation, you are typed and counseled on everything from diet to exercise. Spa staff coordinate with the counselors on a personalized program that you can continue at home.

Along with workouts, try baths matched to your mood. Processed in the spa's lab, mineral salts deposited in desert cliffs by an ancient inland sea are mixed with powdered pearls, pure essential oils, and traces of Vitamin C. Each bath is a sensory experience, color coded to invigorate or relax your spirits, enhanced by matching flowers and candles. The spa's line of skin-care products is called Good Medicine, symbolizing purity and honoring the sacred ways of native cultures.

Red Rock Renewal, Southwestern Style

Green Valley Spa & Tennis Resort
1871 West Canyon View Drive
St. George, UT 84770
Phone: (435) 628–8060
Fax: (435) 673–4084
E-mail: Request@infowest.com
Web site: www.greenvalleyspa.com
Season: Year-round
General Manager: Alan Coombs
Spa Director: Carole Coombs
Reservations: (800) 237–1068
Spa Appointments: (800) 237–1068
Accommodations: Thirty-five single suites and ten two-bedroom suites at Coyote Inn. Oversize suites have four-poster bed or two queen-size beds with feather mattress, goose down comforters, down pillows. Modern bathroom with 6-foot whirlpool tub. Amenities include robes and leisure suit, fax machine, CD and tape player, TV, daily complimentary laundry service. Hospitality lounge with pool table, fireplace, snack bar.
Meals: Three meals daily included in rates. Special diets accommodated with advance request, but choices are limited.
Facilities: Hydrotherapy suite, two aerobics studios, six swimming pools, two saunas, nineteen tennis courts, indoor golf learning center, two racquetball courts, cardiovascular and strength-training equipment.
Services & Special Programs: Massage, reflexology, reiki, mud and herbal wraps, facials, powdered pearl body scrub, mineral bath. Weight management program, tennis/spa package.
Rates: $$
Best Spa Package: Seven-night program includes all meals, daily spa service (fifty minutes), golf and tennis instruction, guided morning hikes, fitness classes, full use of facilities.$3,850 single; $3,675 double.
Credit Cards: American Express, Discover, MasterCard, VISA
Getting There: From Las Vegas McCarran International Airport, scheduled shuttle van (800–933–8320), ninety minutes; car rental; commuter flights to St. George.
What's Nearby: Zion National Park, Bryce Canyon National Park, Pah Tempe Hot Springs, St. George Mormon Tabernacle, pioneer homes.

THE SPA AT SUNDANCE

Sundance, Utah

Sundance is more than a 6,000-acre celebrity-driven ski resort. It is also a 1,200-square-foot freestanding spa. The annual Sundance Film Festival in January is but one aspect of the total Sundance experience—the flip side is a thought-provoking agenda of socially responsive programs that attract more than filmmakers and ski enthusiasts. Healing and nurturing take several paths here, and this intimate spa has been sensitively integrated into the total Sundance experience.

Sundance Village, with ninety-five guest cottages at the base of Mount Timpanogos, is the focal point of a year-round arts program, weekend film screenings, professional theater under the stars, and the Sundance Artisan Center. As you make your way up the winding mountain road, the outside world silently fades away. Originally founded to honor the diversity and artistic vitality of American filmmaking, the Sundance Institute's film festival now generates international publicity. The event is a showcase for independent filmmakers. The Sundance Channel, available in every guest room, features films screened here. It's one of many perks guests enjoy.

At the heart of Sundance is a new spa that, although small in size, has captured the spirit of the spa experience. Treatments honoring Native American influences predominate on the spa menu. Sophisticated skin-care treatments and high-tech equipment are not part of the equation here. You will not find the latest technology nor any attempt to compete with the sophistication of the megaspa trend. Instead you will find a unique place whose construction followed the principles of "green building." Recycled birdseed was used for walls, and the wood was recycled from old railway trestles.

A feeling of timelessness is evident the moment you cross the threshold. As you enter the spa, soft light and music shut out the outside world. This is known in these parts as "the whisper zone." The Sundance lifestyle is evident from the herbal teas that are produced here to the many skin-care products that come from Sundance Farms.

After checking in with the receptionist and leaving the changing area, guests transition into their spa treatment by having a complimentary fifteen-minute foot soak in the waiting area. From here guests are met by their therapist. There are only five treatment rooms, but what this spa lacks in size it makes up for in the purity of its treatments, from the Native Neroli Body Polish (forty-five minutes) to the legendary Honey & Oatmeal Body Blanket (sixty minutes). According to Sundance lore, Native Americans used neroli flowers (orange blossoms) during ceremonies that honored a tribal member's rise to a higher state of understanding and being. The spa uses neroli extracts in a body treatment that starts with a gentle brush exfoliation and concludes with a massage with a neroli moisturizer. Couple this with the brisk mountain air, straightforward cuisine, a walk along wooded trails, and the sheer drama of the majestic scenery, and the result is a well-balanced spa experience. Spa treatments, outdoor sports, and luxurious accommodations accented with a rustic flair make up your spa experience here.

Sundance stands alone in the spa world because of its serious and uncompromising environmental commitment. There are few places in the world with a hands-on program operating year-round. Once you rekindle your creative energy, there are many ways to channel it into a productive project. At the Art Shack, guests are invited to try their hand at activities from jewelry making, photography, and etching to pottery and sculpture. Classes are in session six days a week.

> *To us Sundance is and always will be a dream.*
>
> —ROBERT REDFORD

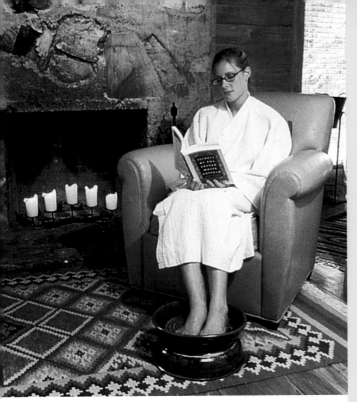

Spirit of the Mountains

The Spa at Sundance
PP3 Box A-1
Sundance, UT 84604
Phone: (801) 225–4107
Fax: (801) 226–1937
E-mail: reservations@sundance-utah.com
Web site: www.sundance-utah.com
Season: Year-round
General Manager: Keith Archibald
Spa Director: Brian Paris
Fitness Director: Brian Paris
Reservations: (800) 892–1600
Spa Appointments: (800) 892–1600
Accommodations: A variety of accommodations (ninety-five) include studios with a queen or twin beds. Sundance suites have a queen bed with kitchenette, fireplace, and patio. Mountain suites have a king or queen bed in the master bedroom and a living room, full kitchen, dining area, and fireplace. Mountain homes with two to five bedrooms can be rented.
Meals: Three choices include the Foundry Grill for breakfast lunch and dinner, the Sundance Deli, and the Tree Room with "earth to table cuisine" for dinner.
Facilities: Spa, art studio, hiking and ski trails, horse stables, mountain biking.
Services and Special Programs: The spa schedules massages, body polishes, and facials and has a fitness center with cardio- and muscle-toning equipment. There are ski and snowboard schools with half- and full-day class lessons. Sundance Gallery and Workshops classes at 10:00 A.M., 1:00 P.M., and 3:00 P.M. are generally $30 an hour.
Rates: $$$$
Best Spa Package: Nurture in Nature includes three nights in a suite, breakfast in the grill, two massages, and two facials. Lodging in the Sundance suite is $1,314; the mountain suite is $1,584.
Credit Cards: Most major
Getting There: By air to Salt Lake City, then a two-hour drive by transfer at $90 per Sundance guest.
What's Nearby: A tour to Sundance Farms; Park City (forty-five minutes) with Zoom's, Robert Redford's trendy restaurant; Soldiers Hollow (twenty minutes), site of the cross-country skiing competition in the 2002 Winter Olympics. Mountain biking, hiking, and fly-fishing are nearby.

Sunscreen Sense

Sunscreens are a necessary part of life, yet they are not all the same. The average sunscreen will protect you from the sun but not necessarily from free radicals. Sunscreens need a higher level of protection than just antioxidants. An ingredient to look for when purchasing a sunscreen is d-alpha tocopherol, or green tea. Kerstin Florian, known in the spa world for skin-care products, recommends a sunscreen with a high sun protection factor (SPF). This helps to build the capillary walls, which keeps the skin protected from free radicals. She urges sun lovers to read the label carefully and purchase a product that has both ingredients, although it could be more expensive. "In the long run antioxidant combination sunscreens are a wise investment," she says. "Permanent sun damage can be reduced by using the right product."

THE GREENBRIER
White Sulphur Springs, West Virginia

Set in the Allegheny Mountains, this monumental Georgian-style hotel is a world unto itself. Founded more than 200 years ago, it is the grande dame of American spa resorts.

Surrounded by 6,500 acres of forest and golf courses, the white-columned hotel is a National Historic Landmark. With its international academy of culinary arts, a private health clinic, tennis academy, and three championship golf courses, a constant stream of activity crosses the marble lobby. The spa emerged in 2001 with a new look and expanded treatment facilities. In addition, there is now a meditation garden—a secluded terrace with a fountain and seats designed to soothe the mind and spirit.

The resort's impressive indoor swimming pool is one of the few parts of the 1913 Greenbrier hotel still in use. Lavishly tiled, the 140-foot pool is grand, and the pool area has a juice bar and lounge with garden wicker furniture. All guests can use the pool without charge.

The famous Greenbrier mineral spring waters flow only in the spa's hydrotherapy baths, where a bubbly soak in the sulfurous water of the Alvon spring is scented with essential oils of krauter herbs from Hungary. Think of it as a cocoon where you are escorted by a personal therapist and treated with cordial Southern care. Select from an extensive menu of services, from body exfoliation to hydrotherapy, facials, and massage. A makeup consultation shop, the Perfect Image, adjoins the spa salon, which offers hair and nail care. Use of exercise equipment and an aerobics studio are charged on an a la carte basis or as part of spa packages.

More than fifty recreational activities are offered to guests. In addition to the Sam Snead Golf Academy, there is indoor and outdoor tennis, Land Rover

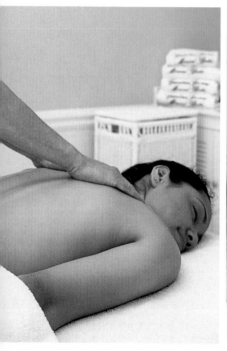
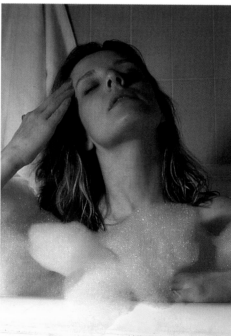
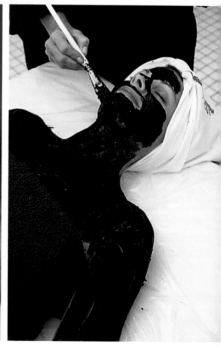

Driving School, croquet, horseback riding, carriage rides, Falconry Academy, skeet- and trapshooting, and fishing. Jogging and biking trails take you into the quiet forest or downtown, where a small business center services the needs of the community. Scattered around the hotel are thirty shops offering sportswear, gifts, kitchen accessories, and books.

The traditional Greenbrier spa experience starts with a private hydrotherapy bath. Next comes a steam inhalation room enhanced with aromatherapy oils to clear congested sinuses. Then more hydrotherapy in a Swiss shower or the Scotch hose treatment, to enhance circulation, which is followed by a body scrub or soothing buff. The finishing touch is a full-body massage with herbal potions.

Medical checkups can be coordinated with a spa program. The fully staffed, privately operated Greenbrier Clinic, located on the resort grounds, has diagnostic, nutritional, and executive health programs.

Ideal for families, the resort has a movie theater, bowling alley, and instruction in shooting and falconry as well as golf and tennis. Staying in one of the seventy-one deluxe cottages and guest houses scattered about the grounds adds privacy and extra space for the kids. Perhaps the most unusual attraction is the once-secret underground bunker built during World War II to be used by the Congress in case of an emergency. Still fully outfitted, the bunker can be toured with a historian leading you through its fascinating history.

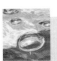

A New Look

Treat yourself to a new look while at the Greenbrier spa. The Perfect Image cosmetic shop is staffed with consultants who can analyze your skin type and suggest the latest shades of eye coloring, lipstick, and sun protection. A signature line of Greenbrier products is available at the spa shop.

Taking the Waters with History

The Greenbrier
300 West Main Street
White Sulphur Springs, WV 24986
Phone: (304) 536–1110
Fax: (304) 536–7854
E-mail: thegreenbrier@greenbrier.com
Web site: www.greenbrier.com

Season: Year-round
General Manager: Jack Damioli
Spa Director: Marie Baumuller
Reservations: (800) 624–6070
Spa Appointments: (800) 624–6070
Accommodations: 637 guest rooms, including forty-six suites and seventy-one estate houses. Traditional furniture and draperies, large walk-in closets in the older rooms, TV, the usual amenities, large tiled bathrooms, air-conditioned. (Greenbrier green is used in carpets and window shades.)
Meals: Two meals are included in daily packages. From morning doughnuts and coffee in the lobby to dress-up dinners with a string quartet in the vast dining room, American cuisine shines. Spa selections are low calorie, with reduced salt and sugar. Alternatives include a cafe called Drapers and Sam Snead's for pub-style food.
Facilities: Full-service spa with hydrotherapy, salon for hair and nail care. Aerobics studio and cardiovascular/strength-training equipment. Indoor and outdoor swimming pools, saunas, steam rooms, whirlpools. Tennis on five covered courts, fifteen all-weather outdoor courts. Golf club.
Services & Special Programs: Executive health checkup, massage, skin care, bodywork. Personal trainers and scheduled group exercise. La Varenne cooking weeks; Land Rover Driving School; Falconry Academy.
Rates: $$$
Best Spa Package: Two-night Healthy Living package with hotel room, two meals daily, unlimited use of exercise equipment, Alvon krauter bath and aromatherapy massage, facial, women's hairstyling or men's scalp massage. Cost includes gratuity, tax: $1,090–$1,153 per person, double occupancy; $1,624–$1,750 single.
Credit Cards: MasterCard, VISA, American Express
Getting There: From Washington, D.C., by car on I–66 west to I–81 south, I–64 to White Sulphur Springs exit (six hours). By train, Amtrak scheduled service, "The Cardinal" (six hours). The closest airport is in Lewisburg, which has scheduled van service to the Greenbrier.
What's Nearby: New River Gorge National River, Lewisburg (Civil War history), Beckley (coal mine museum).

THE AMERICAN CLUB—KOHLER WATERS SPA
Kohler, Wisconsin

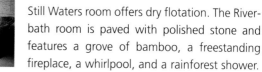

Old-world craftsmanship and the latest technology for hydrotherapy combine to create a unique spa experience in the American heartland at the Kohler Spa. Soothing colors and textures of stone, glass, and wood complement the dramatic design of the treatment rooms, where an amazing array of bathing rituals are offered. The Primal Ritual has a Zen-like setting for bubbling baths. The Still Waters room offers dry flotation. The River-bath room is paved with polished stone and features a grove of bamboo, a freestanding fireplace, a whirlpool, and a rainforest shower.

The Renaissance Bath lets you soak in a slipper-shaped copper tub; you steep in a warm, soothing milk bath with rose petals, then Hollyhock moisturizer is applied to your body.

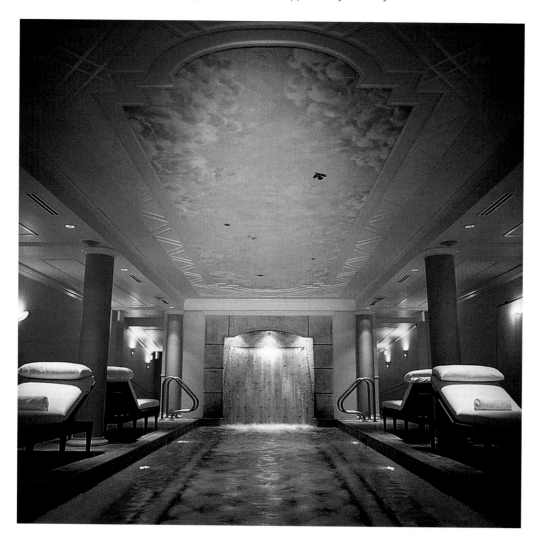

Relax or swim laps in the pool in the central atrium. Elaborate mosaic tile, an 8-foot waterfall, and Roman-style lounges add to the classical look of the pool. Try a water-supported massage, called Watsu, or sit under the waterfall for a natural massage. Tsunami, a ninety-minute combination of massage and hydrotherapy, stimulates your central nervous system with waves of water.

The American Club is the resort that houses the spa, and the resort combines luxury and tradition. Built at the turn of the twentieth century to house the Kohler Company's immigrant employees, the original structure (and the new wings) reflect solid comfort. Guest rooms feature the latest in bath design, and restaurants range from gourmet to tavern-style. In the recently renovated Carriage House, you have direct access by elevator to the bilevel Kohler Waters Spa and salon, plus a private lounge where breakfast and afternoon refreshments can be enjoyed in your spa robe. Next door the Kohler Design Center documents bath design past and present.

Rigorous exercise and group workouts are on tap at Kohler's Sports Core, a private club equipped with trainers and a Cybex circuit, indoor tennis courts, and swimming facilities. Spa guests have access to two 18-hole Pete Dye–designed golf courses and a 500-acre wilderness preserve that offers hiking trails, fishing, and seasonal sports. In a factory town devoted to building better baths, this is a place of comfort and warmth, a restorative and relaxing getaway.

Color Therapy Soothes Moods

The mood-enhancing lighting in treatment rooms at Kohler Waters Spa is adjusted to create effects that range from sunrise to sunset. Said to increase energy and combat depression, color therapy has been effective during long winters typical of the Midwest. Soaking in the spa's sok bath adds a new dimension: Underwater lights change color to suit your mood.

The American Club—Kohler Waters Spa
501 Highland Drive
Kohler, WI 53044
Phone: (920) 928–3777
Fax: (920) 208–4934
E-mail: DKNewsletter@kohler.com
Web site: www.kohlerwatersspa.com
Season: Year-round
Director of Spas and Sports Core: Jean Kolb
Spa Manager: Joan Rogers
Reservations: (800) 344–2838
Spa Appointments: (866) 928–3777 (toll-free)
Accommodations: Fifty-two rooms in the Carriage House with direct access to spa; 237 rooms and suites in main buildings, linked by underground walkway. Wide range of design: four-poster brass bed or modern wood furniture. Suites have fireplace, spacious bathroom with heated towel rack, wet bar. Carriage House rooms feature wood paneling, standard bath and bed with duvet, feather pillows. All have TV, telephone, air-conditioning; on-site check-in, and concierge.
Meals: Light meals are served at the spa relaxation pool. The American Club's signature restaurant, the Immigrant, specializes in Wisconsin seafood and Kohler Purelean beef, served in small rooms representing countries where Kohler Company has roots (jacket required). Nearby, Cucina offers Italian specialties indoors and lakeside; River Wildlife features game, grilled trout, seasonal salads. Pub menu all day in Horse & Plow Tavern. Complimentary continental breakfast for Carriage House guests includes fresh fruit, cereals.
Facilities: Twenty-one treatment rooms, a relaxation pool, fireplace lounge, fitness room, and salon. Sports Core (free admission for spa guests).
Services & Special Programs: Massage, facials and skin care, aromatherapy wrap, baths, mind-body relaxation, makeup and hair styling. Bathroom planning consultation at Design Center. Children's health and fitness at Sports Core.
Rates: $$
Best Spa Package: Three-night Spa Getaway includes four treatments plus bath experience, two spa lunches. Priced from $1,815 for two people in double room, including 18 percent gratuity; taxes are added. Single rate is $1,132.
Credit Cards: All major
Getting There: From Milwaukee, by car I–43 to exit 126, Route 23 west to Kohler (about one hour). Airport Connection (800–236–5452) van from/to Mitchell Airport, Amtrak, and bus stations. From Chicago about two-and-a-half hours).
What's Nearby: Kohler factory tour, shops at Woodlake Center, Lake Michigan, Milwaukee Museum of Art.

ECHO VALLEY RANCH & SPA

Clinton, British Columbia, Canada

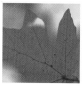

Saddle up for a unique adventure at Echo Valley Ranch. Amid the scenic splendor of the Canadian Rockies, a traditional Thai pavilion shimmers in a stand of pine and maple trees. A bit of the East has come west.

Combining a working ranch with an exotic spa is the kind of trans-Pacific experience that British Columbia seems to inspire. When ranch owners Norm and Nanthawon Dove met the architect who designed a summer palace for the king of Thailand, they conceived a structure that brings both worlds together. Completed in the summer of 2002, the Baan Thai pavilion has two houses equipped for spa treatments. Facing a tiled open-air courtyard, the pavilion is a peaceful place that enhances balance in body and mind.

On the top deck of the Baan Thai you can practice yoga or simply enjoy the scenery. Downstairs, there is an open space for workshops and group workouts. Crafted of teak wood, the entire two-story structure seems to have been transported from Thailand and offers the latest in hydrotherapy and skin care, complete with tradiional herbal treatments. The lavish Baan Thai suite also is available as a Zen retreat.

Staffed by Thai aestheticians, the spa complements the ranch's horseback riding program. Trail rides and training with forty Tennessee Walker thoroughbreds, acres of meadows, 185 head of cattle, falconry flights, and an herb garden add to the feeling that you have entered a realm of nature where all things are in harmony.

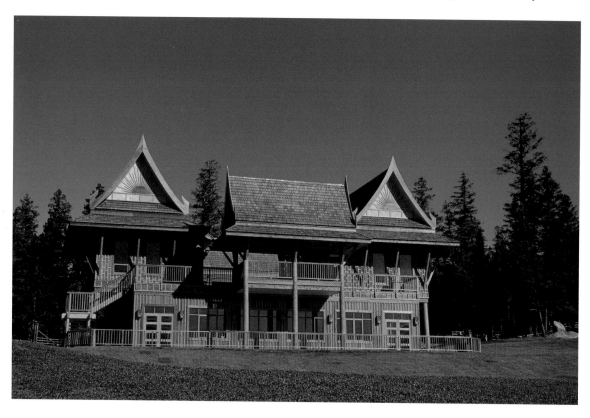

Unwinding after a day on the trail, you can enjoy an indoor swimming pool, sauna, and gym. Three deluxe log lodges and cabins accommodate twenty-six guests most of the time—up to forty as a group.

Forget roughing it; guest rooms feature huge beds with fluffy duvets, modern toilet, and shower. Some rooms have lofts where teenagers (minimum age thirteen) can sleep. Cabins are ideal for families; one has romantic furnishings for honeymooners.

Meals are served in the main lodge, a brawny three-story structure of one-hundred-year-old spruce logs that resembles a ranch house designed for corporate getaways. Ranch host Norm Dove can pilot one of the planes parked on the landing strip, discuss wines of western Canada, and talk international business. On request, ranch hands take you fly-fishing, white-water rafting, and hiking. There are also wildlife expeditions to Fraser River Canyon. In winter snowshoeing, skiing, ice skating, ice fishing, and sleigh rides add to the spa and riding options.

A native of Bangkok, Nanthawon Dove imported Thai silks as well as specialists in Thai massage for the new spa. This is about as authentic as it gets. Think of the experience as a first-class spa hotel with horses, plus a taste of Thailand.

A Lifestyle Match

The focus of the fitness and nutrition programs at the ranch comes from a book titled *Eat Right for Your Type* by R. D. Adamo, M.D. The concept: Your correct diet is a function of your blood group. Chef Kim Madsen, a native of Denmark, brings world-class culinary talent to the ranch kitchen. Honored in New York at the James Beard House, Madsen demonstrates heart-healthy cooking in his big, open-counter kitchen. Understanding your body type helps Madsen match food for maximum energy. Bring medical records with your blood type to set up a special diet.

East Meets West in Canadian Cowboy Country

Echo Valley Ranch & Spa
Clinton, British Columbia V0K 1K0
Canada
Phone: (250) 459–2386
Fax: (250) 459–0086
Web site: www.evranch.com

Season: Year-round, except January and February

General Manager: Norm Dove

Spa Director: Nanthawon Dove

Reservations: (800) 253–8831

Spa Appointments: (800) 253–8831

Accommodations: Deluxe log lodges with private bedrooms for up to forty guests. Choice rooms have private balcony, bathroom with shower or tub, twin or king-size beds with down-filled duvet. Main lodge has large lounge, leather furniture, large-screen TV, billiards, board games, outdoor hot tub. Baan Thai suite and large cabins for couples and families offer luxury and spaciousness.

Meals: Buffet breakfast and lunch, and seated dinner family-style included in daily room tariff. Fresh vegetables and herbs from organic farms; ranch-bred beef and poultry; prized salmon from nearby rivers.

Facilities: Spa complex has hydrotherapy tub, wet table, jet shower, steam room, massage room, fitness center with exercise equipment. Indoor swimming pool with spring water in separate building.

Services & Special Programs: Trail rides included in daily program price. Available a la carte: massage, facials, body wrap, aromatherapy bath. Cooking class and workshop on herbal gardening, falconry demonstration, roping and horse training demonstration are part of all-inclusive package. Wildlife safari, white-water rafting, fly-fishing by float plane (fee) on request.

Rates: $$

Best Spa Package: Echo Valley Ranch Experience, a seven night program with half-day Baan Thai treatment, choice of therapies; all meals included. Ranch horseback rides and adventure outings. From $1,580 to $1,895 per person, double occupancy. Plus 7 percent GTS and 10 percent service charge.

Credit Cards: American Express, MasterCard, VISA

Getting There: From Vancouver by car, scenic route via Fraser River Valley to Highway 97; at Clinton pick up Kelly Lake Road (10 kilometers) to Jesmond Road (seven hours). By air, scheduled flights Saturdays to/from the ranch (one hour) by North Vancouver Air; private plane landing strip.

What's Nearby: Whistler ski area, Cariboo Trail, Fraser River, High Bar Indian Band village, Barkerville ghost town.

FAIRMONT BANFF SPRINGS HOTEL—WILLOW STREAM SPA

Banff, Alberta, Canada

From the moment you enter this well-established icon in the Canadian Rockies, the sheer size of Fairmont Banff Springs will awe you. Built in 1888 and modeled on a Scottish baronial castle, the resort, surrounded by mountains and wildlife, is a statement of grandeur. Canadian hospitality reaches its zenith here, where all is done on a grand scale—from the monumental lobby to the indoor saltwater pool. Hospitable touches include fresh fruit, coffee, tea, and water available in the lounges throughout the day.

The resort's 32,000-square-foot, two-level Willow Stream Spa seeks to create a relaxing, stress-free environment. You enter via a spiral staircase and arrive at the reception area, where there is a boutique, well stocked with Kerstin Florian spa products, and a full-service beauty salon.

Check in and begin your tour of the premises. First you'll visit the extensive pool areas, where you should plan to spend a part of the day. The dome-covered mineral pool with its view of the surrounding natural beauty is a masterpiece of architecture, combining the best of both worlds—spa and wilderness. During the ski season, the idyllic mineral pools of the resort attract even the hard core skiers.

The Willow Stream Spa is a sanctuary amidst one of the finest displays of nature— the setting is one of the most impressive in the world. There are separate areas for men and women, but the gyms are coed. Sixteen treatment rooms offer an excellent range of treatments, from Hungarian moor mud wraps to a chamomile body scrub that produces soft, smooth-looking skin. There are also more esoteric treatments, such as the organic black mud facial, the therapeutic thermal mineral bath, and the spirulina body wrap. The spa brochure describes the facilities and details spa treatments and spa etiquette. The spa alerts guests that "arriving late is a breach of etiquette and will shorten the spa treatment."

Although you might not want to tear yourself away from the slopes or the invigorating mountain hikes, there is an excellent schedule of fitness classes throughout the day, starting around 9:00 A.M. Class offerings fluctuate with the seasons, but examples include sessions focusing on the abdominals, stretch-

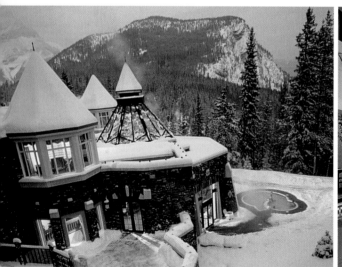
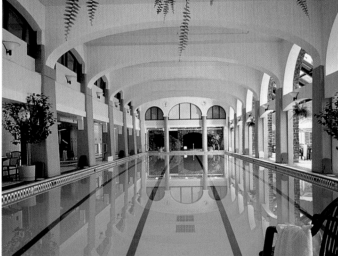

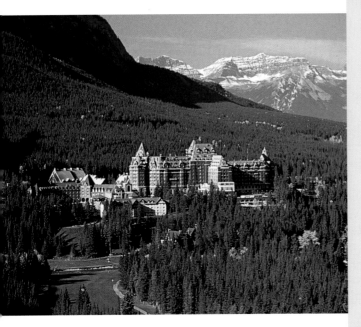

Fairmont Banff Springs Hotel—Willow Stream Spa
405 Spray Avenue
PO Box 960
Banff, Alberta T1L 1J4
Canada
Phone: (403) 762–2211
Fax: (403) 762–4447 (hotel); (403) 762–1766 (spa)
E-mail: banffsprings@fairmont.com
Web site: www.fairmont.com, www.willowstream.com

Season: Year-round

General Manager: Ted Kissane

Spa Director: Karen Vonkeman

Reservations: (403) 762–2211 or (800) 441–1414

Spa Appointments: (403) 762–2211 or (800) 404–1772

Accommodations: 771 guest rooms and suites, offering river or mountain views. Chateau deluxe rooms are suitable for up to four guests; Heritage Premier rooms have chandeliers, mock fireplaces, and traditional decor. Junior and one-bedroom suites are also available.

Meals: There are twelve restaurants in the resort.

Facilities: Willow Stream Spa mineral pool; full-service spa; fitness evaluation; saltwater indoor pool (heated in winter); outdoor whirlpool; indoor whirlpool; cascading waterfall pool; inhalation and sauna rooms; salon for hair and nails; fitness/cardio room; 27-hole golf course; 76,000 square feet of meeting and conference facilities.

Services & Special Programs: Interpretative hiking and guided mountaineering program; horseback riding; guided snowshoeing expeditions; ski trips to Norquay, Sunshine, and Lake Louise ski areas; tours of Banff National Park.

Rates: $$

Best Spa Package: Signature treatments, a one-day Pure Indulgence package for $529. Included are a Wildflower Body Polish, aromatherapy massage, European facial, manicure, pedicure, spa lunch, and hair style (shampoo and blow dry). Accommodations must be reserved separately.

Credit Cards: Most major

Getting There: From Calgary International Airport, transfer by limo, bus, or van. By car, Banff Springs is 80 miles west of Calgary on the TransCanada Highway.

What's Nearby: The Columbia Icefield, Banff National Park, three major ski areas, Banff Center for the Arts.

---

ing, water aerobics, weight training for women, and full-body workout.

There are no evening programs or speakers, but many recreational options are available at the resort's many restaurants and lounges. Fairmont Banff Springs with its Willow Stream Spa lives up to its reputation as one of the world's finest resorts.

Alpine Acclimatization

An alpine environment, although phenomenally beautiful, can provide distinct health challenges. For some, getting acclimated to high elevations can take days or weeks. The problem can be aggravated if visitors unused to the mountains overexert themselves—they may suffer headaches, extremely sore muscles, severe sunburn, shortness of breath, and even nosebleeds. To enjoy the beauty of the mountains and become acclimated gradually, Fairmont Banff Springs recommends taking it easy, increasing water intake, using high SPF sunscreen and lip balm, and limiting caffeine and alcohol consumption.

HALDIMAND HILLS SPA VILLAGE
Grafton, Ontario, Canada

A baronial stone mansion overlooking Lake Ontario is the centerpiece of Haldimand Hills Spa Village. Operated like a destination spa, it's also popular with young Toronto professionals as a day spa excursion. But the laid-back ambience is conducive to long weekends, with sybaritic soaks in the hot tub and sunset walks.

Emerging from hectic traffic on Highway 401, you are suddenly surrounded by the farms and open meadows. The spa village includes suites in former farm houses, a converted schoolhouse, a colonnaded mansion, and the original Ste. Anne's Country Inn and Aveda Spa. Farther east in the picturesque town of Port Hope, Haldimand Hills' sister spa, The Hillcrest, offers romantic escapes, fine dining, and a new menu of treatments with Dr. Hauschka botanical products.

Ste. Anne's features comprehensive skin care, moor mud baths, and the new Maison Santé fitness center with an aerobics studio and indoor swimming pool. Downstairs in the main building, a rabbit warren of treatment rooms and coed steam room leads to the mud bath—the only one of its kind in the eastern part of Canada and the United States. Two specially designed ceramic-tile vats heat moor mud, an organic skin cleanser that soothes muscular pains. Mud baths aren't for everybody. You get either a sense of being connected to nature or claustrophobia.

The Aveda spa menu follows traditional lines: facials and skin care, bodywork, hairstyling, and nail treatments. Using pure essences of flowers and herbs, Aveda products complement this comforting place where body and mind are in balance.

One of the unique features is a "twinning" hydrotherapy room, where wet treatments get an added dimension. As you relax on the table, two therapists synchronize moves to scrub your body with sea salts, followed by application of moisturizer. And there are built-in showers, with piles of fluffy towels stacked in antique wooden cupboards.

Mornings start with guided stretches and meditation. The air has an invigorating quality that's just right for bike trips to nearby villages, hikes, and walks on the estate's trails.

Meals are a combination of country and spa cuisine, featuring local produce and venison, and herbs from the inn's organic garden. Bread is baked daily (and can be wrapped to take home). Calories are not discussed, but the chef accommodates special diet requests. And you can bring your own wine.

Rooms come in many sizes and shapes. Several suites are in small tower wings connected to the manor house. Native stone and slate, topped by copper turrets, give the buildings an old-world look. Recent additions were skillfully blended with the original structures. Some bathrooms have cast-iron soaking tubs.

Join scheduled group exercises and walks at Maison Santé. There is an aerobics studio and exercise

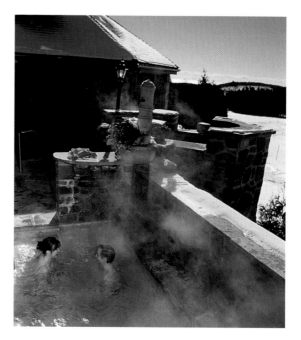

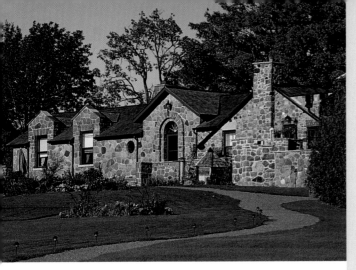

Haldimand Hills Spa Village
RR1
Grafton, Ontario K0K 2G0
Canada
Phone: (905) 349–2493
Fax: (905) 349–3156
E-mail: info@steannes.com
Web site: www.haldimandhills.com

Season: Year-round

General Manager: Jim Corcoran

Reservations: (888) 346–6772

Spa Appointments: (888) 346–6772

Accommodations: Ste. Anne's has nice bedrooms, eleven farmhouse suites, all air-conditioned, with private bathroom. All with fireplace, carved wooden beds or a queen-size four-poster. Completely nonsmoking. Amenities include robes and slippers, TV. The Hillcrest offers seven suites.

Meals: Three meals included in daily tariff. Breakfast includes eggs or egg-white omelette, homemade muesli, country breads. Dinner can be baked Chilean sea bass, wild mushroom and tomato risotto, venison steak, Atlantic salmon or char.

Facilities: Mud baths, aerobics studio, hydrotherapy tubs, steam room and sauna, outdoor lap pools, cold plunge pool, current pool, hot tubs, Vichy shower, Scotch hose.

Services & Special Programs: Scheduled group exercise and hikes. Spa services a la carte: massage (Swedish or Thai, shiatsu, and reflexology), aromatherapy facial, sea salt body scrub, herbal wrap, mud bath, manicure/pedicure.

Rates: $

Best Spa Package: Five night Total Transformation program, with all meals, accommodation, and a $200 allowance for spa services. Cost begins at $1,189 per person, based on double occupancy, plus tax and 12 percent service charge.

Credit Cards: American Express, MasterCard, VISA

Getting There: From Toronto, by car on Highway 401 to exit 487 (Grafton/Centreton), north on Aird Street to Academy Hill Road, left onto Massey Road (ninety minutes); by train, VIA Rail to Cobourg, complimentary limousine transfer.

What's Nearby: Presqui'le Provincial Park (bird-watching, beaches, marsh walk), Victorian Cobourg (Marie Dressler memorabilia museum), marina, Port Hope (antiques), golf courses, wineries, Niagara-on-the-Lake (Shaw Theatre Festival).

equipment—treadmill, bike, rower, ski simulator. Most of the time guests lounge in spa robe and slippers, or soak in the outdoor hot tubs. Swimming pools are heated for year-round use (one has an underwater current). A bottling plant taps into the inn's natural aquifer, which supplies pure drinking water and fills the pools. Three clay-surface tennis courts are available, free of charge, and racquets are on loan. Borrow a bike or drive to nearby vineyards and antiques shops.

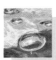

Mud Matters

Thousands of years ago, when the last glaciers melted, the land in what is now the St. Lawrence and Ottawa Valleys was so depressed by the weight of glacial meltwater that salt water flowed in from the Atlantic Ocean, forming an inland sea. Millennia passed as vast deposits of Leda clay were ground into a rocky flour and deposited as sediment on the floor of this inland sea. Naturally rich in minerals and organic trace elements, the mud is processed and sterilized by an Ontario firm, Golden Moor, for bath use. It is mixed with a thickener, sodium betonite clay from Saskatchewan. Maintained at high temperature, and sterilized between treatments, the moor mud soothes sore and tired muscles.

THE HILLS HEALTH RANCH

108 Mile Ranch, British Columbia, Canada

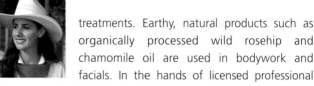

A destination spa within a wilderness ranch, the Hills has pioneered wellness vacations since 1985. Surrounded by 20,000 acres of western high country, the resort boasts the largest staff of health and wellness professionals in all of Canada.

Housed in one of the ranch's woodsy chalets, you join an informal group for daily hikes and rides, as well as workshops on health and fitness. Although discussion topics range from the latest research results on obesity to the benefits of aromatherapy, the emphasis is on learning how to balance stress in your life. Programs focus on athletes and the mature person, including maintaining a healthy heart through exercise and nutrition. You can saddle up for the "horse whisperer" experience or go for weight loss weeks. Also offered are short retreats devoted to hiking, beauty, and executive renewal.

Helping you achieve balance, the spa has an extensive menu of more than fifty healing body and beauty treatments. Earthy, natural products such as organically processed wild rosehip and chamomile oil are used in bodywork and facials. In the hands of licensed professional aestheticians, you gain an immediate sense of relaxation. For longer-lasting results, a take-home program and products are recommended.

All of these activities take place in the main lodge, where sixteen treatment rooms, an indoor swimming pool, an exercise studio, and a restaurant are located. Run like a guest ranch, the family-oriented resort also has stables with thirty riding horses and a resident wrangler, and a ski lodge for winter recreation. You can join morning and afternoon horseback rides most of the year and explore more than 130 miles of trails. Snowmaking equipment assures downhill skiing, snowboarding, and tubing in the night-lit winter play park.

Far from rustic, this is more dude ranch than luxury resort. Bring jeans, boots, and sweaters along with workout clothing, or plan a shopping spree in the nearby town of Williams Lake. In addition to cattle ranches, the area's main industry is logging. Stacks of timber await processing at plants near Williams Lake, which also hosts a major rodeo. Evening entertainment can be line dancing, a hayride, and campfire at a teepee.

Heart-healthy fare is featured in the main dining room, and a cafe in the ski lodge takes care of winter crowds. An extensive menu allows choices of calorie-counted food or typical ranch specialties, from barbecue to steaks and salmon. If you're trying to lose weight, there's a thirty-day package that includes all meals.

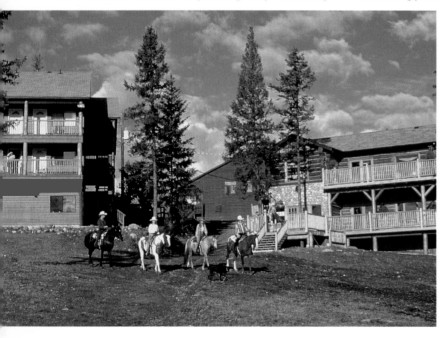

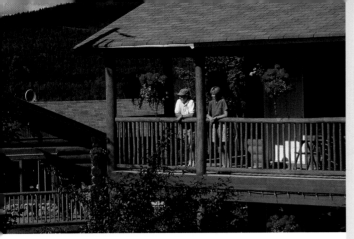

The Hills Health Ranch
P.O. Box C-26, 108 Mile Ranch
British Columbia V0K 2Z0
Canada
Phone: (250) 791–5225
Fax: (250) 791–6384
E-mail: thehills@bcinternet.net
Web site: www.spabc.com

Season: Year-round

General Manager: Patrick Corbett

Spa Director: Juanita Corbett

Reservations: (250) 791–5225

Accommodations: Ranch House with ten deluxe junior suites, sixteen large rooms in two-story manor house, all with balcony, air-conditioning, private bathroom. Pine furniture, country comforters on beds. Families and small groups are housed in twenty private chalets.

Meals: Calorie-counted spa cuisine included in vacation packages, with options for ranch-style food. Lunch can be chicken fajita with sour cream and salsa; dinner choices include baked salmon with asparagus, venison in peppercorn-maple sauce, seasonal vegetables.

Facilities: Indoor swimming pool, aerobics studio, fitness center with free weights, cadiovascular and strength-training equipment. Spa suite with sixteen treatment rooms in main lodge. Full-time riding program on premises; ski lodge open to day guests.

Services & Special Programs: Scheduled group exercise, guided hikes, trail rides. Spa services include massage, reflexology, full-body mud pack, herbal wrap, aromatherapy facial, loofah scrub. Thirty-day weight loss program includes supervised diet, personal training with exercise physiologist. Children's programs for riding and skiing.

Rates: $

Best Spa Package: Six-night Executive Renewal program includes all ranch activity plus daily stress-management sessions and massage. $1,711 single, $1,489 double, plus tax and gratuity.

Credit Cards: American Express, MasterCard, VISA

Getting There: By car through the Canadian Rockies from Vancouver, or points along the U.S. border, Highway 97 to 108 Mile Ranch (five hours). By air, scheduled flights to Williams Lake on Air Canada (one hour).

What's Nearby: Cariboo Trail historic sites, Williams Lake western art gallery.

Having created the first Canadian wellness center, the ranch's resident owners devote a lot of personal attention to guests' well-being. In the homey dining room, staff are always on hand to discuss the day's activities, what's on the menu, and things to see in the area. Offering an all-inclusive program of indoor aerobics and fitness workouts, healthy meals, trail rides and guided treks over rolling ranch land around lakes and forests, the Hills turns "howdy" into a cheerful affirmation of health.

Healthy Hip Rose Harvest

Wild rose bushes grow in abundance on the ranch's Cariboo meadows. July is the best time to enjoy full bloom, but rose hip harvest in fall is when spa guests get the advantage of some of the world's best and richest creams to enhance body and skin conditions. Many gallons of Cariboo rose hips are handpicked, dried, then crushed into powder in a unique grinding process that preserves the vitamin and mineral content of the flowers. Taken as an infusion, rose hips are a ranch remedy for bladder and kidney problems, and prevention of colds. The Cariboo rose hip cream made locally is used in facials to heal broken capillaries and helps with varicose or spider veins on the face and legs. The Hills' special formula adds rose hip powder to cold-pressed grapeseed oil, which is high in vitamin E and niacin—great for skin health and healing.

SPA EASTMAN

Eastman, Quebec, Canada

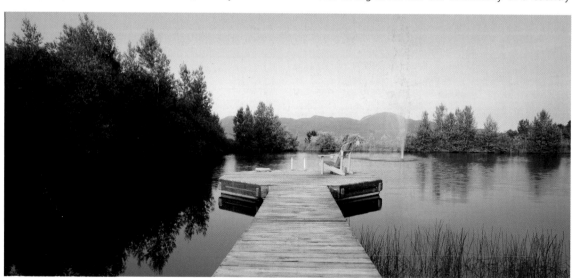

Set among farming villages in the eastern townships an hour southeast of Montreal, Spa Eastman is a unique retreat devoted to health. A crossroad for skiers heading to nearby slopes and summer cottagers, the town of Eastman is on the old stage coach road between New York and Montreal, chemin des Diligences.

Turning off the fast Autoroute 10, you discover a 315-acre nature preserve that harbors Spa Eastman (formerly known as the Eastman Health Center). There is an old barn that no longer stables horses and a new therapy building that looks more like a ski chalet than a spa. Totally secluded among spruce and pine trees, rustic wood lodges offer modern comforts in forty-five guest rooms on ten acres. The natural beauty and quiet are an instant tranquilizer.

Founded in 1977 as a center for naturopathy, Eastman evolved gradually as a full-service destination spa. Under the direction of founder/owner Jocelyna Dubuc, the center's growth climaxed in 1999 with the opening of a two-story pavilion that houses all of the treatment and relaxation rooms, a Watsu pool, a swimming pool, a hammam, steam rooms and saunas, and hydrother-

apy baths. In addition to thirteen guest rooms, the building has a restaurant and lounge.

When selecting treatments (called *soins* in bilingual Quebec), you can opt for European hydrotherapy or California massage. Among the unique experiences here is an invigorating oxygen and steam bath, in which your head pokes out of a covered tub while showers of carbon dioxide, oxygen, and water promote blood circulation and oxygenation. Another way to perk up your skin during the seasonal dryness of winter is to have a body peeling done with sea salts and loofah, followed by an algae wrap, stimulating algae bath, and rubdown with moisturizing cream to finish.

With a naturopathic doctor on staff, the center offers programs that combine fitness and well-being. Shape-ups can start with something as simple as walking mindfully. "It's important to vary the rhythm," explains a trainer. "The heart is a muscle. Keeping one constant rate, as you often do when jogging, isn't very effective." So the morning walks become a test of skills as well as stamina.

The dining room has the informality of a country

inn and a chef who creates spa cuisine with French flair. Menus tend toward vegetarian but include fish, chicken, and even rabbit. Between buffets of home-baked breads and muffins, farm-fresh yogurt and vegetables, fruit and herbal teas, you will not go hungry here.

The serious side of Spa Eastman includes applied kinesiology for rehabilitation after surgery or accidents and workshops on a range of lifestyle issues. Dubuc and her staff (most of whom are English-speaking) present a caring, low-key approach, without a hint of dogmatic preaching on healthy living.

Enjoying the great outdoors is part of the program. Surrounded by gentle hills and woods crisscrossed by trails, with the majestic peak of Mount Orford lording over it all, you can don snowshoes or cross-country skis to explore the winter landscape. There are 8 kilometers of groomed ski trails and 15 kilometers for hikes on the center's property. In fact, walks through the frosty forest are a popular option on long winter nights. If you haven't brought gear, an outfitter named O'Katraventures rents snowshoes and skis (and mountain bikes in summer).

When it's time for a tune-up or self-indulgence, this is a hideaway with a big heart and affordable prices.

Naturopathic Shape-up Taps Energy Naturally

Getting into shape doesn't require strenuous exercise at Spa Eastman. A simple walking technique can be just as effective as many performance sports. Guided by physical fitness professionals, the walking program is part of a fifteen-day package that includes workshops on nutrition and group exercise classes. Supervised by a naturopathic specialist, participants learn healthy food combinations and how to select food rich in nutrients to boost energy. Stretching, posture, and balance are improved through workouts with free weights, FitBalls, and in the pool. Hikes along country roads and on the slopes of Mount Orford are designed to burn fat while increasing cardiovascular capacity. The bucolic charm of Quebec can work wonders.

A Canadian Village of Health

Spa Eastman
895, chemin des Diligences
Eastman, Quebec J0E 1P0
Canada
Phone: (450) 297–3009
Fax: (450) 297–3370
E-mail: courrier@spa-eastman-com
Web site: www.spa-eastman.com
Season: Year-round
General Manager: Jocelyna Dubuc
Reservations: (800) 665–5272
Spa Appointments: (800) 665–5272
Accommodations: Forty-four rooms, including thirteen junior suites with fireplaces in the main building. Guests are housed in nine two-story lodges (pavilions) furnished in simple, modern style; the older units are rustic. All rooms have private bathroom with shower or tub, air-conditioning.
Meals: Three meals daily, plus afternoon break, included in spa package. Breakfast buffet includes cereal, eggs, toast, French toast, coffee, herbal teas, and fruit juices. Lunch menu offers wheat soup with two beans, salad buffet, Norwegian-style cucumber salad, leek quiche. Supper features fettucini or baked chicken with vegetables, roast duckling, or poached salmon.
Facilities: The main building houses twenty-four treatment rooms, indoor swimming pool, Watsu pool, steam room, hydrotherapy tubs.
Services & Special Programs: Hydrotherapy, Watsu (shiatsu in pool), massage, lymphatic drainage, reflexology, shiatsu, shower massage, oxygen bath, aromatherapy, body wraps and peel, pressotherapy leggings, aesthetic care of nails and face. Cure programs for stress, weight loss, body cleansing.
Rates: $$
Best Spa Package: Five nights in a room with a fireplace and mountain view, all meals, daily scheduled walks and fitness classes, two massages, body wrap and peel, facial, two baths, and two underwater jet massages. Rates are $1,031 single, $902 double. Rates are US and don't include tax.
Credit Cards: American Express, MasterCard, VISA
Getting There: From Montreal by car, Autoroute 10, exit 106 to Route 245 toward Eastman, then Route 112 toward chemin du Lac d'Argent, chemin des Diligences (one hour). From New York (six hours) or Boston (four hours) via Montreal.
What's Nearby: Vermont, New Hampshire, New York, St-Benoit-du-Lac Abbey.

FOUR SEASONS RESORT PUNTA MITA—
APUANE SPA
Punta Mita, Mexico

This veritable Garden of Eden is located on the northern tip of the Bahia de Banderas, one of the world's largest natural bays. The Four Seasons Resort, with its stunning Apuane Spa, is a part of a new 2,716-acre development. Punta Mita means "tip of the arrow," and for centuries this deserted stretch of coastline was virtually tourist free. Until construction began at the resort, there was no electricity, running water, or phone lines. Today, the luxury resort coexists beautifully with the surrounding tropical environment.

Offering chic tropical decor in accommodations secreted away in thirteen thatched and red-tiled casitas, Punta Mita is the site of the best surfing beaches along the coast and irresistible spa treatments.

In this lush seaside setting overlooking the Pacific Ocean, the stress of the high-tech world slips away.

What better place to erect a world-class spa offering variations on traditional massage, such as the Punta Mita, a fifty- or eighty-minute treatment that incorporates tequila, indigenous sage oil, and Mexican healing techniques. The fruit scrub and the Punta Mita refresher facial will further convince you that you are in paradise. The full-service Apuane Spa offers massage and skin-care treatments, separate men's and women's steam rooms and dressing rooms, as well as a beauty salon and health club.

The guest rooms and suites are furnished in a style befitting a luxurious Mexican home, all with modern conveniences, including computer modems, color television, and two-line speaker phones. The secluded accommodations range from casita rooms with private terraces to one- to three-bedroom suites.

The distinctive flavors of nuevo latino cuisine, as

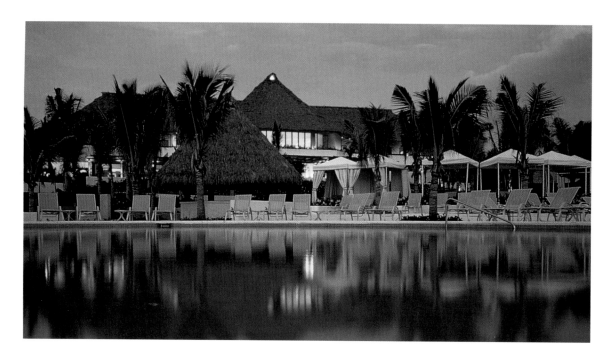

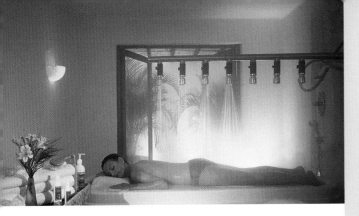

Four Seasons Resort Punta Mita—Apuane Spa
Punta Mita, Bahia de Banderas
Nayarit
Mexico 63734
Phone: 52–329–291–6000
Fax: 52–329–291–6060
Web site: www.fourseasons.com

Season: Year-round

General Manager: Ricardo Acevedo

Spa Director: Holly Beckwith

Fitness Director: Nora Orozco

Reservations: 52–329–291–6000 or (800) 332–3442

Accommodations: 140 guest rooms and suites housed in clay-tile roofed casitas, most with private plunge pools. In-room amenities include fax, terry bathrobes, private bar, TV, telephones, in-room safe, pay-per-view movies.

Meals: Ketsi Pool Restaurant and Bar serves all meals; the Aramara is open for a nuevo latino cuisine dinner.

Facilities: A private 18-hole Jack Nicklaus–designed golf course; four night-lit tennis courts; large free-form pool with whirlpool; white-sand beach. Apuane Spa: eight massage rooms, two wet-treatment rooms, skin-care treatments, beauty salon, separate men's and women's sauna and steam rooms and locker/dressing rooms; health club with equipment.

Services & Special Programs: Airport transportation; complimentary children's services; nonsmoking rooms; twenty-four-hour concierge; sailboat and powerboat charters, deep-sea fishing trips, surfing trips; seasonal whale watching and sea turtle hatching tours.

Rates: $$$

Best Spa Package: El Dia de Belleza (Day of Beauty) starts with a Swedish massage, followed by a deep cleansing facial. The three-and-one-half-hour package ends with a manicure and pedicure. Cost is $311. Accommodations during the high season, October 1–June 30, start at $590 single or double occupancy; during the low season, July 1–September 30, the rates start at $390.

Credit Cards: American Express, MasterCard, VISA

Getting There: The resort is a thirty-minute ride northwest of the Puerto Vallarta International Airport. The concierge can arrange transportation.

What's Nearby: Deep-sea fishing and other water sports; Los Veneros Beach Club with ecological park and artisan center; a horseback tour of Mismalya jungle.

well as a range of seafood and international dishes, dominate the menus at Punta Mita. Spa-goers will delight in the Four Seasons's own alternative cuisine menu choices, which limit cholesterol, sodium, and calories. The Ketsi Pool Restaurant and Bar, located in the pool area, offers spectacular ocean views. The Aramara Restaurant, with an outdoor bar/terrace, has live music beginning each night at sunset.

The Four Seasons's deluxe touches are found everywhere. If you yearn to indulge your senses in a quiet corner of Mexico, this is the place to make it happen.

More Than One Way to Sip Your Tequila

Some men are reluctant to experience the more esoteric spa treatments, but those offered here in an ultraprivate ambience are too tantalizing to resist. The Man for All Seasons Facial, a cleansing and nutritive facial designed to neutralize the impact of stress, sun, and sports, as well as the harsh abrasives the male skin endures, will leave the skin feeling younger than springtime. El Dia del Guapo (the Handsome Man) package starts with a salt scrub followed by a relaxing Punta Mita massage. Men, if you think most lotions and potions don't pack a punch, this massage is your answer—the secret massage ingredient is tequila! The Volcanic Mud Wrap is another serious step for men on the verge of loving spas; the black mud stimulates metabolic functions and rejuvenates skin and body. Olé!

JW MARRIOTT CANCUN RESORT & SPA

Cancun, Mexico

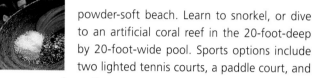

Set in the heart of beachfront action on Cancun's hot hotel strip, the new spa at JW Marriott Cancun Resort is a cool oasis. Mayan-inspired treatments use healing properties of fresh fruit, stone and crystal, incense, mud, and milk for a rejuvenating experience.

Overlooking the Caribbean, this three-level sanctuary is the largest resort spa in Latin America. Among its distinctive features are an indoor lap pool and Jacuzzi, juice bar, dedicated aerobics room, and sixteen treatment rooms. Enjoy spectacular views while working out in the fitness center or getting a massage.

Mexican traditions enhance treatments created exclusively for resort guests. Based on cleansing rituals to prepare brides and pregnant women, ancient Mayan ceremonies have been updated with state-of-the-art materials. The body is wrapped with self-heating clay or rose petals; hydrotherapy baths are infused with milk serum; jade crystals are said to help drain excess fat from your body.

Sybaritic recreation comes with spa seclusion. The resort's free-form fantasy pool and dive pool, and a freshwater lagoon with waterfalls are set right on the powder-soft beach. Learn to snorkel, or dive to an artificial coral reef in the 20-foot-deep by 20-foot-wide pool. Sports options include two lighted tennis courts, a paddle court, and nearby golf courses.

With a choice of five restaurants, from Mexican to Italian, you can be as casual as you want or get into the salsa beat. The spa offers complimentary juices, teas, and fruit throughout the day and has a small cafe where meals and smoothies pamper the calorie-concerned. For a change of scene, cross the "Skywalk" to the adjacent Marriott CasaMagna Cancun Resort. Or explore the shopping village in Old Cancun, complete with bullfight arena.

Accommodations also set a new standard for Cancun resorts. Opened in 2001, this is the first JW Marriott built "offshore" to honor the founder of Marriott Corporation, J. W. Marriott Sr. Elegant luxury distinguishes contemporary guest rooms, and personal service creates a milieu that combines legendary Mexican hospitality and flair. Ideal for discerning travelers, this is a resort where families and spa-goers can enjoy the best of Cancun.

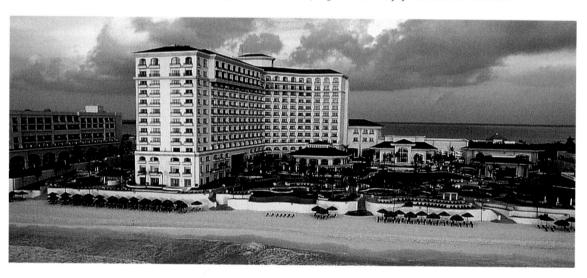

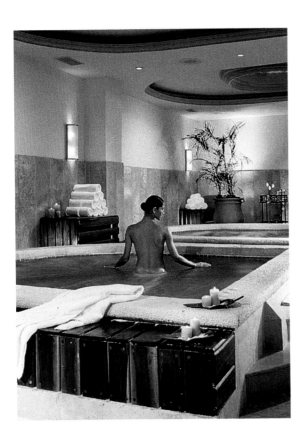

JW Marriott Cancun Resort & Spa
Boulevard Kukulcan, Lote 41 Zona Hotelera
Cancun, Quintana Roo
Mexico 77500
Phone: 52–998–848–96–00
Fax: 52–998–848–96–01
E-Mail: info@offshoreresorts.com
Web site: www.offshoreresorts.com
Season: Year-round
General Manager: Chris Calabrese
Spa Director: Cynthia Claudia Graf
Reservations: (800) 223–6388
Accommodations: 449 guest rooms including seventy-five suites, each with spacious private balcony and ocean view. Bathrooms have double-vanity dressing area, bathtub, separate shower stall. Amenities include bathrobes and slippers, coffeemaker, iron and ironing board, hair dryer; TV with Spanish networks and U.S. cable, two phone lines. Purified water systems and climate control throughout the hotel. Nonsmoking and wheelchair-accessible rooms available.
Meals: Spa packages include buffet breakfast featuring tropical fruit and eggs cooked to order. The Spa Cafe serves healthy, low-fat food throughout the day. Cafe Salsa has indoor and outdoor dining overlooking the sea; Gustinos Italian Beach Grill offers seafood and specialty cuisine. Poolside service and gourmet deli.
Facilities: 35,000-square-foot, three-level spa with sixteen treatment rooms, fitness center, aerobics studio, beauty salon, indoor lap pool, Jacuzzi, and juice bar. Also freshwater swimming pool, ocean beach, lighted tennis courts, water-sports equipment rental, children's play area.
Services & Special Programs: Mayan rituals, massage, body scrubs and polishes, manicure and pedicure, facials, hydrotherapy bath, hair treatments and styling, sauna and steam rooms, personal trainers.
Rates: $$
Best Spa Package: The Mayan Essentials Spa Package includes accommodations in a premier oceanview room, two treatments per room per stay, daily admission to spa, and buffet breakfast. Seasonal rates range from $195 to $325 per room/per night based on double occupancy.
Credit Cards: Most major
Getting There: Located 11 miles from Cancun International Airport, the hotel is on the beach boulevard. Airlines include American, Continental, Delta, USAirways, Mexicana, and Aeromexico. Visitors need proof of citizenship and photo ID.
What's Nearby: Mayan ruins, Xcaret and Xel Ha ecological parks, Palencar reef at Cozumel.

Mayan Makeovers

Spa Director Cynthia Claudia Graf, a native of Mexico, researched historic Mayan rituals and ceremonies to develop treatments for the new Marriott spa. Experience the Sihi Na Queen bodywrap that firms the skin with self-heating clay. Real Mayan jade crystals enhance the Jade and Rose Sculpture treatment, which encases you in a mud mask and rose petals. Although not promising to help you discover the fountain of youth, the spa's hydrotherapy treatment uses milk serum for a bath that helps combat certain physical and emotional ills. Preparing your skin for intense tropical sun may be the best reason to take advantage of the latest in spa products.

LAS VENTANAS AL PARAISO

Cabo San Lucas, Mexico

As you enter this stunning golf and spa resort, passing through the gates, your senses are confronted by "The Windows of Paradise," the translation of this aptly named enclave. Located at the southern tip of Mexico's 1,000-mile-long Baja Peninsula, where the desert meets the Sea of Cortez, this flower-filled retreat offers a distinct personality. Forget cookie-cutter, high-rise hotels, because once you experience the sheer drama of this Mexican Mediterannean-style getaway, you will never think about resorts in quite the same way. Original works of art are showcased throughout Las Ventanas. Woodcarvings, raised pebble walkways, and hand-painted accents adorning furnishings and fireplaces add charm and beauty.

The heart of this stunning resort is its spa, where out-of-the-ordinary treatments are the norm—such as the nopal anticellulite and detox wrap (featuring the special powers of Mexico's nopal cactus), the volcanic clay purification treatment, and the Tepezcohuite healing wrap. There are ample choices in facials, a half-dozen massage therapies, and eight exfoliation treatments. Hippocrates himself, the father of medicine, reputedly said, "The way to health is to have an aromatic bath and scented massage every day." Taking that seriously, the healing waters include a milk whey bath (said to be Cleopatra's secret weapon), which is prescribed for healing and restoring dry, sensitive skin. You can also partake in an old-fashioned mustard bath, an antioxidant green tea bath, and a milk and honey wrap. Lovers are often seduced by the massage for two. New Agers are inclined toward the holistic crystal healing massage, which uses ancient Shamanistic purification techniques to induce relaxation and generate healing memory patterns.

Adjacent to Las Ventanas is Cabo Real Golf Course, designed by Robert Trent Jones II, which winds down from the desert hills to the white-sand beaches of the Sea of Cortez, offering eighteen holes of dramatic natural beauty.

The restaurant provides bounty from the sea, with a wide variety of fish and seafood entrees, such as grilled snapper, Baja shellfish, and seared rare tuna. Light fare is included on the menu as well, with spa-compatible salads, low-fat yogurt soup, and a tomato-coriander glazed chicken breast. Room service is available twenty-four hours a day.

Spacious guest rooms and suites all open to the ocean, the coastline, or the golf course. The decor is handcrafted and features raised bed platforms, dressing areas, and glass doors to private terraces. Suite ter-

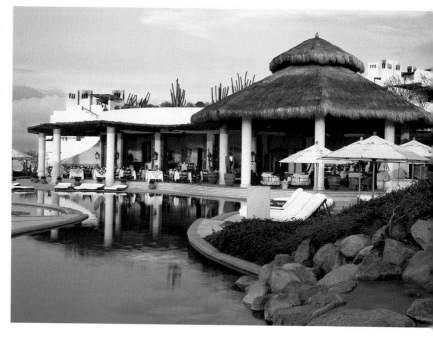

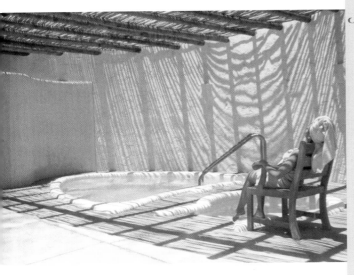

Las Ventanas al Paraiso
KM 19.5 Carretera Transpeninsular
Cabo San Lucas, San Jose del Cabo
Baja California Sur
Mexico 23400
Phone: 52–114–40300
Fax: 52–114–40301 or (310) 824–1218
E-mail: lasventanas@rosewoodhotels.com
Web site: www.rosewoodhotels.com

Season: Year-round (warm, arid climate; about 350 days of sunshine)

General Manager: Edward Steiner

Spa Director: Carole Spellman Sullivan

Reservations: 888–525–0483

Spa Appointments: 888–525–0483

Accommodations: The sixty-one guest accommodations include fifty-six suites, four one-bedroom superior suites, and a three-bedroom suite with three baths, private pool, and rooftop terrace.

Meals: The Sea Grill offers open-air patio dining, indoor dining, and dining in the guest room or suite. Twenty-four-hour room service.

Facilities: Full-service spa; a **Fit Plus** package with a fitness profile, lifestyle assessment, body composition analysis and instruction; cardiovascular machines and resistance equipment; personal trainers; beauty salon.

Services & Special Programs: Snorkeling and scuba diving; sportfishing; sailing; kayaking; windsurfing; desert excursions; horseback riding; sunset cocktail cruises; whale watching; and marine wildlife expeditions.

Rates: $$$

Best Spa Package: The Spa Discovery Package is a three-night program for two that includes accommodations (in a junior suite), round-trip airport transfers, breakfast and dinner daily, private mind/body evaluations, program planning session, and personally designed essential oils; sage foot bath; neck/shoulder massage; aromatherapy loofah salt glow; aromatherapy facial; moisturizing aloe; tea tree and lavender wrap; aromatherapy massage; hot-oil scalp massage; foot reflexology; two fifty-minute stretch/yoga classes; and use of the spa and gym facilities. $3,300 for two; tax and service additional.

Credit Cards: Most major

Getting There: Major airlines, such as America West, serve the San Jose Del Cabo International Airport.

What's Nearby: Cabo San Lucas with nightclubs, shops, cafes on the sand, and a variety of restaurants.

races host combination splash pools/Jacuzzis.

Bringing an unprecedented level of luxury to Los Cabos, Las Ventanas is a charismatic spa and golf resort with mesmerizing views, nearly perfect weather, and enchanting treatments to lift mind, body, and spirit.

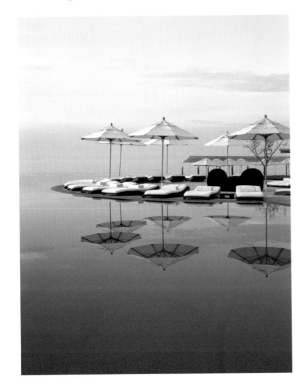

RANCHO LA PUERTA

Tecate, Baja California

Rancho la Puerta, in a small Mexican border town 45 miles east of San Diego, has endeared itself to three generations of health enthusiasts since it was established in 1940 by Edmund and Deborah Szekely. Today this spa, which resembles a quiet Mexican village, accommodates up to 150 guests within its 575 lush acres of gardens and paths.

"Siempre mejor" (always better) is the key to the Rancho's success; there is always something new and better on the agenda, such as the labyrinth, where guests can take a guided meditation walk. Guests come here from all walks of life and from all social and economic levels. Breakfast and lunch are served buffet-style; dinner is served by the waitstaff. You may be seated at a table with an astounding range of spa-goers, from a movie star to a psychiatrist and everyone in between. The ambience is informal; guests dress casually throughout the week-long program, which begins every Saturday.

Each fitness week offers as many as eighty activities. The early-morning hike and exercise program form the cornerstone of the Rancho. There are ten options, including the early-bird hikes, two 6:30 A.M. hikes, and a meadow hike at 7:00 A.M. It's best to view this as a progressive week. Guests are encouraged to start at their own level and partici-

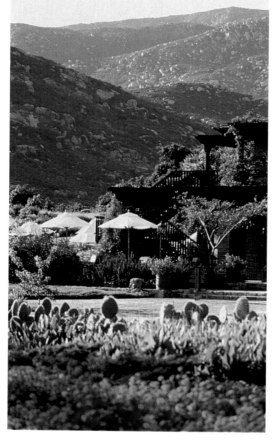

pate gradually in more challenging choices. Many fitness classes are scheduled for the morning so that by lunch you can pat yourself on the back for having already participated. Among those from which to choose are aerobics, power walking, and weight-training. After lunch, which showcases recipes developed by chef Bill Wavrin, it is time to relax with a massage, herbal wrap, facial, or the latest on the massage menu, called the Hot Stone. The new Health Center features spacious treatment rooms, original art, an immaculate locker room, and well-trained therapists.

Guests congregate in the main lounge to sign up for their favorite activities, ranging from an hour with Grandfather Raven (a Native American who talks about casting bones and stones) to the 4-mile vegetable garden breakfast hike, both offered once a week.

The unique accommodations are scattered throughout the property. Rancho La Puerta seems immense at first, but every structure is well lit and signed (although new guests still ask directions the first few days). The villa studios and suites, in a lush garden setting, are at the high end of the price range; they include in-room breakfast service in the winter and poolside breakfast service in the summer. The rancheras and haciendas are

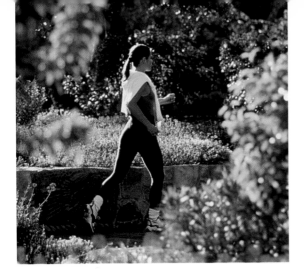

Rancho La Puerta
Tecate, Baja California
Mexico
PO Box 463057
Escondido, CA 92046
Phone: 52–665–654–9155
Fax: 52–665–654–1108
Web site: www.rancholapuerta.com

Season: Year-round

General Manager: Jose Manuel Jasso

Fitness Director: Phyllis Pilgrim

Reservations: (760) 744–4222 or (800) 443–7565

Accommodations: Cottages (rancheras and haciendas) with studio bedrooms, private patios and gardens. Villa studios and villa suites are cottages in a parklike garden setting with nearby swimming pool and hot tub; all have fireplaces.

Meals: All meals and snacks are included. Fresh fish twice daily, vegetarian dishes, plenty of greens, legumes, whole grains and other fibers, little fat or salt, and no white flour or refined sugar.

Facilities: The spa offers a comprehensive hiking program on 3,000 acres of rolling, natural terrain; seventy fitness classes; spiritually focused classes in meditation, tai chi, yoga, and more; tennis; volleyball; basketball; gyms; swimming pools; men's and women's health centers with steam rooms, whirlpools, and saunas.

Services & Special Programs: Garden tours and cooking demonstrations; men's fitness program; Pilates; evening programs and movies; couples weeks. Regular services include Hot Stone massage; water massage; salt glows; herbal, seaweed, and aromatherapy wraps; reflexology; facials; beauty salon services; tennis lessons; craft classes.

Rates: $$–$$$

Best Spa Package: The spa offers only one package; the one-week stay includes accommodations, classes, gourmet meals, evening programs, and use of all the facilities, and runs from Saturday to Saturday. Price varies depending on type of accommodation: from $2,460 single occupancy or $1,790 per person double occupancy to $3,505 single occupancy or $3,349 per person double occupancy.

Credit Cards: MasterCard, VISA

Getting There: Charter buses operate on Saturdays to and from the San Diego Airport at no charge. If you do not wish to take the bus, other arrangements can be made.

What's Nearby: Beyond its natural setting at the foot of Mount Kuchumaa, sightseeing from Rancho la Puerta is limited to nearby Tecate or other Baja towns. San Diego is only forty-five minutes away; Tijuana is thirty minutes.

designed in Mexican colonial style and, in keeping with all of the buildings, are accented with local arts and crafts. There are single accommodations in this category.

Rancho la Puerta has a loyal following. You might meet guests who've been here twenty times or more (they're recognized at the final dinner). The spa glow seen on the Rancho's guests stems from a harmonious flow of activities, healthy dining, and the upbeat attitude of a caring staff.

An Inner Journey to Personal Bliss

The fitness director at Rancho la Puerta, Phyllis Pilgrim, met the Dalai Lama in 1999. The knowledge she gained from this experience has influenced the tone she sets for her popular class, the "Inner Journey," offered at 4:00 P.M. daily. "Life is short so you must make the most of it," she says. "Think about what you are going to do that will make you feel good at the end of the day. Open your senses daily to appreciate what is around you." Pilgrim encourages guests to appreciate the aromas, the gardens, and the tranquillity of the moment. She believes that a "great metaphor for life" is practicing choice. At the ranch this happens the first day, as the guest may choose among seven group workouts. Pilgrim believes this is practical training for life.

EUROPE

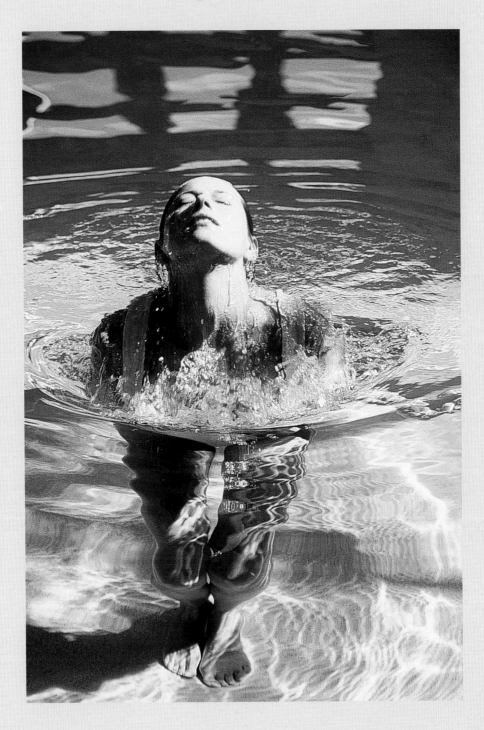

ROGNER-BAD BLUMAU

Bad Blumau, Austria

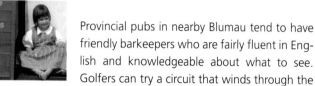

Creating harmony between body and mind, nature and art, the unique health resort of Rogner-Bad Blumau is both a destination and day spa. Its ten buildings, opened in 1997, are the work of Friedensreich Hundertwasser, an internationally renowned architect. Contemporary inside and out, the spa draws on ancient traditions of an Alpine region richly endowed with thermal waters and cultural centers.

The multicolored, curved buildings initially seem to clash with the pristine meadow in which they are set. Their shapes suggest recumbent dinosaurs; their swooping roofs are covered with grass. Windows are placed haphazardly: rectangles, circles, and squares, their frames painted in natural colors and neon tints. Think of it as the Guggenheim Museum meets EuroDisney. Though disorienting at first, the purpose becomes clear as you explore and experience this architectural wonder.

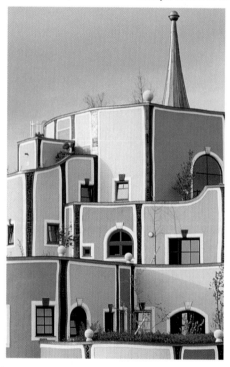

Treatments and activities, some in English, most in German, include such classics as moor mud wraps, nutrition for natural healing, revitalization therapies through sound, and the traditional water cure for purification and detoxification. Because accommodations and spa services are separately priced, your best bet may be to sample what's available on an a la carte basis.

Vacationing here includes all of the above, plus enchanting villages spread out in the direction of Graz (an hour's drive north) and Vienna (two hours south).

Provincial pubs in nearby Blumau tend to have friendly barkeepers who are fairly fluent in English and knowledgeable about what to see. Golfers can try a circuit that winds through the valley, playing nine different 18-hole courses. And, naturally, there are miles of well-tended hiking trails.

As a day spa, Bad Blumau is more thermal water theme park than holistic retreat. Developer Robert Rogner sought to capitalize on thermal springs that gush enough hot water to fill pools that hold the equivalent of 250,000 bathtubs. At times during the summer and holidays, it seems as if that many people are bathing in the outdoor pools, leaping into man-made waves, and enjoying the whirlpool recessed within the main swimming pool. A freshwater pool for children and babies draws lots of families, who are on day trips and have nothing to do with the spa.

But there are private places for spa treatments. You may escape to Meditation Island, where you have a choice of saunas—Finnish, Swedish, Turkish, herbal aroma—and a bar called the Klimbin. Or try the FindeDich center, to balance health and mind, or the beauty tower, Wunderschon, with skin care by Biodroga and Decleor.

Staying in the Kunsthaus, you are challenged by the artist/architect's aversion to straight lines. Some rooms, with their smooth, curved walls, evoke a modern-day version of Fred Flintstone's lair. Small but efficient, they are furnished in a modern kind of country style. Foyers hold charming pine armoires, matched by pine-plank floors.

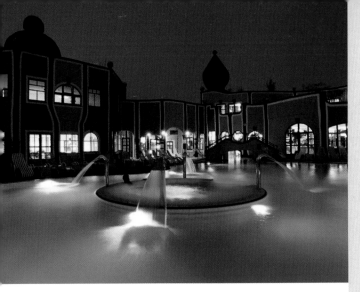

Rogner-Bad Blumau
A-8283 Blumau 100
Austria
Phone: 43–3383–5100–9444
Fax: 43–3383–5100–808
E-mail: spa.blumau@rogner.com
Web site: www.blumau.com
Season: Year-round
General Manager: Alfred Hackl
Spa Director: Wolfgang Kolbl
Reservations: (800) 650–8018 (United States and Canada); 800–13–67–46–81 toll-free from parts of Europe.
Spa Appointments: E-mail: resm@blum.rogner.com
Accommodations: 247 double rooms, fifty-nine suites, twenty-four apartments. Individually detailed, each includes tiled bathroom with shower or tub. Interiors feature unvarnished wood and natural fabrics. Amenities include bathrobe.
Meals: Buffet breakfast, included in room rate, offers muesli, yogurt, fresh fruit, country breads. Lunch and dinner are a la carte, feature local farm produce, Styrian specialties. Vegetarian menu and health food available.
Facilities: Holistic health center with extensive selection of hydrotherapy, wraps, and massage; thermal water park; beauty salon for bodywork, skin care; Roman bath, saunas, steam rooms; indoor and outdoor swimming pools; gym with Spinning bikes.
Services & Special Programs: Extensive selection of therapies and water cures. Body wraps include choice of grape residue, hay, aromatherapy oils, or fango. Massage can be Esalen-style, Thai or TuiNa, shiatsu or Swedish. Sound therapy for stress management; kinesi-therapy for muscular or bone problems. Special weeks: ayurveda, biking, walking.
Rates: $$
Best Spa Package: Discover Yourself; $200 includes Thalasso bath, body cocoon, Shiatzu massage, and Esalen bodywork. Unlimited use of the thermal spa and saunas, bathrobe and towel, and use of the sports and leisure program. Weekday all-day spa passes for the thermal spa and sauna facilities are $18; weekends, $20. Daily tax $2.00.
Credit Cards: American Express, MasterCard, VISA
Getting There: From Vienna or Graz, by car or taxi on Autobahn A-2, exit Sebersdor; by train, complimentary transfer.
What's Nearby: Graz, Salzburg.

The walls curl gently around corners and archways, painted a restful off-white. Apartments have a balcony and a bathroom with thermal water. Special rooms are reserved for allergy sufferers, nonsmokers, and the physically challenged.

At dusk, steam rises from the outdoor pool, adding to the fantasy of the buildings. With day-trippers gone, a meditative mood sets in. Couples cuddle on the concrete banquette that encircles the whirlpool, watching the sun set behind an iridescent golden-onion spire. Natural healing doesn't get much better.

Musical Meditation

Sound therapy with holistic doctor Wolfgang Kolbl gives you a sense of release. It is an intriguing inner adventure accompanied by the sounds of bells and gongs. You lie on a couch while the doctor moves around you, banging huge gongs and tubular bells, waving a buzzard's wing, setting Tibetan prayer bowls resonating on your chakra points, and strumming a monochord under the couch. The fifty-string monochord sends vibrations through your body. The copper bowls on your forehead and stomach vibrate. This symphony of sound is a virtuoso performance, harmonizing body and soul.

LE MERIDIEN LIMASSOL SPA & RESORT

Limassol, Cyprus

The legend of Aphrodite, the goddess of love and beauty, is alive and well on Cyprus in the eastern Mediterranean. According to Greek mythology, Aphrodite was born from the sea near here, emerging from the foam to earn her niche as a celebrated figure symbolizing femininity, beauty, and love. The Greek gods and goddesses chose Cyprus as their destination of choice for indulging pleasure and sport, and Cyprus continues to build on this theme.

The mystique of the gods flourishes on this romantic island. The spa was designed to reflect the spirit of the past but uses state-of-the-art engineering to harness the mineral-rich seawater for use in its spa treatments. The seawater, used in treatments with Thalgo Marine products, is thought to have a therapeutic effect on joint and back problems, arthritis, osteoporosis, and water retention. Skin care, facials, and massages feature Elemis products.

Le Spa opened just in time to host participants in the Donald Trump Miss Universe 2000 Pageant. With seven seawater pools (three outdoor), an aquarium plunge pool, a heated freshwater pool, an algaeotherapy center, and thirty-two treatment rooms, this is truly a sybaritic dream.

Enhancing Le Spa are thirteen renovated garden villas with a swimming pool built exclusively for their use. Four villas have private pools. Le Meridien also has two floodlit tennis courts and a multipurpose, all-weather training area for football, volleyball, and basketball. Children enjoy the Penguin Village Children's

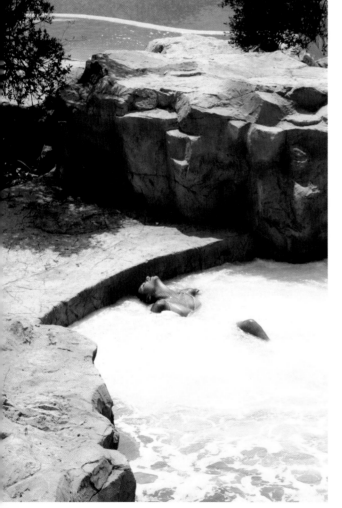

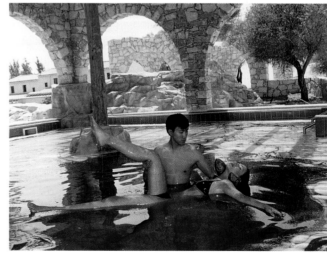

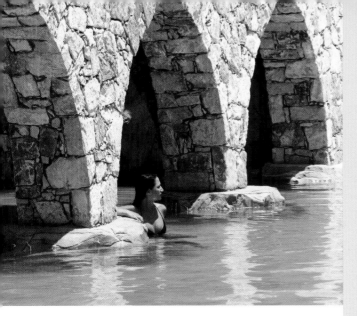

Le Meridien Limassol Spa & Resort
Old Limassol-Nicosia Road
P.O. Box 56560
CY-3308 Limassol
Cyprus
Phone: 357–25–862–000
Fax: 357–25–634–222
E-Mail: lespa@lemeridien-cyprus.com
Web site: www.lemeridien-cyprus.com

Season: Year-round

General Manager: Andreas Christopoulides

Spa Director: George Tavelis

Reservations: (800) 543–4300 (Meridien Hotels) or (800) 742–4591 (Amelia International)

Accommodations: 329 rooms, including fifty-six garden villas and suites. Amenities include air-conditioning, balcony or terrace, direct dial telephones, in-house movies, Jacuzzi bath tubs in suites, minibars, safe deposit boxes, and satellite TV.

Meals: Six restaurants at the resort and six bars; French gourmet fare at Le Nautile, the open-air Le Vieux Village, sushi at Kojima Lagoon restaurant, and all-day dining at Le Café Fleuri, a poolside restaurant and terrace with specialty buffets. All have no-smoking sections.

Facilities: Le Spa with four outdoor seawater pools, saunas, whirlpools, plunge pool, three heated indoor pools, algaeotherapy center, and thirty-two treatment rooms; two tennis courts and an all-weather area for various sports; children's area; art gallery; games room; shopping arcade.

Services & Special Programs: Thalassotherapy, medical checkup, massage, fango, facials.

Rates: $$

Best Spa Package: The six-day Equilibrium and Purity package includes a medical evaluation, six thalassotherapy programs, nutritional consultation, body fat measurement, lunch and dinner daily, personal exercise program, lime and ginger salt glow, two aroma spa ocean wraps, two detox ocean baths, affusion shower, two fennel cleansings, cellulite and colon therapy, strawberry herbal back cleanse, aroma-pure facial, sea shower, well-being massage, Japanese silk booster facial, Japanese silk eye-zone therapy, and daily herbal tea. Starts at about $2,200 per person.

Credit Cards: Most major

Getting There: The resort is on the south side of the island, fifteen minutes from Limassol city center, forty-five minutes from the Larnaca International Airport, and fifty-five minutes from Paphos International Airport.

What's Nearby: The resort sits directly on the beach and is fifteen minutes from the center of the city of Limassol.

Club with new waterslide and climbing apparatus.

Le Meridien Limassol Spa & Resort has a new "residents only" policy, providing guests total exclusivity, privacy, and personal service. It's a fitting tribute to the goddess of love and beauty, born from the sea.

Vive La Difference!

More men are enjoying the benefits of spa treatments, according to a study by the International Spa Association. It must be right. Just listen to one of our spa colleagues, who, after considerable reluctance, experienced a pedicure and facial for the first time. "I felt so relaxed and wonderful after having my face worked on. I couldn't believe a facial could make my entire body so relaxed. Most men are into their heads and not their bodies. They don't think of their face, feet, or hands. I guess I carry a lot of tension in the facial muscles. The same can be said for feet. We abuse those poor things all day in tight airless shoes, covered with socks. I was proud I had the treatments and felt very good about myself. I looked years younger and felt very relaxed. I should have been enjoying facials and pedicures years ago."

GRAND HOTEL PUPP—HARP SPA CLINIC

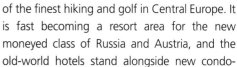

In the grand tradition of the original European spa hotels, the Grand Hotel Pupp in northern Bohemia exudes the charm and grace of the nineteenth century. Elegantly restored, the ballroom and marble atrium create the feeling that crowned heads dance the night away in this magnificent structure.

Privatization and a new government in Prague have encouraged preservation of the traditional water kurs along with new facilities for advanced treatment of stress-related illness. One of the best examples of this new breed is the Harp Spa Clinic at the Grand Hotel Pupp. Housed on two floors of the hotel's garden wing, the clinic offers a full range of treatments under medical supervision. Facilities include underwater massage tubs, mud therapy, massage rooms, facial rooms, and electromagnetic muscular stimulation. Your kur can include lymphatic drainage, reflexology, acupuncture, and hydrotherapy. Hotel guests also have access to the Roman Bath Spa and a beauty salon.

Beyond its façade of Mitteleuropa luxury, Karlovy Vary (better known in the West as Karlsbad) offers some

of the finest hiking and golf in Central Europe. It is fast becoming a resort area for the new moneyed class of Russia and Austria, and the old-world hotels stand alongside new condominiums and remnants of communist-era buildings. If you're not under a doctor's supervision, typically for a three-week kur program, the place to stay is Hotel Pupp. It's a return to the pleasures of a bygone era, with freshly decorated rooms that feature antiques and modern amenities. There are vast restaurants and bars serving Czech and international specialities, not spa cuisine. Concerts are held in the hotel's ballroom, originally opened in 1907, as well as in the city's newly refurbished theater, an 1886 architectural confection. During the annual International Film Festival Karlovy Vary in July, it's not unusual to see Hollywood stars at the Hotel Pupp.

The hotel's spa is replete with marble columns and mosaic floors and is modeled after ancient Roman baths. There are daily massages, saunas, steambaths, whirlpools, and fitness classes. Prices for spa services are about half what you'd pay at an American spa; appointments can be made by the hotel's concierge when you arrive.

The thermal waters still attract throngs to the town's public springs. According to test results, the warm mineral water contains all the vital minerals your body requires. Said to improve digestion and offer immunity from disease, a daily dose of the waters has been effective in reducing inflammation and for treating lipid disorders. Souvenir mugs with long sipping handles are sold in shops that line the promenade in front of the colonnades, where spring water is freely dispensed. Sipping water and strolling along the riverside is a daily ritual here. Visitors snack on waffles—first created in Karlovy Vary in 1788—and Viennese pastry. There is a museum of handmade glass from the Moser factory just outside town, where outlet shoppers can find bargains, and a brewery that offers

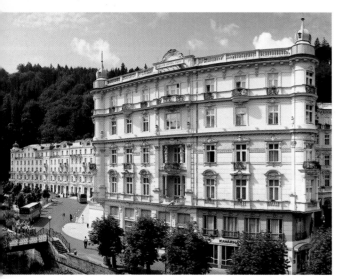

herbal liqueur samples. Surrounded by forested slopes, the central district of Karlovy Vary conveys a comforting sense of being set apart from the world, a place of health and healing.

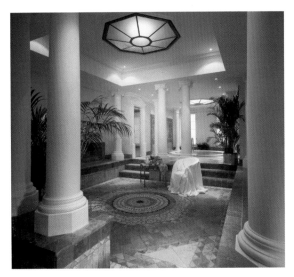

Spa Redefines Wine

Symbolizing beauty and harmony, the sculptured harp atop Hotel Pupp celebrates the pleasures of music, food, wine, and health.

"Wine is highly suitable for man if, in sickness and in health, he takes care to drink it with purpose and in proper measure, according to his individual condition." So said Hippocrates, the father of modern medicine. He advocated white wine as a diuretic. This belief in the beneficial powers of wine persists today. According to Michel Montignac, author of *Dine Out and Lose Weight,* wine has been proven to be beneficial to cardiovascular ailments. One glass of wine at the end of a meal is therapeutic, he says. He recommends champagne for rheumatism, pinot noir for weight loss, and dry champagne for bloating. Some spas serve a glass of wine occasionally. Perhaps Hippocrates would say what better way to enjoy spa dining!

Bohemian Traditions Meet Modern Medicine

The Grand Hotel Pupp—Harp Spa Clinic
Mírové námestí 2
360-91 Karlovy Vary
Czech Republic
Phone: 420–353–109–111
Fax: 420–17–323–44–88
E-mail: drsarova@atlas.cz
Web site: www.pupp.cz

Season: Year-round
General Manager: Jaraslav Sára
Spa Director: Dr. Milada Sarova
Fitness Director: None
Reservations: 420–353–109–631 (hotel); (800) 457–4000 (U.S.)
Spa Appointments: www.karlsbadspa.cjb.net
Accommodations: 112 luxury guest rooms rebuilt between 1994 and 1996. Some rooms are air-conditioned.
Meals: The hotel's main restaurant serves Czech and international specialties.
Facilities: Full-service spa with Roman baths; the Harp Spa medical center; tennis; squash; swimming; horseback riding; volleyball; basketball; conference facilities.
Services & Special Programs: Kur programs for metabolic, digestive, muscular disorders; oxygen therapy; antistress with acupuncture and homeopathic therapy; dental care; anticellulite series; cosmetician; facials, manicure, and pedicure. Kur Spa Course (in English) each May, two-week study tour including treatments. Information: phone (210) 822–7238; fax (208) 279–7596.
Rates: $$
Best Spa Package: The Harp Spa and Medical Therapy is custom designed to meet individual needs. It includes treatment for digestive, metabolic, and motor problems. The cost of the package is relative to the length of stay. The clinic offers a two-hour "rejuvenator" for $55. A day at the salon costs $98.
Credit Cards: Most major
Getting There: From Prague by car, Highway 6 West (ninety minutes); by train or bus; airport bus (two hours).
What's Nearby: Golf Resort Karlovy Vary; Moser Glassworks; Thun Porcelain; Zen Garden; horse racing course; Dvorak Autumn Music Festival; Marienbad; Plzen (Pilsen Brewery).

NAANTALI SPA HOTEL & RESORT
Naantali, Finland

Come aboard the world's only spa ship! Overlooking the blue Baltic Sea, the Naantali Spa Hotel's Sunborn Yacht symbolizes the rebirth of a Finnish maritime tradition. Since 1723, health-seekers have come by boat to enjoy the curative powers of the hot springs in Naantali. By combining a yacht with a modern resort, a unique destination for health conscious travelers has been created.

With the arrival of its magnificent Sunborn Yacht Hotel (launched 1998), the resort got a new lease on life. Although treatment facilities are centralized in Naantali Spa Hotel (opened in 1984), guests now have full use of both the yacht and a waterfront complex of shops and restaurants. Staying aboard Sunborn is like being on a deluxe cruise without waves. Permanently docked in the bay, the ship has a covered walkway that leads directly into the spa center. Each of the 102 staterooms is deluxe, similar to small luxury liners built at Finnish shipyards. For the ultimate sauna experience, stay in one of the royal suites that have a private veranda attached to the sauna.

Water is the theme at the main hotel, which has a thermal pool complex stretching toward the sea. You can swim outdoors year-round, even when it's snowing, duck into the hotter Roman pools, two Turkish baths, and four saunas. The fitness center has state-of-the-art exercise equipment, with trainers on hand for personal instruction. In the same area are a gym for group exercise and a sports hall where basketball, volleyball, and badminton games are organized by the activity directors. Don't worry about language problems; English is spoken by all staffers.

Water also invigorates the spa's treatments. For an antidote to winter darkness, try the Polar Night Bath, a soothing soak in herbal oils that includes bright-light therapy to boost your mood. Arctic plants and natural blue clay from the region's lakes and forests are used in body treatments to detoxify your body and stimulate your metabolism.

Southwest Finland and its capital city Turku have always had connections with the sea. Located about fifteen minutes by bus or taxi from Naantali, the ancient port has excellent ferry connections with Sweden. A university town, Turku's concert halls and museums add a lively dimension to enjoying the area's natural attractions.

The spa hotel is a world of its own, but a short stroll to Naantali's timbered Old Town reveals the romantic side of Finland. Rows of wooden houses are perfectly preserved, painted in bright colors, with attractive shops offering handcrafts and antiques.

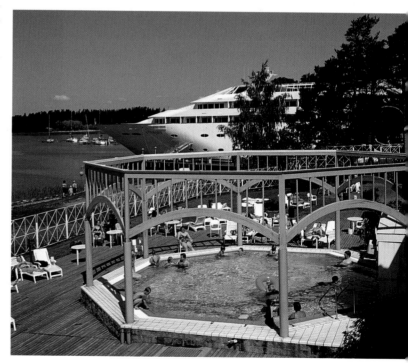

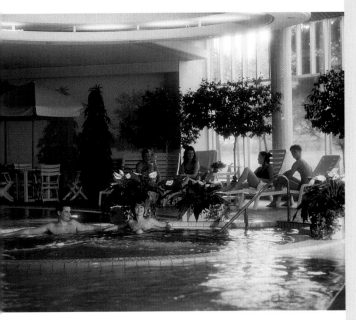

The old Monastery Church, where a summer festival of chamber music is held, and the gardens of the Finnish president's summer retreat, Kultaranta, are open to visitors.

The Baltic Sea's soft embrace makes Naantali an ideal escape from stress.

Sauna's Spiritual Side

The Finns have a spiritual as well as social connection with the sauna. It is not simply a place to sweat and douse yourself with water; it is also a place of healing. Babies were born in saunas, and the dead were laid out in them. To exorcise the devil, the possessed were taken into the sauna and beaten with a vihta—a whisk made of small birch branches—until the evil spirits departed. Today the sauna ritual is alive and well. Families gather in them to talk and meditate. After a pause for refreshments and a cooling shower or roll in the snow, it's back to the sauna (pronounced *sownah*) for another session of healthy sweating.

A Sea Change at Nordic Springs

Naantali Spa Hotel & Resort
21100 Naantali
Finland
Phone: 358–2–44–55–660
Fax: 358–2–44–55–623
E-mail: info@naantalispa.fi
Web site: www.naantalispa.fi

Season: Year-round

General Manager: Heli Virtanen

Spa Director: Ritva Niemi

Spa Appointments: 358–2–44–55–800

Accommodations: 331 rooms and suites, including 227 in the main hotel, 104 on Sunborn Yacht Hotel. All have private bathroom with shower, hair dryer, bathrobes, TV, telephone; most have balcony or sea view. Royal and presidential suites come with private sauna and large terrace.

Meals: Four restaurants and Cafe Roma provide Scandinavian and European specialties. An extensive buffet breakfast is included in hotel rates. Seafood, salads, and organic vegetables are featured. Also available: reindeer steak, pizza, Danish pastry, traditional Finnish rice cake. Special Diet Week with daily menu totaling 1,000 calories.

Facilities: Pool complex indoors and outdoors, saunas, steam baths, hydrotherapy bath, beauty salon. Balneotherapy remedial and galvanic baths, underwater massage, water gymnastics. Solariums.

Services & Special Programs: Aromatherapy massage, zone therapy, lymphatic drainage, reflexology, shiatsu, facials, body wraps and peels. Salon for skin, hair, and nail care. Medically supervised programs for physical rehabilitation, obesity, stress management, and fitness evaluation.

Rates: $$

Best Spa Package: Three-day Pamper Yourself holiday includes accommodations at Yacht Hotel, half-board, two treatments, use of facilities. Price per person $370, double; single room supplement $109. (Arrive Sunday or Wednesday.)

Credit Cards: Most major

Getting There: From Helsinki, by train or car to Turku. Take bus numbers 11, 110, or 111; taxi (twenty minutes).

What's Nearby: Turku, Helsinki, Valley of the Moomins.

INSTITUT DE THALASSOTHERAPIE LOUISON BOBET AT HOTEL MIRAMAR—CROUESTY

Port Crouesty, Arzon, France

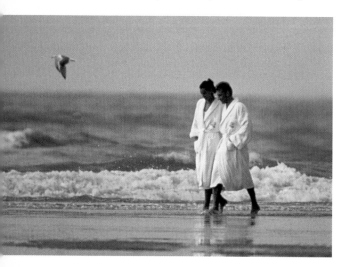

Tour de France champion cyclist Louison Bobet experienced a sea change thanks to thalassotherapy forty years ago. Amazed at the good it did his joints after an accident, Bobet and his brother Jean developed a health institute on the coast of southern Brittany. Taking seawater therapy to a higher level, the Institut de Thalassotherapie Louison Bobet at the Hotel Miramar has a cure for all seasons.

Step inside the Miramar Port Crouesty and you might think it's an oceangoing liner. Every detail of the hotel's design suggests a ship, decked out for a luxury cruise. Even the five floors are numbered "ponts," meaning decks, as on a French liner. The color scheme of your "cabin" echoes the blue of the sea and sky, and there's a deck chair on the balcony.

This "liner of Good Health" may resemble a ship architecturally, but it is beached in an artificial lake created by recycled seawater from the hotel's thalassotherapy center. Located on a peninsula jutting into the Atlantic Ocean, the sandy beaches at Arzon are protected by environmentalists, so the Miramar's designers came up with a system to naturally filter

water through the sand after it has been treated.

Taking the seaside cure begins with a medical evaluation. A sports medicine doctor checks your heart and general condition, then you head for the Institut to schedule treatments and exercise sessions. Occupying an entire deck of the hotel, the Institute has treatments for chronic aches and pains, fatigue, stress-related disorders, and postnatal body shaping as well as overall fitness programs. Whirlpool baths, jet showers of various kinds, exercise in the water, and massages—plus long walks along the beach and windy cliffs—leave you as tingly-pink as the cheeks of the Bretons.

The hotel has a diététique restaurant offering satisfying seafood dishes calculated at about 300 calories per meal. On the other hand, there is classic cuisine on the *pont supérieur* (the top deck) in a first-class dining room reminiscent of ocean liners. The dazzling Friday night seafood buffet spreads around a top-deck swimming pool—just like being on a cruise.

Thalassotherapy centers come in many sizes and styles—there are nearly fifty on France's Atlantic and Mediterranean coasts—and French law sets the standards. Built in the early 1990s, the Bobet Institute and its sister spa in Biarritz are among top-rated facilities. The nautical ambience at Miramar Crouesty sets it apart from others we have visited, and its location is a plus. Arzon has ancient history and a huge marina at Port Crouesty.

A "cure" requires a week or more, but you can come for a few days and enjoy the beach and indoor seawater swimming pool. The hotel has a well-equipped gymnasium, beauty salon, and sauna. Outings "sportif" by bike and boat are available. Part health club, part seaside resort, the Miramar is managed by Groupe Royal Monceau, known for its prestigious flagship hotel in Paris, Hotel Royal Monceau.

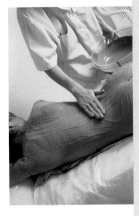

Padding about in bathing suits and fluffy white robes, guests follow the prescribed routine or relax at the rooftop pool, where the glass roof opens on warm days. Everyone carries a tote bag issued at the reception desk; it's likely to be filled with books for reading between bubblings and hosings, sunscreen, and perhaps a pet. After a few days, you'll feel part of the crew, swept away by the beauty of Brittany.

The Seaside Cure

For many people, the scent of sand, sun, and surf is a natural sedative, according to Dr. Alan Hirsch of the Smell and Taste Research Foundation in Chicago. He suggests some reasons for this: Vacations mean lower anxiety levels; odors evoke positive memories via chemical reactions in the brain; and odors may work like olfactory Prozac. Another factor may be negative ions. Studies have yielded conflicting results. Some suggest negatively charged ions wafting off the sea interact with the outer layers of our cells, which in turn alters brain chemistry and is subtly intoxicating. Thalassotherapy, which evolved in France from studies by Dr. Rene Quinton in the late 1800s, combines all these elements in a structured program under medical supervision. The application of seawater and algae to the body, and the simultaneous experience of a bracing seashore climate, has been found to be very beneficial. Thus the French used a Greek word *thalassa*—meaning the sea—to describe the course of treatments in thalassotherapy. Twenty-five centuries ago Euripides wrote: "The sea cures the maladies of man."

Sea Changes in Brittany

Institut de Thalassotherapie Louison Bobet at Hotel Miramar–Crouesty
Port Crouesty
Rue Leen-Vihan (BP 32)
56640 Arzon
France
Phone: 33–2–97–53–49–00
Fax: 33–2–97–53–49–99
E-mail: reservations@miramar-crouesty.com
Web site: www.miramarcrouesty.com

Season: Year-round

General Manager: Jacques Zartarian

Spa Director: Odile de Lescar

Accommodations: 120 rooms, twelve suites, all with balcony, contemporary furniture, modern bathroom. Amenities include robe and slippers, TV, radio, minibar. All air-conditioned, with sea view.

Meals: Separate dietetic and gourmet dining rooms, fixed-price menu or a la carte. Dinner starters can be fish soup, salad with sea scallops, smoked salmon, or fresh oysters. Grill choices include grilled swordfish, sole, steak, sea scallops, salmon. Specialties include Breton lobster, shellfish, and presalted lamb raised on seaweed and salted herbs. Desert is fruit tart, flan with plums, savarin. Herbal teas and espresso at pool bar.

Facilities: Thalassotherapy exercise pools, indoor seawater swimming pool, hydrotherapy tubs, Vichy shower, foot and hand baths, jet showers, ultrasonic baths, sauna, hammam (steam room), ionization spray, pressotherapy. Beauty salon, gymnasium, medical clinic.

Services & Special Programs: Weight loss, anticellulite week; ayurvedic cure prasama week. Aromatherapy, seaweed skin care, lymphatic drainage, physical rehabilitation. Postnatal program (seven days). Skin care with LaPrairie products, hair treatments using Rene Furterer method, pedicure, relaxation sessions.

Rates: $$

Best Spa Package: Remise en Forme Six-Night Package Croisière with room and half-board. Price: $1,260–$1,502 per person, double; $1,608–$1,966 single. VAT services included.

Credit Cards: American Express, Diners Club, MasterClub, VISA

Getting There: From Paris, by TGV train to Vannes (two hours), by car Autoroute D–780.

What's Nearby: Belle Isle, Nantes, Vannes.

LES FERMES DE MARIE

Megeve, France

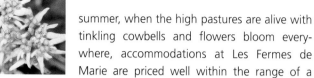

At first sight, the town of Megeve is beyond-belief picturesque: narrow, winding cobble-stone streets, tiny squares lined by ivy-covered buildings, and a fourteenth-century church with bulbous bronze-green bell tower. Megeve bans autos in the town center but has hiking trails and a cable car that ascends to breathtaking 12,600-foot views of Mont Blanc.

A cluster of chalets above a stream outside town, Les Fermes de Marie is more like a mountain village than resort hotel. Created by the owner/manager team of Jean-Louis Sibuet and his wife Jocelyne, it looks ancient but opened in 1989. Collected from farms in the area, 300-year-old lumber, carved wooden columns, and antique furniture conceal the resort's concrete infrastructure. There are eight lodges, the restaurant Grand Salle, and a spa building complete with an indoor swimming pool. Furnished in a mix of Savoyard and Ralph Lauren styles, no two rooms are alike.

It's easy to see why the king and queen of Sweden stay here in a private chalet during the ski season. In

summer, when the high pastures are alive with tinkling cowbells and flowers bloom everywhere, accommodations at Les Fermes de Marie are priced well within the range of a four-star hotel. What you don't get are crowds, organized fitness classes, and Americans. Summer clientele are an international mix of Italians, French, and British; only about 4 percent are American. The main attractions are pure mountain air, warm, dry climate, and great food. Families are welcome, although there is no program for kids other than hikes, sports, and a six-day climbing course offered by the Megeve tourism office.

Mountain herbs and flowers fill "the beauty farm" with sensory pleasures while you are enjoying an aromatherapy massage or facial. The all-natural treatments use beauty care products made from plants, essential oils, and biologically neutral bases. There are ten private treatment rooms in a rabbit warren below the reception area, all done in wood logs, stone, and terra-cotta tile. For exercise, a small gym offers bikes and treadmills, and there is a glass-walled swimming pool that overlooks an herb garden.

Men are treated to a personalized regimen at Les Fermes. The six-day fitness package alternates sessions of relaxing massage with skin care, hydro-massage baths, and seaweed wraps. Other programs for men and women include hydrotherapy and skin care. Altogether, forty-five different treatments are available a la carte.

Lodged in one of the wood-paneled chalets, you will find an array of antiques plus a big soaking tub in the bathroom. Fluffy white bathrobes are provided for lounging on the sunny terrace or balcony. The hotel compound is on several levels, surrounding a small garden where aperitifs and meals are served. The main dining room, a cozy grill, and a specialty restaurant offer enough variety that you may never need to request the dietetic menu.

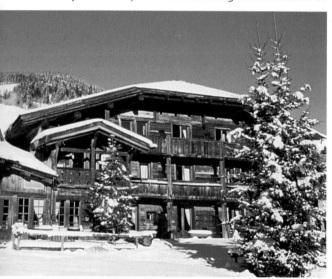

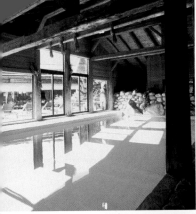
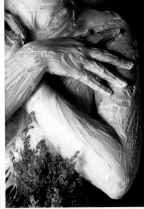
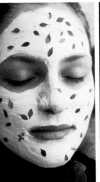
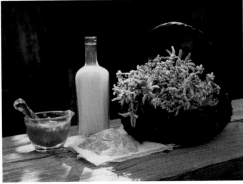

Les Fermes de Marie
Chemin de Riante Colline
74120 Megeve
France
Phone: 33–04–50–93–03–10
Fax: 33–04–50–93–09–84
E-mail: contact@fermesdemarie.com
Web site: www.fermesdemarie.com

Season: December 15–April 15; June 15–September 5

General Manager: Jocelyne Sibuet

Spa Director: Brigitte Flament

Accommodations: Sixty-nine rooms in Alpine lodges for 150 guests. All have private bathroom with modern amenities. Furniture is French-country antiques, wooden armoire, walnut table, rustic bedspread, lounge chairs. TV, telephone, clock/radio are standard; no air-conditioning needed. Dogs and children allowed.

Meals: Gourmet menu served in three restaurants. Breakfast buffet includes eggs cooked to order, cereals, cold meats, cheeses, coffee. Lunch and dinner feature nouvelle cuisine. Dietetic menu on request.

Facilities: Hydrotherapy tubs, Jacuzzi, sauna, steam room, Vichy shower, pressotherapy, exercise studio, indoor heated lap pool.

Services & Special Programs: Swedish massage, Thai massage, shiatsu, reflexology, seaweed wrap, mud packs, body gommage, G5, lymphatic drainage, hydrotherapy bath, jet sprays. Yoga class, excursion for Alpine luncheon, workshop on mountain plants led by a naturalist.

Rates: $$

Best Spa Package: Six-day Balance Program combines skin care and hydrotherapy, two treatments daily, teaching how to take care of yourself. Includes accommodations; buffet breakfast and dinner; lunch at mountain chalet; fitness program; free entrance to pool, sauna, and Jacuzzi; and a basket of beauty products. $986–$1,051 (summer); $1,078–$1,235 (winter). Rate is per person, double occupancy.

Credit Cards: American Express, Diners Club, MasterCard, VISA

Getting There: From Geneva, by car on Autoroute A–40 via Sallanches (sixty minutes). By train from Paris, TGV to Lyon, connection to Sallanches (three hours).

What's Nearby: Chamonix, Le Montenvers, Mer de Glace glacier, Mont Blanc.

Fight Jet Lag with Ginger Tea and Mountain Flowers

Mountain flowers and herbs grow wild in the fields around Les Fermes de Marie. Taking a nature walk with Clotilde Boisvert, founder of L'École des Plantes, a school for nature studies in Paris, you can learn about the healing properties of plants and flowers. As a booster for your immune system, fresh herbs are used in infusions you can sip while awaiting spa treatments.

Kim and Cary Collier, an American couple who developed Jamu herbal rituals while living in Indonesia, recommend ginger tea to fight jet lag. They find it helps digestion and improves systemic blood circulation, served hot or iced. "Sipping ginger tea while relaxing in a warm bath filled with flower petals is truly one of life's irresistible pleasures," they say.

LES PRÉS D'EUGÉNIE—LA FERME THERMALE

Eugénie-les-Bains, France

When food cravings get the better of your fitness program, this is the place to combine both passions. Michel Guérard's three-star restaurant rates among the best in France. A pioneer of *cuisine minceur*, his 500-calorie meals taste like 2,500. Matching the menu's excellence are thermal baths and country-chic accommodations that give new meaning to taking the waters.

La Ferme Thermale at Les Prés d'Eugénie, as the thermal resort complex is known, includes two spa treatment buildings, three hotels, two restaurants, and a cooking school. Clustered on forty acres of parkland planted with an herb garden and shaded by magnolia, plane, and tulip trees, it's in Eugénie-les-Bains, a Belle Époque village that seems to be in a time warp. Each of Les Prés d'Eugénie's hotels has a distinct look and mood, a result of antiques hunts through surrounding farms by Christine Guérard.

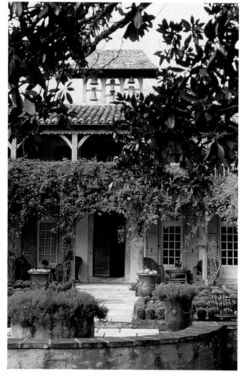

La Maison Rose is exclusively for guests who sign up for minceur meals and spa treatments. More modest than lodging at the Couvent des Herbes (a converted convent) or the main hotel, Les Prés d'Eugénie, the thirty-one-room Maison is a shuttered mansion, not a full-service hotel, so the price of accommodations is lower. By 9:00 A.M. spa-goers are up and about, clad in cheerful pink bathrobes and heading across the garden for their morning session. By noon, they will have been tub soaked, water massaged, steam bathed, and mud packed—a regimen designed to blast away cellulite, eliminate stress, and alleviate a host of other ailments.

The secret of this water therapy is in sulfurous springs that so enthralled Empress Eugénie that she convinced her husband, Napoleon III, to build a posh resort where her society friends could take the waters and be pampered in style. Cold drinking water flows from the *Imperatrice* spring; warm water used for external treatments and baths comes from "Christine Marie"—named after Madame Guérard. There is also a clay bath along with the latest in hydrotherapy, skin care, and antiaging programs.

Designed in the style of a provincial farmhouse, the thermal spa has a covered courtyard tiled in terra-cotta, where you sip a lemon-balm infusion while awaiting treatments. An herbal bath is activated with sprigs of lavender, chamomile, and hawthorn fresh from the garden. In a different version of aromatherapy, oils of lemon, orange, and grapefruit are added to the bath, plus a sachet for scrubbing, filled with rinds of the same fruit—all with thermal spring water that flows at a natural temperature of 102 degrees Fahrenheit.

Although the standard cure at La Ferme lasts six days, with four to five daily treatments chosen from a menu of thirteen in consultation with a staff doctor, you can also opt for a single treatment or packages designed for relaxation. The spa complex has a beauty parlor, gymnasium, indoor and outdoor swimming pools, tennis courts, and bowling.

Located 75 miles northeast of Biarritz, this pastoral pleasure palace is for hedonists who relish good food and the art of the bath.

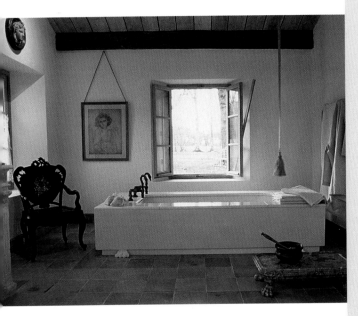

Chef's Special: Minerals and Mud

Experiments in his kitchen led Michel Guérard to recast more than spa food. A new signature treatment is the mud bath enriched with thermal plankton, said to be an effective skin toner and hair conditioner. Dipped into the vat of white clay, you float weightlessly. The active ingredient is kaolin, a fine-grained clay used to make porcelain and known for its ability to draw toxins from the body. Post treatment, you recline on a Louis XV daybed amid walls adorned with scenes of French pastoral life.

Cuisine minceur active **combines hunger-staying fiber with slow-burning carbohydrates. Grains, peas, beans, and lentils appear in various dishes; eggs, cream, sugar, and butter are dirty words. Transferring minerals to food by using Eugénie's thermal water as a cooking medium is another innovation.**

La Ferme Thermale at Les Prés d'Eugénie
40320 Eugénie-les-Bains
France
Phone: 33–5–58–05–05–05
Fax: 33–5–58–51–10–10
Season: Mid-February–end of December
General Managers: Christine and Michel Guérard
Director: Olivier Pollard
Reservations: 33–5–58–05–05–05
Accommodations: Seventy-four rooms and four suites with antique Turkish rugs, Louis XVI armoires, four-poster beds, and modern tiled bathrooms. The main hotel, Les Prés d'Eugénie, has rows of French doors opening to fanciful wrought-iron balconies. The eight-room Couvent des Herbes, a former convent, is most romantic. French-English colonial antiques, formal restaurant, and billiard room. La Ferme aux Grives, once a farmhouse, has four suites and country kitchen restaurant.
Meals: *Cuisine minceur* served at La Maison Rose, table-d'hôte fixed menu: salmon en gelée with capers, eggs with caviar, carpaccio of duck, vegetable risotto, roast venison with spicy quince, crepes with lemon sauce or lemon verbena mock ice cream garnished with strawberries and raspberries. Gourmande meal (included in seven-day package) can begin with morsels of lobster in eggshell or grilled prawns, asparagus tips, osetra caviar, salmon escaloppes with a carrot mousse, ends with pear soufflé.
Facilities: Thermal therapy pool with underwater whirlpool, Vichy shower, mud bath and mud packs, gym, sauna and steam room, beauty parlor, indoor and outdoor swimming pools.
Services & Special Programs: Dietetic drinking cure; weight management weeks; medical team for muscular, arthritis, and rheumatism treatments; massage; beauty parlor. Cooking school seminars.
Rates: $$$
Best Spa Package: Semaine Prive (week of peace and quiet), an all-inclusive package with three meals daily, room at Prés d'Eugénie, spa, leisure, sports, outing to local places of interest, optional car rental. Cost: $2,130–$2,725 per person (double).
Credit Cards: Most major
Getting There: From Paris by car, Autoroute A–10 via Bordeaux, Le Muret exit (715 kilometers); by Air Inter to Pau; by train, TGV to Pau.
What's Nearby: Lourdes, Biarritz (Atlantic beach resort, Hotel du Palais), Toulouse, Pyrenees mountains, Spain.

LES SOURCES DE CAUDALIE

Bordeaux-Martillac, France

Wine lovers have a new reason to visit Bordeaux: a grape escape right in the middle of a Grand Cru vineyard, Chateau Smith Haut Lafitte. With grapevines adorning the lobby, baths in wine barrels, and vintage wines accompanying spa cuisine, this is vinotherapy.

Rising amid undulating vineyards, Les Sources de Caudalie looks more like a winemaker's storage barn than a luxury spa. But that's part of the charm that Mathilde Cathiard-Thomas and Bertrand Thomas achieved by scouring the countryside for battered barn timbers, stone fountains, and handwoven linens. Drawn inside by the overpowering scent of grapes, you discover a "cure" straight from the vines. Spa treatments utilize grapeseed extract from the chateau's cabernet sauvignon crop; mineral water from the estate's thermal spring fills a swimming pool set among the vines; and there are two restaurants overseen by a chef with Michelin star credits. As a bonus, you can tour the cellars of two of France's most honored wineries, Chateau Smith Haut-Lafitte (owned by the Cathiard family) and Chateau Lafitte-Rothschild, which have produced fine vintages since the fourteenth century.

The theory behind vinotherapy is a recent scientific discovery that polyphenols in red grapes help reduce the free radicals responsible for skin aging. Red grapes are rich in polyphenols; voilà, le grape cure!

Mornings begin with walks in the hills of Bordeaux, then a massage with grapeseed oil extract, followed by full-body exfoliation scrub with grapeseed powder. After a high-pressure hosing to reduce cellulite, your therapist suggests rest in the *tisanerie,* where you sip herbal tea infused with red wine. Next comes a wine-and-honey wrap. Slathered in a gooey paste of wine yeast extracts, you are wrapped in warm blankets to sweat out toxins. The final touch: a bubbling bath in a *barrique* (tub shaped like an oaken barrel), spiked with freshly pressed grapeseed extract.

The wooden-shuttered pavilion housing the spa contrasts with elegant accommodations in the hotel. Amid eighteenth-century antiques and rich fabrics, you can savor the lifestyle of a wine baron. No two rooms are alike, but all have warm provincial furnishings, fluffy duvets on the beds, and Caudalie skin-care products in the big bathroom.

Meals are a la carte or part of the spa package. There are two restaurants (open to the public): Table du Lavoir, which serves brasserie food like steak Bordelaise, and La Grand Vigne, showcasing chef Didier Banyols's new take on spa cuisine. Dinner choices can be lobster with rice and chestnuts, or a health menu that adds up to 500 calories. Nobody counts calories with food this good: sautéed sea bass with steamed asparagus and a shaving of truffle as a main course;

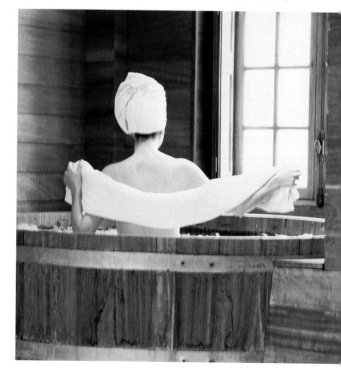

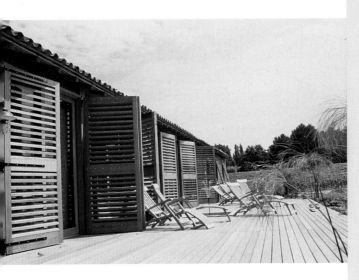

Les Sources de Caudalie
Chemin de Smith Haut-Lafitte
33650 Bordeaux-Martillac
France
Phone: 330–5–57–83–8383
Fax: 330–5–57–83–8384
E-mail: sources@sources-caudalie.com
Web site: www.sources-caudalie.com

Season: Year-round

General Manager: Mathilde Cathiard-Thomas

Spa Director: Delphine Duffours

Reservations: (888) 465–8383

Accommodations: The hotel has forty-nine rooms, including suites. Individually decorated, all have private bathroom, air-conditioning.

Meals: Southwestern French cuisine served a la carte in two restaurants. Health menu for spa program guests.

Facilities: Barrel bath (*barrique*), indoor and outdoor swimming pools, 3-hole golf, tennis, bicycles, jogging trail, Turkish bath, marine shower.

Services & Special Programs: Grapeseed wet and dry body care, facials, massage. Grape diet detoxification program, one to seven days (September, October, November). Antiaging, slimming programs, cooking school, wine tastings.

Rates: $$$

Best Spa Package: Two-day Vinotherapy Vintage, with four daily treatments, half-board (two meals), $641 per person, double occupancy.

Credit Cards: American Express, MasterCard, VISA, Eurocard

Getting There: Bordeaux airport (twenty minutes); TGV train from Paris to Bordeaux (three hours). By car, Autoroute A–10 (five hours from Paris). Located 10 miles south of the city.

What's Nearby: Vineyards, Bordeaux museum, opera, Arachon chateaux.

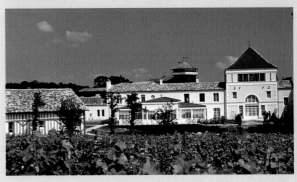

fruit sorbet accented by strawberry coulis for dessert. Traditional dishes from southwestern France are featured, but portions have been reduced. After dinner, there's conversation and wine by the glass in the Cigar Tower. English is spoken by most hotel staff and spa aestheticians, so the non-French guests have no problem meeting an international mix of spa-goers.

City lights are close enough for a night at the Bordeaux Opera or one of the restaurants for which the area is celebrated along with its wines. Even if you don't take vinotherapy seriously, a glass of vintage cabernet or barrel-aged *Graves* may be just what the doctor ordered.

Vinotherapy vs. Vitamin E

Polyphenols, the basis of vinotherapy, are antioxidants—similar to but more effective than Vitamin E—that help keep arteries in shape and enhance your skin's resistance to free radicals. Although a ton of grape seeds yields only two pounds of polyphenols, Caudalie uses them in skin-care products as well as wraps and baths. Said to be part of the beauty regimen for Madonna, Princess Caroline, and actress Catherine Deneuve, the line can be purchased at Sephora, Bergdorf Goodman, and Barney's.

ROYAL PARC EVIAN—BETTER LIVING INSTITUTE

Evian-les-Bains, France

Bien-être. It's French for "well-being," and catering to your well-being is what this legendary spa at a world-class resort is all about.

Nestled between the mountains and Lake Geneva on a forty-two-acre site with private golf course, century-old trees, and gardens, the Domaine du Royal Club Evian is legendary. Built in 1907 during the Belle Époque for the pleasure of King Edward VII, this 127-room resort at the foot of the awesome Alps has been updated to fulfill the desires of today's spa-goer.

Evian has become a household word for pure drinking water, and this scenic locale in France is its source. Evian has become synonymous with the ideals of youth, fitness, and beauty, but it takes more than sipping this crystal-clear water to turn back the years. All of the ingredients for a spa elixir are found at the Better Living Institute, where treatments include global sensory massage, shiatsu, Thai massage, marine mud wrap, Dead Sea salt peels, hydromassage baths, and fangotherapy.

The wisest way to take in the extensive spa offerings is to select one of the spa packages, which is added on to the cost of accommodations. The resort is a popular venue for conferences and special events, from golf tournaments to music festivals, so it is best to reserve spa packages in advance. Once you've checked in to one of Evian's comfortable rooms, many with mesmerizing pastoral views, it becomes apparent there is much more to do than "spa." There are dozens of activities, depending on the season of your stay. The spa year is basically divided into three seasons: the club season (February through March), the privilege season (April through July), and the royal season (August), which is the most expensive because August is France's traditional vacation month. Highlights at the club include eight restaurants, the Casino Royal Evian on the shores of Lake Geneva, and a multitude of sports.

The mother-baby program, established more than ten years ago, is designed for new mothers with babies between three and nine months old. It includes twenty-six health appointments spread over six days, with such opportunities for bonding as discovering music and swimming. Other classes for new mothers exclusively include a nutrition workshop, gentle massage, fun gym, and exercises to restore muscle tone.

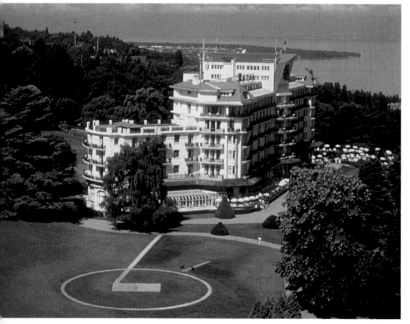

New treatments are regularly added: Try the sensorial touch massage, a hands-on approach for rediscovering energy and body suppleness. The new Turkish-style steam room is for those who enjoy immersing themselves in purifying heat.

The Royal Club Evian may be housed in a nineteenth-century structure, but the spa programs are anything but vintage!

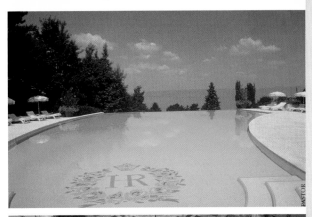

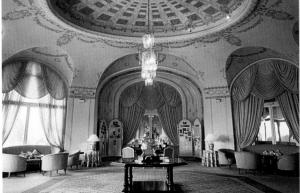

Royal Parc Evian—Better Living Institute
South Bank of Lake Geneva
74501 Evian-les-Bains
France
Phone: 33–4–50–26–8500
Fax: 33–4–50–75–61–00
Web site: www.royalparcevian.com

Season: Year-round

General Manager: Roger Mercier

Spa Director: Dr. Sylvie Sheerens

Reservations: (800) 223–6800 (Leading Hotels of the World); (800) 888–4747 (Concord Hotels) or reservations@royalparcevian.com

Spa Reservations: Same

Accommodations: The resort has 154 guest rooms, including nine suites. The comfortable accommodations offer generous views of Lake Geneva and the park.

Meals: Eight restaurants are on property, including the new La Veranda Rotisserie; the Cafe Royal Gourmandin; Liberta; Le Jardin des Lys, an elegant dietetic restaurant next to the Better Living Institute; and Le Barbecue-Piscino.

Facilities: Full-service spa; 18-hole golf course and club-house; five tennis courts; four swimming pools; the Casino Royal; archery; squash; climbing; jogging.

Services & Special Programs: The Evian Music Festival; intensive golf program; children's and junior golf; children's clubs; teenagers' club; horseback riding, four-wheel drive tours, paragliding, helicopter trips, cross-country skiing, alpine skiing, dogsled excursions, canoeing, waterskiing, sailing, lake cruises; cooking and patisserie school; gardening classes. A shuttle bus links the hotel to the golf course and casino.

Rates: $$$

Best Spa Package: A two-day, two-night package includes accommodations with a view; breakfasts; choice of two lunches or dinners; facial treatment; mud treatment with trace elements; foot reflexology; water massage; jet shower hydro-massage bath; Chinese massage or a shiatsu or a flexibility massage; and unlimited access to swimming pools, steam room, sauna, Jacuzzi, gym, cardiotraining, stretching, fitness classes, and jogging in the park with a coach. All inclusive per person in double room is about $850.

Credit Cards: Most major

Getting There: The resort is 28 miles from the Geneva Coitrin International Airport and 360 miles from Paris.

What's Nearby: Chateau de Chillon; the Grange au Lac.

The Diététique Cocktail

The latest rage at European bars is the *diététique* cocktail, thanks to the success of the International Diététique Cocktail Competition, an extravaganza showcasing nonalcoholic cocktails held at the Royal Club Evian. At the competition, creative bartenders whip up more than a hundred cocktails splashed with everything but alcohol! In 1994 the winner was Simon Bogarelli, a twenty-three-year-old barman from Switzerland who named his frothy winning cocktail for his mother, calling it "The Carla." You can easily stock your home bar with fresh ingredients such as those used at the Royal Club Evian—pineapples, passion fruit, mango, blueberries, melons, and garden veggies from carrots to cucumbers—to invent your own diététique cocktail.

THALGO LA BAULE THALASSOTHERAPY CENTER

La Baule, Brittany, France

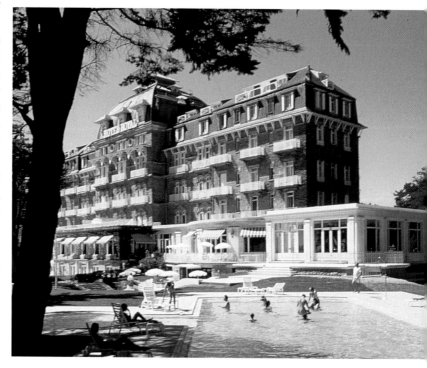

One of the gems among the thalassotherapy centers that lie along the Atlantic Ocean on the northwest coast of France, the ultra-modern Thalgo La Baule, which is linked to the Royal-Thalasso Barrière Hotel, provides a seaside cure par excellence.

Set between the ocean and pine woods, Hotel Royal and the Thalassotherapy Center bring together all the elements for a healthy vacation. Known for its tonic and calming effects, the salty air coming off tidal flats is a taste of things to come when you begin the daily schedule of treatments. Typically the morning includes a bubbling bath in fresh seawater heated to body temperature, exercise in a seawater pool, and massage. Additional water therapies, such as a high-pressure shower of salt water, may be prescribed by the center's medical staff. Following an evaluation, you are pretty much on your own to enjoy the charms of Brittany.

Overlooking the ocean, the spa's saltwater swimming pool is light and airy, no matter what the weather is like. A corridor connects the center with the hotel, so you need only to dress in the terrycloth robe issued to all guests. But bring your own swimming cap, along with suit and slippers. French sanitary habits require men and women to wear a cap in the pool. A separate exercise pool has underwater jets that work on muscles while you follow an instructor's movements. During warm weather, group exercises on the beach are scheduled.

Afternoons are open for swimming, walking, and touring the area. Bicycles are free for hotel guests, and there is a complimentary car service to the casino and other resort attractions. Throughout your stay the hotel offers golf, horseback riding, tennis, and sailing. The restaurants command a view of the outdoor swimming pool and gardens that slope down to the beach, where windsurfers can be rented for a spin on the bay. Considered one of the most beautiful white-sand beaches in Europe, La Baule is close to small fishing villages and upscale vacation centers that draw families throughout the summer. The rest of the year, beaches are largely deserted, and you can enjoy peace and solitude on walks.

Managed by the Lucien Barrière Group, this four-star hotel has a golden patina associated with Belle Époque hospitality. Meals range from gastronomic to dietetic—the choice is yours—and the services of a nutritionist are available to plan your menus. The Royal Dietetic Restaurant has a special menu of light cuisine, whereas La

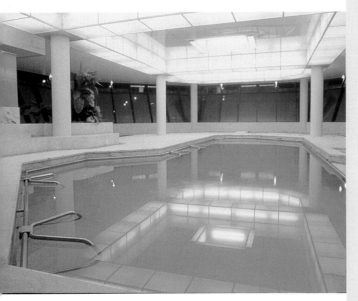

**Thalgo La Baule Thalassotherapy Center
Royal-Thalasso Barrière Hotel**
6, avenue Pierre Loti
44504 La Baule Cedex
France
Phone: 33–2–40–11–48–48
Fax: 33–2–40–11–48–45
E-mail: royalthalasso@lucienbarriere.com
Web site: www.lucienbarriere.com

Season: Year-round; Thalasso Center open daily.

General Manager: Didier Le Lostec

Thalasso Center Director: Yves Treguer, M.D.

Reservations: www.lucienbarriere.com; (800) 457–4000 (U.S.)

Accommodations: One hundred traditional rooms, three junior suites, six suites. All with private bathroom, air-conditioning.

Meals: Continental or buffet breakfast. Separate dietetic and gastronomic restaurants, beach restaurant.

Facilities: Indoor and outdoor seawater swimming pools, hydrotherapy; access to golf, horseback riding, windsurfers; free bikes, golf lesson, tennis.

Services & Special Programs: Medical consultation, nutrition evaluation, group exercise, massage, sauna, facials, hair and nail care.

Rates: $$$

Best Spa Package: Two-night Thalasso Discovery with three treatments per day, $253.59–$320.61. Six-night Thalasso Freedom, includes medical examination, four treatments per day, breakfast and dinner, free round of golf, $970–$1,241.

Credit Cards: American Express, MasterCard, VISA

Getting There: From Paris, TGV Atlantique (just under three hours); Autoroute Oceane A11 (462 kilometers); Air Inter to Nantes.

What's Nearby: Casino (theater, disco), St.-Nazaire Sea Museum, La Brière Nature Park, Ker Anas Bird Park, Guerande (medieval town), Nantes.

Rotonde is devoted to traditional French gastronomy and regional dishes. Naturally the cuisine here features fresh seafood, and the chefs display their talents with a Sunday brunch seafood plateau. Perhaps this will put you in the mood to attend cooking classes at a nearby inn. Whether taking thalasso treatments or simply enjoying a seaside break, you will discover a beautiful side of Brittany.

Seaweed Sources Beneficial Minerals

Marine algae harvested from the sea off Brittany are considered the purest form of minerals and trace elements that can be absorbed by the human body. Selected fucus and lithothammions algae are processed by Thalgo's patented micronization technique for use around the world. In France, however, only fresh seawater and seaweed can be used at certified thalassotherapy centers. Thalgo La Baule earned the distinction of Qualicert, meaning that it is authorized by the French government for the standards of its treatment. The signature treatment is a nine-step Aquaminceur® course.

BAD WOERISHOFEN: SPA TOWN
Bavaria, Germany

Credited with originating the herbal wrap and a restorative kur program based on hydrotherapy, Sebastian Kneipp then developed a health center in this Bavarian village during the nineteenth century. Kneipp's legacy is alive and well today, thanks to a medical establishment that combines modern technology with botanical knowledge. Completely devoted to Kneipp cures, Bad Woerishofen brings the healing power of nature into the twenty-first century.

Looking like a prosperous resort in the pastoral heart of Bavaria, about an hour's drive from Munich, the village of Bad Woerishofen has dozens of kur hotels, guest houses, campsites, and a shopping mall. There is a country club for golf and tennis, a central park with lake and ducks, and extensive gardens of herbal plants—all designed to get visitors in tune with nature.

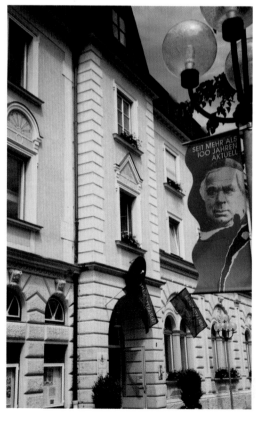

The teachings of Pastor Kneipp resonate in the **Sebastianeum,** his original clinic, which is now part of a modern treatment center and hotel, where water therapies, nutrition, and exercise are prescribed for a healthy lifestyle. Forget strenuous exercise—barefoot walks in dewy grass and pools of alternately warm and cold water are the favored therapy for circulatory problems. Guided walks, bicycle tours, and dancelike gymnastics are part of a weeklong program for persons with leg problems. Along with massage, relaxation training, and fresh country food, Kneipp's naturopathic therapies are as modern as any New Age holistic health retreat.

In Germany, and throughout the world, Kneippness means wellness. Even if you don't speak German, the message is clear: Believe it, we know it works. So when a therapist enters your bedroom at five o'clock in the morning with a hot sack of hay for an herbal wrap, there's little to do but sweat out toxins as you rest. Balancing your nervous system is better done in a resting mode, the doctor explains during a mandatory examination to prescribe your kur course of treatment. Some treatments alternate cold and warm water, either with a high-pressure hose or simply by dipping your arms in basins. Warm baths are infused with essential oils of rosemary, spruce, pine, chamomile, and linden. Strollers in the lovely parks stop at stone fountains to soak their arms and legs. But taking the waters does not mean drinking foul-smelling mineral water; what comes out of the tap here is refreshing, pure, and free.

Kur hotels in Bad Woerishofen are privately owned, but all have similar treatment facilities, outfitted from clinical style to the level of a luxury spa. Standouts among traditional five-star hotels: the **Fontenoy, Tanneck,** and **Residenz.** Family-run, small (averaging sixty rooms), each has private garden with swimming pool, indoor exercise pool, and gymnasium, with

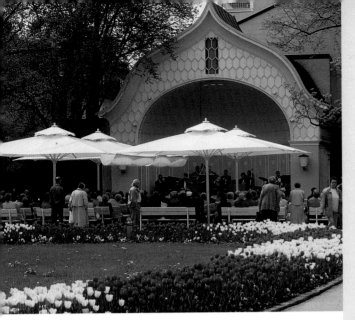

full-board meal plan. The old-world **Sonnenhof** has a new 200-room resort wing and condominium suites, plus conference facilities managed by Steigenberger. Others specialize: Family-oriented **Hotel Park** treats children and mothers; the **Kurpark Hotel** offers chiropractors, psychologists, and treatments for the ear. At the budget-priced **Sebastianeum,** men and women are housed in separate sections, and there is a chapel for daily prayers; otherwise, the facilities are similar to first-class hotels. Retreats with original Kneipp treatments are also available at a historic monastery in the center of town. You can stroll to the Kurhouse for daily concerts and swim at Thermal Bathhouse. Cafes serve Bavarian specialties and Kneipp herbal teas; there's a rose garden and several pharmacies that offer Kneipp nutrition supplements, herbal and vitamin tablets, and bath products.

Private medical consultation with Kneipp specialists provides an opportunity to learn how natural medicine complements mainstream therapies for aging and chronic disease. Leading researchers include Heinz Leuchtgens, M.D., and Tassilo Albus, M.D., who are part of a European network devoted to classical natural cures for prevention and rehabilitation of degenerative and stress-related diseases. Under their care, language barriers disappear as you focus on feeling healthier.

The Healing Power of Nature

Bad Woerishofen
Kurverwaltung
Postfach 1443
86817 Bad Woerishofen
Germany
Phone: 49–8247–993310
Fax: 49–8247–993316
E-mail: info@bad-woerishofen.de
Web site: www.bad-woerishofen.de

Season: Year-round

Spa Director: Alexander von Hohenegg

Accommodations: The central reservation service of the cure administration (Kurdirektion) offers packages that include accommodations at hotels, guest houses, apartments, the sanatorium, or campsites. Information about specific hotels and programs can be secured by e-mail. At a five-star hotel like the Residenz, standard junior suites include a sitting area with TV, balcony, and full bathroom with tub and shower. Two single beds are small but comfortable.

Meals: All five-star hotels include breakfast buffet, lunch, and dinner prepared according to heart-healthy guidelines.

Facilities: Kneipp clinic with hydrotherapy showers and tubs; indoor and outdoor swimming pools, gymnasium.

Services & Special Programs: Daily treatments, Kurhouse concerts, lectures. Excursions to nearby sites by bicycle and guided walks. Special weeks for leg therapy include medical consultation, group exercise, demonstrations of wrapping technique and Kneipp therapies for home use.

Rates: $$

Best Spa Package: Sample Kneipp's natural health concept in a weeklong program that includes accommodations for seven nights, two or three meals daily, medical examination, and transfers from/to Munich Airport. Priced from $700, with upgrades for five-star hotel.

Credit Cards: Most major

Getting There: By train from Munich, Augsburg, Memmingen, or Lindau. By car from Stuttgart and Wurzburg by way of Ulm (the Autobahn B–18 toward Munich merges into A–96). The nearest international airport is Munich (72 miles/120 kilometers), where limousine, car rental, and taxi service are available.

What's Nearby: The Bavarian Alps (Allgaeu); Munich museums, opera, and historic churches; Neuschwanstein and Hohenschwangau castles (1868–1886) built for King Ludwig II (1845–1889); the Musical Theater Neuschwanstein production of Ludwig II; Fuessen; winter sports in Schwangau; Lake Constance.

BRENNER'S PARK-HOTEL & SPA
Baden-Baden, Germany

Secluded in a fifteen-acre park overlooking the Lichtentaler Allee, Brenner's Park-Hotel dates back to 1872. Over the years there have been additions—a medical clinic and a glass-walled swimming pool—but nothing quite like the spa recently added to the hotel. Forget taking the waters; Brenner's is all about beauty of body and mind.

A personalized program tailored to your needs and time combines elements of new and traditional spa regimes. Themed to the town's Roman origins, the Relaxarium has two whirlpools just big enough for one person; you choose aroma additives to suit your mood. The Frigidarium is an open-air cold-water plunge pool. The fitness center provides cardiovascular workouts on equipment with German and English control panels. Personal trainers staff the fitness area, conducting classes in a mirrored aerobics studio and one-on-one stretches outdoors. The fitness lounge has a sports bar that is a comfortable spot for lunch in your spa robe, especially on pleasant days when the garden terrace is open.

Feeling romantic—or want to get away from it all? The luxurious spa suite includes personal attention from a spa butler. For about $500 per day you and up to three guests enjoy pampered privacy: marble bath, radiant-heat Roman sauna with heated benches of green quartzite, and a vitalizing shower where rain, mist, aroma, and light sensors create a relaxing mood. Shoji screens and photos by Helmut Newton set the stage for an East-West indulgent interlude. Relax in a Japanese steam bath, enriched with jasmine and orchid blossoms, and gaze at the Japanese garden on your private terrace. It's perfect for a candlelit dinner and nude sunbathing.

Brenner's remains among the world's truly grand hotels. The new, intimate Park restaurant, aglow with rose pink damask linens and crystal, offers classic dinners. The breakfast buffet that comes with the daily tariff is huge, an array of fresh fruits and breads, eggs, and smoked salmon, as well as Bavarian ham and local farm cheese. Staff members remember your name and

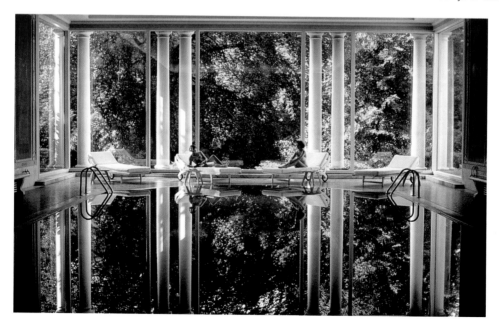

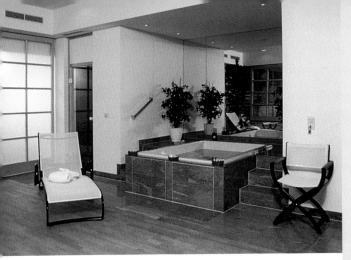

your drink preferences in the lounge, a dress-up place where sedate couples take tea and business deals are made over cognac.

Evenings are made for exercising your luck at the gilded casino or enjoying opera and concerts at the Festpielhaus. Surrounded by the natural splendor of the Black Forest in southwestern Germany, Baden-Baden retains an old-world ambience while looking to the future as a world-class wellness center.

Thermal Traditions

Being rich and famous isn't necessary in today's mass-oriented Baden-Baden. Sweating at the Roman-Irish Bath appeals to traditionalists who enjoy the ornately tiled saunas and pools of thermal water at the Friedrichsbad. Opened by the emperor in 1877, it looks much the way it did when Bismarck and Brahms came for a healthy sweat and scrub. House rules require bathing au natural, so throw modesty to the wind and see one of the grandest bathhouses in the world. Next door, the modern Caracalla Bath was built over a Roman campsite (excavations are visible beneath the building). Busy night and day, this is a waterpark for families who frolic in the steamy open-air pools. Admission tickets are modestly priced; appointments can be made for massage and other treatments.

A Twenty-first Century Wellness Center in the Black Forest

Brenner's Park-Hotel & Spa
4–6 Schillerstrasse
76530 Baden-Baden
Germany
Phone: 49–7221–900–0
Fax: 49–7221–38772
E-mail: info@brenners.com
Web site: www.brenners.com
Season: Year-round
Managing Director: Frank Marrenbach
Spa Director: Peter Droessel
Reservations: (800) 223–6800, Leading Hotels of the World
Accommodations: One hundred high-ceilinged rooms and suites, individually appointed with antiques and rich fabrics, chandeliers and walnut armoires; each with private bathroom, most with balcony and park view. Amenities include robes and slippers, Anne Sémonin bath products.
Meals: Restaurants include the Wintergarden (conservatory) for lunch and dinner in a more informal environment, Salon Lichtentál for breakfast, and the Park Restaurant for gastronomic cuisine.
Facilities: Spa suite; LifeFitness cardio and strength training, indoor swimming pool with Finnish sauna, Turkish and bio steam baths, whirlpools, sports bar. Beauty salon.
Services & Special Programs: Jet-lag treatment with seaweed and trace elements, facials, massage (Swedish, lomi-lomi, shiatsu), lymphatic drainage, reflexology, G5, body peeling, packs, makeup, hair and nail care.
Rates: $$$
Best Spa Package: Four-night Stroll in the Park includes half-day spa suite, beauty treatments, fitness training, pool exercise, gymnastics. Breakfasts, tea, dinner for two, and hotel accommodations. $1,085 per person double; $1,517 for single. Taxes and service included.
Credit Cards: Most major
Getting There: From Frankfurt, by car on Autobahn A–4 (two hours), by train from airport (two hours).
What's Nearby: Strasbourg (French Alsace), Heidelberg; traditional dining in nearby restaurants featuring local specialties.

TOSKANA THERME

Bad Sulza, Germany

An architectural masterpiece completed just in time for the millennium, the Toskana Therme takes spa-going to new heights. Located in an old spa town near Weimar, the complex includes the Hotel an der Therme, a wellness clinic, and a training school for spa therapists. Both a day spa and a destination spa, this high-tech therme makes taking the waters a unique experience.

Star Trek comes to mind as you approach the domed Toskana Therme. Spanning an entire hillside, the glass-walled structure is a work of art that combines water therapies with music and underwater sound. With six interconnected pools, the main hall is flooded with light, colors, and music. At night, it turns into an aquatic opera house, with dance and band concerts. The audience often gets into the act, floating along rivers of light to the bottom-level swimming pool.

Set amid verdant hills of Thuringia, an area often called the Tuscany of the East, Bad Sulza has been a healing center for more than a century. The saline waters rise from an ancient seabed at 92 degrees Fahrenheit (32–34 degrees Celsius) right under Toskana Therme, constantly circulating fresh, warm mineral water in the pools and baths. Spa-goers can arrange treatments or simply relax. There are saunas, some with panoramic views, and lounges on balconies overlook the pools. Massages and beauty and kur treatments are available in a wellness center staffed by professionals. Meals and snacks are available on the garden level, where Ristorante il Toskana provides pasta inspired by the chef's homeland.

Orchestrating the various elements of this extraordinary new pleasure palace is a husband-wife team, Klaus Boehm and Marion Schneider. Their arts events turned Bad Sulza from a sleepy East German backwater into a center for integrative art. Close to the fountainhead of German modern design, the original Bauhaus University in Weimar, the area, with its nature-oriented buildings and festivals, attracts lovers of the avant-garde. Performances in the new Toskana Therme have included a water ballet and live concerts of electronic music as well as works by Bach and Handel's *Water Music*.

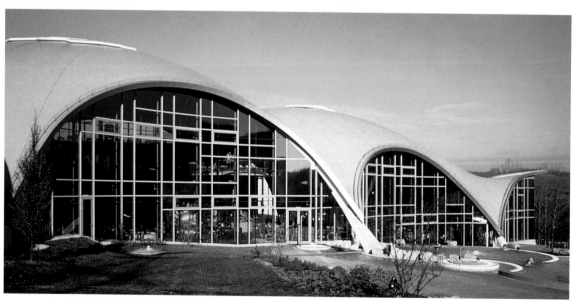

The ultimate experience comes in the domed Liquid Sound Temple. Multimedia artist Micky Reimann worked with the architects on an integrated system of under-

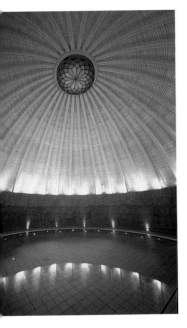

water sound and projected images that fill the dome. A session of aqua wellness in the hands of a trained therapist leaves you float-ing in a sea of color, your body gently moving and vibrating to the rhythms of underwater music. Special evenings are devoted to both live and electronic concerts.

The three-day relax-ation program includes accommodations at Hotel an der Therme, a holdover from the days when Bad Sulza served the medical needs of the East German government. This is without a doubt a wellness water-park for the twenty-first century.

The Art of Liquid Sound

Beneath warm, salty water in a domed pool, a unique technology transforms bathing into a mystical experience. Invented by media artist Micky Reimann, the idea was inspired by encoun-ters with orca whales in the Canadian Pacific. As you float weightlessly in salt water at body tem-perature, sounds, music, and colors surround you, creating a feeling of release from earthly stress. Video images and colored lights fill the futuristic dome as music wells up from the water. Opera arias, tangos, New Age music, even the ur-sound of whales, mix in a burst of creative energy. Blur-ring the lines between therapy, wellness, and entertainment, the Liquid Sound experience stim-ulates a relaxation response and a sensory high.

Liquid Sound and Light in a Thermal Springs Temple

Toskana Therme
Wunderwaldstr 2a
99518 Bad Sulza
Germany
Phone: 49–36461–91080
Fax: 49–36461–92835
E-mail: toskana@kbs.de
Web site: www.toskana-therme.de
Season: Year-round
General Manager: Klaus Boehm
Spa Director: Marion Schneider
Reservations: E-mail to hoteltherme@aol.com; phone 49–36461–92836
Accommodations: Eighty modern rooms with private bath in Hotel an der Therme have direct access to the spa. Simply furnished, rooms are air-conditioned, have woodland view. Some are equipped for people who are physically chal-lenged; some have four beds. All with TV, phone. Some two bedroom apartments; sixty room annex.
Meals: The spa cafeteria features Italian specialties from Tuscany, pasta, pizza, and veal. Hotel guests are served breakfast and dinner in a private dining room. Produce from organic farms is used for vegetarian dishes. Seasonal spe-cialties include venison, fish, and modified regional special-ties that are low in fat, salt, and sugar.
Facilities: Thermal water pools (four indoor, two outdoor), hydrotherapy baths, fango, foot- and armbaths, exercise studio, saunas, steam bath, medical clinic, and beauty salon.
Services & Special Programs: Aqua Wellness (floating water movement and massage); Liquid Sound sessions. Massages, body wrap, mud packs, Kneipp herbal and water therapies; medical consultation. Stress management kur.
Rates: $$
Best Spa Package: Health & Happiness, includes classic fifty-minute massage, fango mud pack, foot reflexology ($90). Available only with three-night stay at Hotel an der Therme.
Credit Cards: VISA, Mastercard
Getting There: From Frankfurt, by car on Autobahn A–4 to Apolda exit, Route B–87 to Bad Sulza turnoff (three hours). From Berlin by train (three hours) via Naumberg.
What's Nearby: Weimar (Goethe house, Bauhaus Univer-sity), Dresden, Nuremberg, Hanover, Berlin, Leipzig.

THERMAE SYLLA SPA WELLNESS HOTEL

Edipsos, Evia Island, Greece

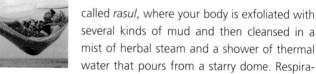

Known by Aristotle, Plutarch, and health-seekers throughout the early Hellenistic period, the waters of Edipsos rise from volcanic springs in the sea. Full of minerals, this constant source of hot water is utilized with state-of-the-art equipment and medical supervision to provide revitalization and wellness programs at the new (1999) Thermae Sylla Spa.

Set on the tip of a popular seaside resort, about 150 kilometers from Athens, Edipsos has connections by ferryboat with some of the most important archaeology sites in Greece. What it does not have is a sandy beach. The new spa makes up for this by mixing seawater with thermal water in the outdoor swimming pool. The water is constantly circulated and requires no chlorine, and the pool can be used year-round.

Given the island's subtropical climate, eucalyptus trees and palms are abundant: they shade the pool and are used in spa therapy. Relax in a wooden sauna as steam infused with essential oils bathes you. A most magical treatment is the mud chamber ceremony called *rasul*, where your body is exfoliated with several kinds of mud and then cleansed in a mist of herbal steam and a shower of thermal water that pours from a starry dome. Respiratory problems are treated by inhaling steam of ionized water mixed with extracts of eucalyptus, chamomile, and other plants grown on the island.

All things natural is the key to Thermae Sylla. Geothermal springwater heats the buildings as well as the swimming pools and relaxing whirlpool baths. Physiotherapy under supervision of the spa team takes place in the warm pools. Calming showers are combined with massage, and mud mixed with thermal water relieves pain of arthritis, rheumatism, and muscular ailments.

Designed around a secluded garden pool, the new spa complements the original Thermae Sylla Grand Hotel, which first opened in 1897. Newly restored, the hotel offers four-star accommodations with sea views and new spa rooms overlooking the garden. With interior access to all facilities, this is a self-contained resort, offering destination spa programs and day spa packages for guests at dozens of hotels nearby.

Mediterranean cuisine comes naturally in the Greek islands, and the Grand Hotel offers a choice of two restaurants with traditional healthy cooking. Special diets for slimming also take advantage of the local seafood and farm products. Combined with massage and physiotherapy, the spa doctors design personalized programs to show results that you can take home.

Nature lovers can explore the Sporades, home of rare seals, and Chalkida, a fishing village noted for restaurants overlooking a rush of tidal waters. Excursions to the Byzantine monasteries of Meteora,

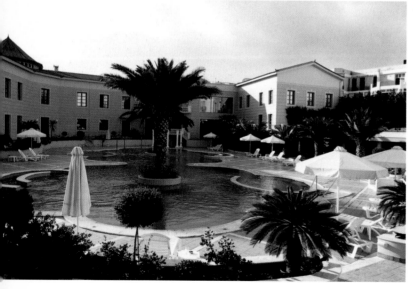

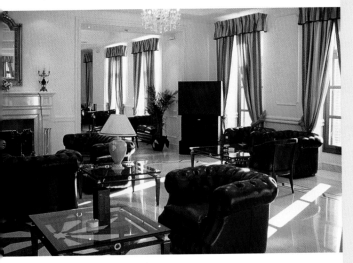

which cling to rocky cliffs, offer hospitality from the monks. In winter, there is skiing at Mount Parnassos.

Surrounded by the Aegean sea, Thermae Sylla Spa brings healing waters together with modern technology on an island where time stands still.

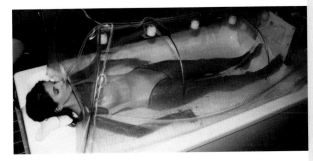

Natural Thalassotherapy

Thalassa is the Greek word for the sea. A French doctor, Rene Quinton, conceived thalassotherapy with fresh seawater and algae. Here seawater is mixed with thermal mineral water. Two layers of water meet in front of the hotel, where steps in the rocks allow you to bathe in the sea. Or have a body wrap with seaweed and special creams said to be effective for body firming. This is thalassotherapy of a different kind.

Thermae Sylla Spa Wellness Hotel
Edipsos, North Evoia
Greece
Phone: 30–22260–60100
Fax: 30–22260–22055
Web site: www.thermaesylla.gr

Season: Year-round

General Manager: Nikos Trikourakis

Accommodations: 110 rooms in a seafront complex that includes a modern wing adjoining the spa and the original Grand Hotel with high-ceilinged rooms, French doors opening to small balconies. Completely air-conditioned, rooms have king-size or double beds, modern bathroom, some with marble tub. Amenities include robes and slippers, TV, radio, safe, refrigerator.

Meals: Seafood, from giant shrimp to lobster, lamb herbed and cooked with olive oil, are features of the traditional Greek cuisine served in the hotel's two dining rooms. Local farms supply fresh produce year-round, and fruit comes from Mediterranean orchards of Israel and Spain.

Facilities: Gymnasium with exercise equipment; private treatment rooms for clay, mud, and seaweed body masques and facials; Cleopatra Bath with milk and oils; mud bath; underwater massage tubs with ozone; Vichy shower; herbal steam bath; volcanic steam bath; inhalation therapy.

Services & Special Programs: Massage, reflexology, aromatherapy, body wraps, facial, pedicure, manicure. Physiotherapy program, anti-stress program. Tennis, biking, fishing, and water sports. Evening concerts.

Rates: $$

Best Spa Package: Thermae Sylla Energy, a three-day program that integrates exercise and relaxation with beauty treatments. Price: $182.84 per person includes half board (buffet breakfast and lunch), taxes, medical exam. Room for two from $118.94 to $288.74.

Credit Cards: Most major

Getting There: From Athens by car, the Lamia Highway to Arkitsa, ferryboat to Edipsos (three hours).

What's Nearby: Delphi, Mount Parnassos, Meteora, Epidaurus Roman coliseum and healing center.

BUDAPEST: SPA TOWN

Budapest, Hungary

In a city where "taking the waters" is a daily ritual for traditionalists, spa culture can take many forms: medicinal, restorative, or simply recreational. Therapy-seeking voyagers have trekked here since the time of the Roman Empire. Elaborate bathing establishments built by the city's Ottoman rulers are now open to the public. The waters certified medicinal are used to treat rheumatic diseases and for physical therapy. A relaxing soak in the buoyant, slightly sulfurous water is an effective antidote to tourist fatigue.

Back in the 1930s, guests at the St. Gellert Hotel tested the latest in aquatic entertainment: a wave pool where bathing beauties accompanied by a gypsy band faced artificial waves. Every fifteen minutes, a whistle signaled the start of a series of waves pumped from natural hot springs under the hotel. Destroyed by Nazi bombs in 1945, the art deco hotel was rebuilt after the war, complete with wave pool. Now known simply as the **Gellert,** the spa complex has grown to include a family pool and two separate baths, one for men and one for women, each with three plunge pools of varying temperatures, a sauna, and a steam bath. Hotel guests have direct access and can come in bathrobes; the public entrance from a side street is busy day and night. Facilities for massage and nail care aren't fancy, but the elaborate domed pools are a

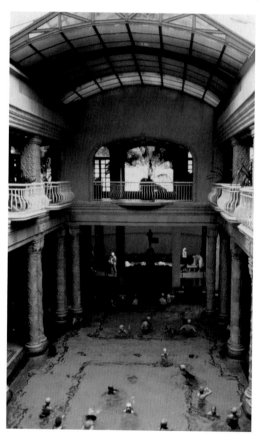

sybaritic fantasy right out of a Fellini movie. Located on the Buda side of the Danube, the hotel looks a bit faded, but is scheduled for a major facelift.

Budapest, with its tree-shaded boulevards and Danube venues, retains an air of sophistication. On the Pest side of the river, the city's past splendor is visible in the restored Opera House and the City Park, where a major art museum and famed Gundel restaurant are close to the **Szechenyi Baths** (Allatkerti ut 11). One of Europe's largest bathing establishments when it opened in 1927, Szechenyi offers pools of thermal water inside and out, set among grandiose statuary. Apart from the health care and medical section, its popularity as a recreation center continues today.

The **Kiraly Baths** (Fo ut 84) were built in the mid-1500s on a Roman road still busy with city traffic. Topped by a golden Turkish crescent and domed roof, the interior is dark and foreboding. Pinpricks of colored glass permit light through the dome. Alternate days are allotted for men and women, and unlike the Gellert, bathing is au naturel. Ask for a massage and you will be soaped, pummeled, rubbed, and smacked, and leave feeling good!

Modern thermal hotels cluster around **Margaret Island** (Margitsziget), where you have a choice of destination spa or day spa programs.

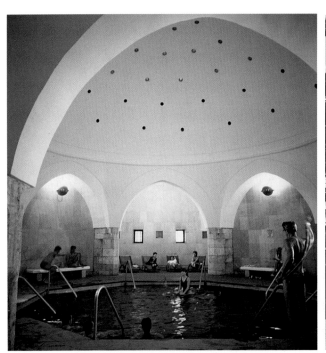

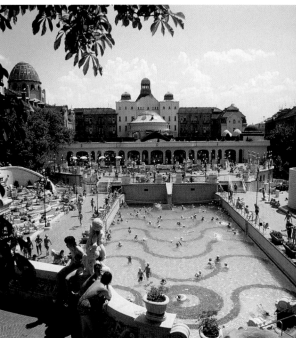

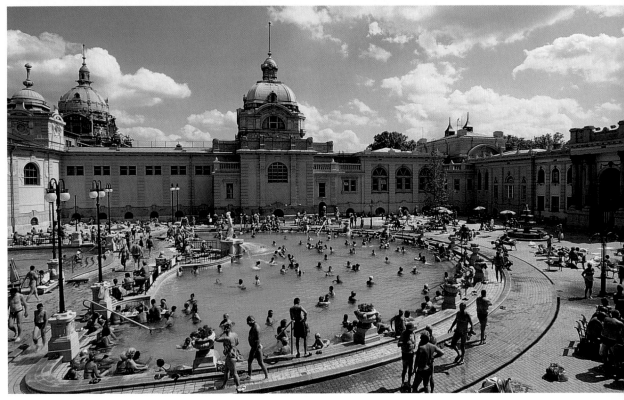

A giant park in the Danube, with rose gardens and jogging paths, Margaret Island's two spa hotels are linked underground to thermal pools of such intensely hot waters that a checkup with the medical director is required before you bathe. The 206-room **Danubius Thermal Hotel Margitsziget,** rated five-star, has full medical and dental clinics; the more charming, 163-room **Danubius Grand Hotel Margitsziget** dates from 1873. Both hotels feature dietetic and Hungarian cuisine. Sharing the island's spring water and facilities, **Danubius Thermal Hotel Helia** (262 rooms) on the Pest embankment offers a Finnish sauna, gymnasium, indoor swimming pool, massage, and salon.

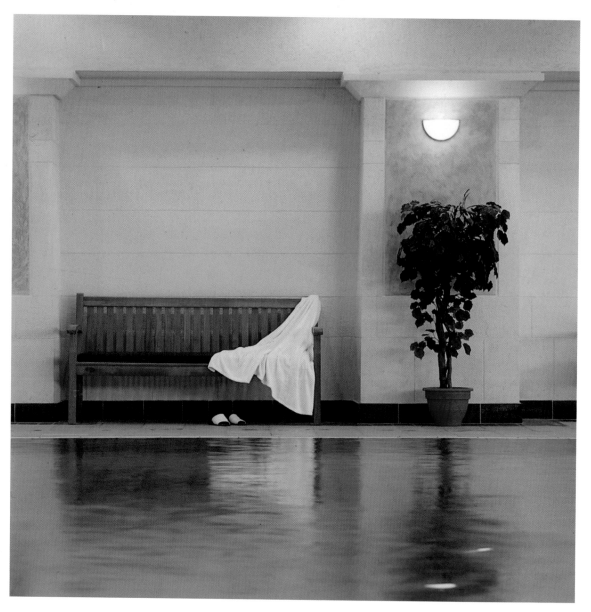

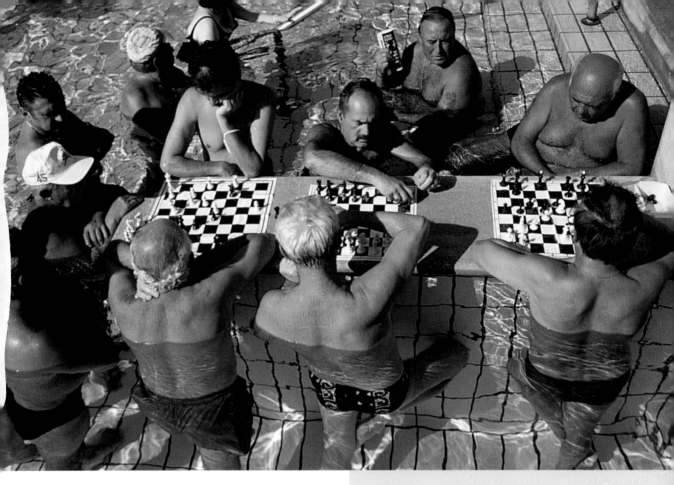

Forget Modesty

Bathing au naturel is the traditional way to get in touch with your outer self at the old bath-houses. Tickets for the furdo (baths) cost about $3.00; if you want massage, point to a menu posted over the ticket booth. Bring a bathing cap (mandatory); modesty is served by an apron available in the locker room. No matter what shape you're in, all are equal when naked. Get a free neck massage under spouts of water that constantly refresh the pools. Exposure to thermal water can't hurt you, but skeptics question medical benefits. Simply soaking, however, will put a spring in your step.

Taking the Waters in an Ancient City of Thermal Springs

Hungarian Hotels
6033 West Century Boulevard
Los Angeles, CA 90045
Phone: (310) 649–5808
Fax: (310) 649–5852
E-mail: Tradesco@earthlink.net
Web site: www.tradescotours.com

Reservations: (800) 448–4321

Rates: $$

Getting There: International airlines serving Budapest include Malev, British Airways, and Lufthansa. Train service from the airport to downtown, then taxi.

What's Nearby: Lake Heviz (thermal springs); Lake Balaton (sailing, camping); Sarvar (thermal springs); Eger (wineries, Lippizan horse farm).

THE LODGE & SPA AT INCHYDONEY ISLAND
West Cork, Ireland

If you enjoy walking along a secluded beach, listening to the sounds of crashing waves, and inhaling brisk ocean air, then the Lodge & Spa at Inchydoney Island is the spot for you. The pristine environment on this mystical island off the coast of West Cork is the perfect location for a thalassotherapy spa—it is free of pollution, offers expansive areas for exercise and relaxation, and, importantly, has an abundant supply of seawater. This is a retreat where the word *stress* is unwelcome and virtually unknown.

This luxury spa, opened in 1999, is a full-service thalassotherapy center, Ireland's first and only such center. Perched on a headland above two pristine beaches, which have received the exclusive Blue Flag eco-label and which benefit from Gulf Stream waters, the spa is a natural choice for a thalassotherapy cure.

The lodge was designed to reflect the environment in subtle ways. Natural simplicity is evident in all areas of the building, from the foyer, with its stunning natural slate floor and limestone fireplace, to the guest quarters.

The stunning heated seawater pool has a geyser, a waterfall, a countercurrent swimming area, underwater jets, an aqua gymnastic area, neck showers, and microbubble seats. The sheer delight of the wondrous edifice to seawater should be experienced in a leisurely fashion.

The pool serves as an introduction to the thalassotherapy treatments, which are based on the fundamentals of the French seawater cure. The spa has eleven treatment rooms offering a complete range of therapies, including balneotherapy, brumisation, hydrojet therapy, and algeotherapy. ESPA products are used for facial, body, scalp, foot, and nail treatments.

The diet plan is creative and ambitious. Executive Chef Chris Farrell has designed a sensible program based on 50 percent carbohydrates; 30 percent fat

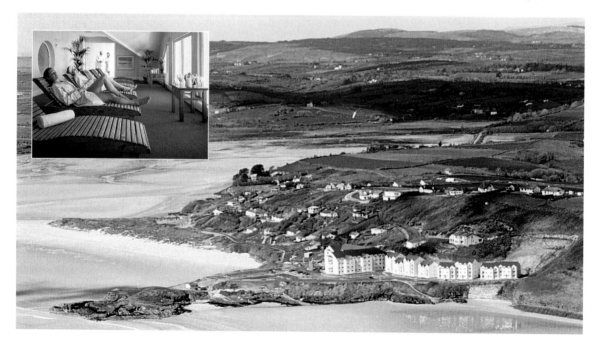

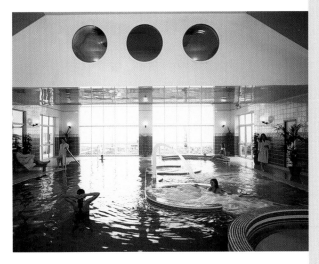

(with olive and fish oils, avocados, and nuts); and 20 percent protein. You will find fresh fruits and vegetables, plus cereals and grains on the menu, which includes information on calorie and fat content.

The lodge's guest rooms and suites are spacious and comfortable, and all capture majestic views of the ocean. They are equipped with satellite television and direct-dial phones. Fortunate spa-goers here enjoy the benefits of a thalassotherapy cure at one of Ireland's premier resorts.

The Seawater Cure Comes of Age

To specialize in thalassotherapy, a spa must meet six rules that were established by the French government in June 1997. The thalassa spa must have an exceptional location by the sea; it must use natural seawater and elements derived from the sea, such as seaweed, sea mud, and sand; there must be permanent medical supervision; there must be professionally trained staff; there must be permanent concern for hygiene and security; and there must be specialized, well-maintained equipment. Thalassotherapy has been known to be effective in treatments for headaches, menopause, leg problems, stress, and insomnia; it also induces relaxation and slimming.

Spa Setting an Inspiration for Poets

The Lodge & Spa at Inchydoney Island
Clonakilty
West Cork, Ireland
Phone: 353–23–33143
Fax: 353–23–35229
E-mail: reservations@inchydoneyisland.com
Web site: www.inchydoneyisland.com

Season: Year-round

General Manager: Michael Knox-Johnston

Spa Director: Dr. Christian Jost

Reservations: 353–23–33143 or (800) 888–4747 (from the United States only) or by e-mail (above)

Accommodations: Sixty-three double- or twin-bed ocean-view rooms; three suites with conservatory sitting rooms overlooking both beaches; one junior suite; eighteen two-bedroom apartments and two four-bedroom apartments. All accommodations face the famous Inchydoney beaches.

Meals: The resort has two restaurants, the Gulfstream Restaurant and Contented Plaice at Dunes Pub.

Facilities: Hydrotherapy; skin care; fitness center; lounge and library; snooker room; gymnasium.

Services & Special Programs: Wellness week, weight management; golf at Bandon and at the unique Lisselan 6-hole course; horseback riding at Clonakilty Equestrian Center; deep-sea fishing; salmon and trout fishing; off-road driving; clay pigeon shooting and archery; diving; and twenty-four-hour room service.

Rates: $$

Best Spa Package: The Sejour Specifique Experience is seven nights and includes accommodations, seven Irish breakfasts, seven dinners, and eighteen thalasso treatments. The rates start at $1,950, double occupancy (per room) in the low season, September through April. Add to this a 10% service charge.

Credit Cards: Most major

Getting There: British Airways to London with a connecting flight to Shannon. Three-hour drive to Inchydoney Island.

What's Nearby: Golf at the Old Head of Kinsale Golf Links; fishing in the Gulf Stream waters; Mallow races; wreck of the *Lusitania,* thirty minutes offshore; the West Cork Museum; Animal Park; Park Collins Memorial Homestead; Lisselan Gardens.

CAPRI BEAUTY FARM AT THE PALACE HOTEL

Capri, Italy

Since ancient times, Capri has been considered the ideal place to reunite with nature. Thanks to the island's mild Mediterranean climate and lush surroundings, the Capri Beauty Farm provides the perfect environment for a memorable spa vacation.

Perched atop one of the highest hills on Capri, the Palace Hotel is surrounded by stunning views of the Gulf of Naples, Vesuvius, and the Amalfi coast. After breakfast in a garden suite or on your balcony overlooking the sea, stroll to the hotel's intimate Capri Beauty Farm for a morning of ritual renewal. Water therapies are emphasized here: Seawater invigorates your workout at the indoor pool; there is a hydrotherapy bath with seaweed and algae and a saltwater Kneipp circuit. Hydrotherapy baths are prescribed for inflammations or chronic problems associated with muscular and bone structure, plus a full range of hydrokinestherapy (motion and exercise), electrical

stimulation, and massage. Personal trainers and a medical staff work as a team with each guest.

Treatments feature thalassotherapy based on French technology and marine products.

Housed in a recently expanded two-story wing of the hotel, serenely quiet and private, the Beauty Farm is a favorite hangout of Hollywood celebrities (Julia Roberts and Harrison Ford), fashion designers from Milan, Saudi royalty, and the king and queen of Sweden.

The highly professional staff at Capri Beauty Farm is led by Francesco Canonanco, a medical doctor and specialist in food science, immunology, and aesthetic medicine. With a full range of face and body treatments prescribed in what the doctor describes as a logical and progressive sequence, aesthetics becomes a science here. The terme marine program offers fango treatments with sea mud, inhalations, and seaweed body wraps.

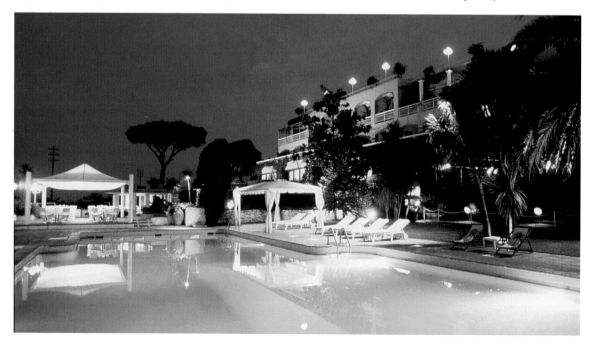

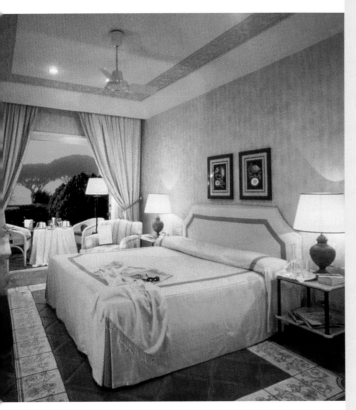

Capri Beauty Farm at the Palace Hotel
Via Capodimonte, 2
80071 Anacapri
Capri, Italy
Phone: 39–081–978–0111
Fax: 39–081–837–3191
E-mail: info@capri-palace.com
Web site: www.capri-palace.com

Season: March–November, December 27–January 1.

General Manager: Tonino Cacace

Spa Director: Francesco Canonaco, M.D.

Reservations: (800) 223–6800

Accommodations: Eighty rooms, including twenty-two junior suites (four with private garden and heated plunge pool) amid Moorish arches, whitewashed walls. Mediterranean-modern look of bedrooms features tile floor, baldachino-style beds (four-poster draped in white linen), wicker, and wood furniture. Travertine marble bathroom with robes, full-size bathtub, shower. Completely air-conditioned, rooms have ceiling fans, minibar, safe. Penthouse suite has hanging gardens, private swimming pool.

Meals: Buffet breakfast included in room rate. Main dining room serves a la carte lunch and dinner with salad bar, a selection of heart-healthy food, and a low-fat Mediterranean diet that uses lots of grains, olive oil, and fish.

Facilities: Beauty farm with private hydrotherapy tubs, indoor exercise pool with salt water, outdoor Kneipp walk, pressotherapy leggings, Turkish steambath, solarium, hair salon, gymnasium. Medical clinic for laser therapy, electro-cardiogram, laboratory tests.

Services & Special Programs: Cosmetology facials, aerosol inhalation, marine algae baths and body wraps, hairstyling, manicure/pedicure, massage, shiatsu, Vodder manual lymphatic drainage, ayurvedic massage. Special program for tired legs includes massage, diet food, medicated wraps.

Rates: $$$

Best Spa Package: Beauty Program, a seven-day program with full board (dietetic meals), medical checkup, Kneipp therapies for vascular system, algotherapies, massage, seawater aerosol inhalations, clay facial and hair treatments, gymnastics in pool, guided walks. From $3,000 per person, double occupancy. Service and VAT included.

Credit Cards: Most major

Getting There: From Naples or Sorrento, slow ferries or fast hydrofoil to Marina Grande (forty minutes). Hotel sends porter and car to pier on request.

What's Nearby: Blue Grotto, Villa San Michele museum, the island of Ischia.

The island's sun-splashed environment gets you in the mood to relax once your medical checkup is complete. Located in Anacapri, steps from a hiking trail and cable cars on Monte Solaro, the Palace is a convenient base for sightseeing. Unless you're trying to escape paparazzi, take a taxi or a public bus down hairpin-curved roads to the port. After the last ferries full of day-trippers leave Marina Piccola, walk along a cliffside path to Fontelina, a club set in the rocks of an ancient Roman landing place. Among yachts and cafes is a swimming hole called Da Luigi. Night is the best time to explore Capri town, midway up the mountain, and to people-watch on Capri's version of Rodeo Drive.

A style-setter in the 1960s, the five-star Palace Hotel has gotten a new lease on life under owner Tonino Cacace, whose parents liked the location even though it was on the unfashionable side of the island. Beyond the souvenir stands and pizzerias, this is a small gem where even the police wear designer shades.

GRAND HOTEL TERME ABANO

Abano Terme, Italy

Surrounded by the Euganean hills an hour from Venice, Abano is a spa town like no other. Fango, a medicinal mud dug from the hills, is the main attraction. More than 135 hotels in the valley offer fango treatments for arthritis, rheumatism, osteoporosis, gout, and sciatica. Doctors use mud therapy for patients recuperating from surgery and accidents. Mixed with hot thermal mineral spring water to simmer and mature in open-air vats, fango's ingredients include algae, minerals, and trace elements. It's as natural a cure for aches and pains as you can find.

Following a routine prescribed by the hotel's resident doctor, fango treatments are relaxing and help to sweat out toxins. The mud is spread on linen sheets by a fanghini therapist, who tucks you in and then applies a cool cloth to your sweating brow. The warm mud opens pores, allowing heat and minerals to penetrate the body. With little to do but meditate, think about the Romans who discovered this place, named *aponus* from the Greek for "to relieve pain." Legend says temples to Hercules were built here, and some archeological sites have been excavated in the center of town.

The doges of Venice had villas in the valley, and Lord Byron visited in the 1800s. Just when you feel stuck in the mud, it's time to shower off and soak in a bathtub full of bubbling ozonated mineral water. Following a rest period and massage, you're ready for breakfast.

A personal program is planned by a coordinator at the hotel. First, your heart is checked and medical condition discussed with a staff doctor. Contraindications: Fango is not allowed for pregnant women and people with certain medical conditions. Diet and nutrition complement the cure program, and consultation can be arranged to set up special meals. Alternative therapies also are discussed by the doctor before you begin a "cure." Recommended for best benefits: twelve-day stay with daily treatments.

At the five-star Grand Hotel Terme Abano, traditional fango cures mix with today's spa trends in beauty and well-being. Set in landscaped, semitropical gardens, the hotel has an atmosphere of elegance and exclusivity. Crystal chandeliers, marble floors, and Oriental rugs decorate the lobby. Created by the privately held GB Hotels Group

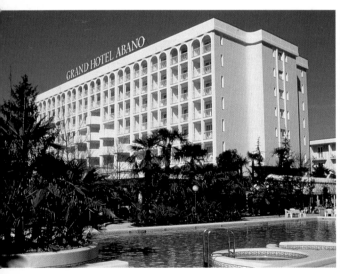

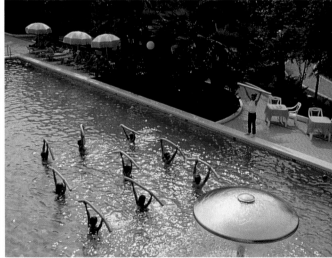

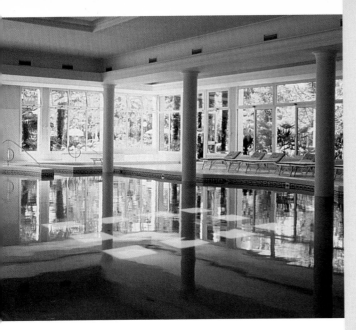

Grand Hotel Terme Abano
Via V. Flacco, 1
35031 Abano Terme (Padova)
Italy
Phone: 39–049–8248100
Fax: 39–049–8669994
E-mail: ghabano@gbhotels.it
Web site: www.gbhotels.it

Season: Year-round
Managing Director: Chiara Borile
Spa Director: Maurizio Grassetto, M.D.
Accommodations: 189 rooms, twelve junior suites, and eight suites. Some are nonsmoking. All have balcony, full modern bathroom with tub and shower, hair dryer, decorated in marble. Furnished with antique reproductions, rooms are air-conditioned, have TV, telephone, spacious closet, linens and robes by Frette.
Meals: Full board includes breakfast buffet with eggs to order; lunch and dinner in the main dining room. Health menu at no extra charge, based on 1,000 calories.
Facilities: Thirty-three private rooms for fango thermal therapy; beauty salon; gymnasium; two outdoor swimming pools (one with whirlpool and jets) with thermal mineral water; indoor swimming pool and whirlpool; Kneipp water walk; sauna grotto; steam room.
Services & Special Programs: Massage, shiatsu, Thai massage, facial mud pack, inhalation therapy, ayurvedic scalp treatment, lymphatic drainage, hydromassage. Programs include antistress, anticellulite, body firming.
Rate: $$$
Best Spa Package: *Remise en Forme,* a week with varied treatments daily, including facial gommage, body peeling, collagen treatment, massage. The program starts with a medical examination at the hotel and includes checkups as needed. Daily group gymnastics in the swimming pools or gymnasium, plus an evening infusion drink. Priced from $2,005 per person, this package includes meals and six nights accommodations.
Credit Cards: Most major
Getting There: By car from Milan, Autostrada (highway) A–4, exit Padua west. By train to Terme Euganee or Padua stations; taxi, car rental, or bus. Nearest airport: Venice.
What's Nearby: Four championship 18-hole golf courses; Venice, Verona, Padua; Palladio's Vicenza villas.

and managed by the Borile family, this is more than a hotel. Two floors are dedicated to health and beauty. Separate from the fango department and not requiring medical supervision, one floor is devoted entirely to beauty treatments. All guests have access to the fitness equipment, gymnasium, steam room, and huge sauna designed to resemble a mountainside grotto.

Excursions by private bus are scheduled, and the hotel has bicycles for guided trips in the region. Concerts in the town garden and opera evenings at the hotel are free of charge.

Doing the Fango

All mud therapy sessions are composed of four fundamentals: the body wrap; bathing in mineral water; the sweat reaction; and, finally, massage, with its tonic action on the muscular and nervous system. The therapeutic properties of the mud combine with the mineral water's chemical composition (bromine-iodine) and temperature to benefit the skin. The doctor may also prescribe sessions in a steam bath or "sweat grotto" for treatment of obesity, gout, and diabetes.

GROTTA GIUSTI TERME SPA HOTEL

Monsummano Terme, Tuscany, Italy

Beneath this hillside hotel is a grotto called the Inferno. This ancient natural vapor cave, the largest thermal grotto in the world, provides a place to cleanse body and mind.

Terme in Tuscany come in many sizes, from traditional hot springs to sophisticated resorts. Grotta Giusti is neither the largest nor the grandest, but it has a combination of comfortable lodging and affordable treatments that make it among the best buys in Italy. Basics include thermal mud baths and facials, consultation with dermatology specialists, and choice of treatments designed to activate musculoskeletal and circulatory systems. Add the grand country villa ambience and the personalized service of a four-star hotel and you have an affordable escape.

Both a day spa and destination spa, Grotta Giusti offers revitalization packages with the adjoining hotel of the same name. Guest rooms are functional and modern, rather than posh old world. Surrounded by extensive gardens, tall parasol pines, and chestnut trees, the hotel itself is an enchanted place where time seems to stand still. The villa's history goes back to the nineteenth century, when the poet Giuseppe Giusti had the hillside estate created. Today you don a spa robe in your room and walk down the hall directly into the reception area and thermal swimming pool.

A physical checkup is in order before any heat-based treatment, so an English-speaking hostess escorts new arrivals to the medical department. Once your appointments are programmed into the computer, red-coated hostesses help you get oriented. Spa clothing appears in your room: a long white cotton tunic for relaxing in the grotto, a hooded woolen robe for warmth, and plastic shower shoes.

Group activity is minimal, but meeting people is no problem. The dining room host speaks four languages and seats you in a section of the room where menus are in the appropriate language. Join a morning exercise group or walk in the park to make new friends. In the palestra, an airy aerobics studio with sprung-wood floor, aerobics, tai chi, and back muscle stretches alternate with sessions of yoga. Your daily routine might include a sweat in the grotto, a massage, or inhalation therapy.

Save one morning to take the waters in Montecatini at the grandest spa park in the world, Tettuccio Springs. As an orchestra plays operatic arias and waltzes under a classical rotunda, stroll to ornately tiled fountains and try

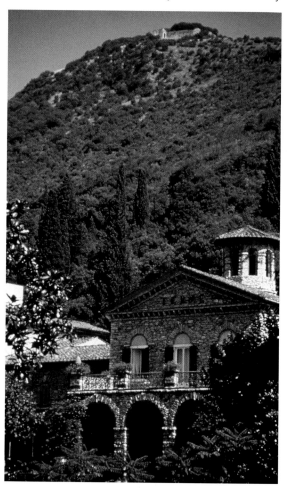

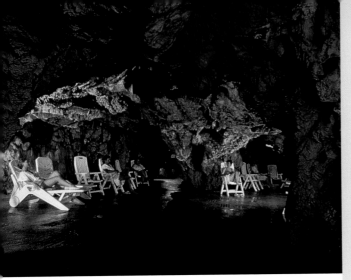

Grotta Giusti Terme Spa Hotel
Via Grotta Giusti, 1411
51015 Monsummano Terme
Italy
Phone: 39–0572–90771
Fax: 39–0572–9077200
E-mail: info@grottagiustispa.com
Web site: www.grottagiustispa.com

Season: March 16–January 8

Owner and director: Leandro Gualtieri

Spa Medical Director: Giusto Tintorini, M.D.

General Manager: Mario Patechi

Spa Appointments: 39–572–51008

Accommodations: Sixty-four air-conditioned rooms (six suites) with stylish furniture, marble bathroom with shower or full bathtub. Room rate varies according to view: park or hillside, standard or superior. Amenities include satellite color TV, direct-dial telephone, minibar, safe.

Meals: Breakfast buffet included in daily hotel room rate. Lunch and dinner offer low-calorie alternative menu, typical Tuscan dishes. Specialties include gnocchi in tomato sauce, veal scalloppini with braised fennel, and risotto. Salads, fish, and steak included in the fixed menu. Dessert can be cream cake or baked apple.

Facilities: Hydrotherapy, inhalations, indoor thermal exercise pool, aerobics studio, thermal steam grotto.

Services & Special Programs: Body wraps, facials, massage, shiatsu, reflexology, facials. Dermatology clinic and medical consultation.

Rates: $$

Best Spa Package: Seven-day antistress revitalization program with three-night hotel accommodation and full board. Treatments by dermatologist include glycolic acid peeling, rebalancing, and cellular therapy. Two physiotherapy massages, shiatsu, and daily thermal steam bath. Take-home gift of antifatigue bath gel made with Grotta Giusti thermal water. From $1,359 double, $1,423 single. Tax and service included.

Credit Cards: MasterCard, VISA

Getting There: From Florence or Pisa by car, Autostrada E–76 to exit Montecatini-Monsummano. By train, commuter service Florence-Montecatini.

What's Nearby: Pisa, Florence, Lucca, Viareggio beach resorts.

a cup of sulfurous, salty water. Famous for helping to repair the damage of overindulging in the good life, Tettuccio's waters have been praised for their purgative powers. Because all shops and spa services shut down each day from noon to 3:00 P.M., and all day on Sunday, complimentary van service is provided by Grotta Giusti to get you back to your hillside hideaway in time for lunch, a swim in the thermal pool, and perhaps a nap before dinner.

Antidote to la Dolce Vita

As an antidote to la dolce vita, the grotto at Grotta Giusti ranks among the best spa experiences. Robed and hooded, you join a monklike group on stone ramps leading to subterranean caves and an underground lake. Handed towels, you recline on wooden chairs, meditate, and sweat out toxins. An eerie beauty pervades the vaulted rocky chambers of Inferno. Heat increases as you descend past dripping stalactites and a transluscent pool called Lake of Limbo, where scuba divers explore on weekends. Arriving at Purgatorio, your tunic soaked in sweat, it's hard to keep track of time. But an attendant brings towels and a dry tunic just in time to head back up for a shower and massage. Paradiso!

PALAZZO ARZAGA HOTEL—SATURNIA SPA

Brescia, Italy

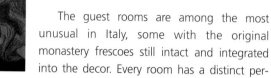

Imagine having an herbal wrap in a fifteenth-century monastery just twenty-five minutes outside of Verona. An ambitious renovation has transformed the Palazzo Arzaga, a once austere abbey, into a luxurious golf and spa resort.

Designed with golfers in mind, there is a morning warm-up and stretch program endorsed by PGA Europe, as well as a variety of massage therapies under medical supervision designed especially for golfers. For those who want to assess their muscle contraction and posture (which might affect swing or cause pain), a kinesiologist is on staff to solve the problem. And for those who simply wish to "spa," the holistic skin and body treatments span the Saturnia product range, with antiaging facials, biopeeling, reflexology, and aromatherapy.

The Palazzo is for those who are comfortable at a resort where the outside world is held at bay (thanks in part to excellent security). In many ways the ambience is that of an upscale American spa and golf resort. There are year-round tournaments at the Jack Nicklaus II 18-hole, par-72 golf course and a golf academy for those who want to improve their game.

The guest rooms are among the most unusual in Italy, some with the original monastery frescoes still intact and integrated into the decor. Every room has a distinct personality: eighteenth-century Venetian and nineteenth-century Lombardy furnishings, sumptuous fabrics, marble bathrooms, fireplaces, hand-painted and timbered ceilings, and such modern amenities as satellite television, minibars, and hair dryers. Guests choose not only from a superb collection of rooms in the hotel but also from thirteen chapel rooms near the church and others that overlook the golf course. From their windows, guests may view the serene inner courtyard and chapel, the original orchard behind the hotel, or the Palazzo's terrace.

Pistachio gelato and penne pasta aside, there is a weight program integrating the Arzaga light menu (low sugar and low-fat ingredients) with a personalized exercise program. Together they afford a gentle way to induce weight loss.

Unique in Italy, the resort's Slim & Tonic Pool contains water formulated with mineral, marine, and thermal salts that are thought to have an impact on metabolism and circulation. Magnesium, potassium, bromine sodium, and iodine are added to the pool to stimulate venous and lymphatic circulation, important for the treatment of cellulitis and general circulatory problems, according to spa director Dr. Marco Merlin.

Situated in the tranquil Italian countryside combined with a beautifully restored palazzo, Saturnia Spa, championship golf courses, and acres of gardens, the Palazzo Arzaga is one of Europe's

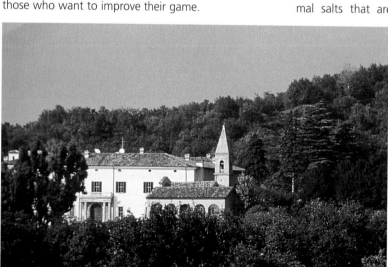

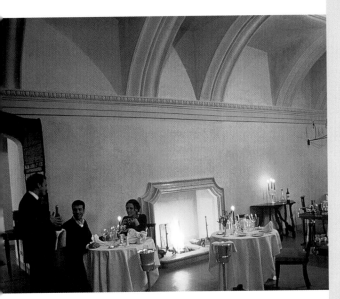

Palazzo Arzaga Hotel—Saturnia Spa
25080 Carzago di Calvagese della Riviera
Brescia
Italy
Phone: 39–03–068–0600
Fax: 39-030–680–6270
E-mail: info@palazzoarzaga.it
Web site: www.palazzoarzaga.com

Season: Year-round

General Manager: Giampaolo Burattin

Spa Director: Marco Merlin, M.D.

Reservations: (800) 323–7500 (Preferred Hotels & Resorts Worldwide)

Accommodations: Eighty-four guest rooms and five suites. Antiques, hand-painted walls, some fireplaces, marble bathrooms, minibars, in-room safes, air-conditioning, satellite TV.

Meals: Five restaurants and bars. La Taverna, the hotel's original fifteenth-century cellar, specializes in Italian wines.

Facilities: Full-service spa; indoor mineral pool; cardiovascular equipment; aerobics and water exercise classes; indoor and outdoor swimming pools; massage; herbal wraps and beauty treatments; professional trainers; hiking trails; jogging track; 18-hole Jack Nicklaus II course and 9-hole Gary Player course; driving range; golf academy; two tennis courts; boutique; pro shop.

Services & Special Programs: Physician-guided program for golfers; cooking school; chapel concerts; day trips (wine tastings, tea in Venice); sailing; biking on site through seventy acres of hills and gardens; concierge; twenty-four-hour room service.

Rates: $$$

Best Spa Package: The Spa Vacation package includes six nights' accommodation with breakfast and dinner; daily water and low-impact aerobic classes; use of tennis courts, fitness center, sauna, and pools; and choice of two spa programs: the twelve-treatment Arzaga Face and Body or the ten-treatment Arzaga Oriental Sensation. $1,600 to $2,000, depending on season, per person double occupancy.

Credit Cards: Most major

Getting There: Fly into Brescia or Verona (twenty-five minutes). The concierge can arrange for a car to meet you at either airport. Rental cars available as well. Those arriving in Milan should request a private car transfer.

What's Nearby: Cremona, where Stradivarius made his violins, home of Torrone nougat candy; Lake Garda, water sports and lakeside activities.

finest resorts, one where the spa experience has been taken "religiously."

An Italian Olive Oil Bath to Soften Skin

Roman aristocrats did more than cook with olive oil. When they reclined in their lavish marble bathtubs in about A.D. 212, it was olive oil they used to soften their skin. Roman soldiers, who often returned from battle with dry skin, added olive oil to their baths, too. Today olive oil is an ingredient of many skin-care products, but you can recreate an authentic olive oil bath at home or when you travel by following this easy recipe. Betsy Morscher, author of *Heal Yourself the European Way*, recommends the following as an excellent skin moisturizer: ½ cup of sesame oil, ½ cup of olive oil, 1 tablespoon of liquid detergent or shampoo, and ½ teaspoon of your favorite perfume or essential oil. Pour the oil, shampoo, and perfume or essential oil into a bottle and shake vigorously. Add two tablespoons to your bath as the warm water is running. Add a few scented candles, play some soft music, and relax.

SPA'DEUS
Tuscany, Italy

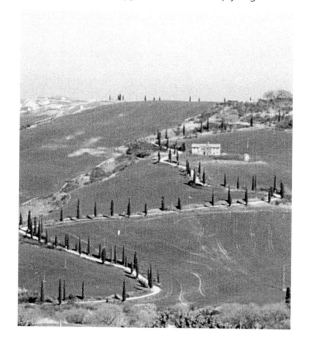

Inspired by visiting California health spas, Christina Newburgh created Italy's first and only American-style wellness program in Tuscany. Located in Chianciano Terme, a town noted for medicinal mineral water therapy, Spa'Deus offers hydrotherapy treatments, aquacize, and lots of mineral water daily. This unique destination spa program teaches that doing away with old habits and learning to move freely are the keys to living well.

The main attractions at Spa'Deus, which sits atop the town's highest hill, are walks in the scenic hills of Tuscany, with meals to match. Serious workouts are balanced by relaxation time, pampering treatments, and excursions to historic hill towns.

What makes Spa'Deus a true destination spa is the camaraderie that develops among the guests. Coming from many nations and backgrounds, they form a happy group of hikers. English is a common bond; the program attracts single women and men, a sprinkling of Milanese and Manhattan fashion models, London business executives, and couples from Rome. Personal attention by the multilingual staff, including American and European fitness trainers, helps newcomers learn where to go for treatments and exercise classes. Awaiting you are a sweatsuit, robe, and slippers, so the main thing to bring is walking shoes.

Every day starts with stretches and aerobics to get you revved up for an hour-long walk. Driven to backroads and private estates, you discover the real Tuscany. Vistas of vineyard-covered hills, ancient towns, and valleys covered in a patchwork of flowers and farms make each morning an adventure. Sometimes the hike ends at a country inn where the spa's kitchen has sent breakfast.

Returning to the hotel in high spirits, the group splits into three aerobics studios, where Spinning sessions on stationary bikes, stretching, dance exercise, and FitBall training are scheduled. Everyone gets basic treatments as part of the spa package, such as compressed air massage in pneumatic leggings to improve lymphatic circulation. Scheduling treatments from an extensive menu of beauty and skin-care services requires a visit with the spa programmer, which is charged to your account. Choices include ayurvedic massage synchronized by two therapists, massage with hot and cold stones placed on your body's pressure points to relieve stress, rhythmic lomi-lomi massage from Hawaii, and water-borne massage. Several of these treatments are exclusive to Spa'Deus and are not available elsewhere in Italy. Others require attention by the resident doctor and nurse, such as a water cleansing of the colon or juice fast.

Getting weighed and measured daily encourages progress in shedding pounds (kilos here), which proves surprisingly easy if you stick to the spa menu. The dining room manager suavely offers choices: diet or maintenance, with pasta, eggs, and fish, or simply vegetarian.

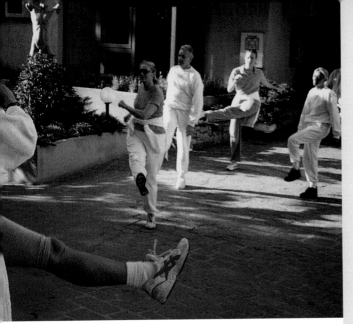

Some meals include salad; most of the time you are served the posted menu, plus fruit drinks, herbal teas, or coffee substitutes. One day lunch might be at a farm villa, complete with piano player; another outing takes in a wine tasting. Tuscany couldn't be better.

From Tip to Toe

Cracked, dry feet need not prevent you from showing off your latest sandals or strapped shoes. Keep your feet supple and moisturized by using creams with ingredients that do the job. Lactic acid, glycerin, and eucalyptus oil have proven results, according to Michael Vandermeersch of CCS by Nordic Cares (www.nordiccare.com).

He says that daily application of a moisturizing cream will gradually reduce the appearance of unsightly heels. Spas are the perfect venue for showing off your smooth-as-silk feet. Take time before bedtime to massage your feet with a potent cream and see the difference after a week or two of application. Spas often provide slippers at check-in, so prepare your feet to look their best when you arrive.

California Inspires an
Italian Masterpiece

Spa'Deus
Via le Piane, 35
53042 Chianciano Terme
Italy
Phone: 39–05–78–63232
Fax: 39–05–78–64329
E-mail: info@spadeus.it
Web site: www.spadeus.it
Season: March–October
General Manager: Christina Newburgh
Accommodations: Thirty spacious rooms with private bathroom and balcony in three-story hotel furnished in an eclectic mix of antique rugs and contemporary Italian art. Amenities include robe and workout clothing. All rooms have TV, phone, air conditioning.
Meals: Three meals daily are served at communal tables. Breakfast can be fruit, an egg, multigrain bread, and plum jam. Lunch features include Tuscan baked chicken, salmon baked in a bread crust, and homemade pasta with tomato sauce. Salads, yogurt, herbal tea, and coffee substitute available at all times.
Facilities: Gymnasium with extensive selection of exercise equipment, large indoor swimming pool, climbing wall, spinal traction pool, underwater exercise equipment, hydrotherapy tubs, sauna, steam.
Services & Special Programs: Massage, shiatsu, reflexology, facial, thalasso bath, CO_2 bath to promote circulation, underwater massage bath, oxygen inhalation, yoga. Medical checkup, colonic, juice fast. Mud wrap, gommage, aromatherapy, ayurvedic massage, hot stone massage, lymphodrainage NIA (Neuromuscular Intergrative Action), rebirthing, Watsu, Tae Bo, Pilates floorwork.
Rates: $$
Best Spa Package: All-inclusive rejuvenation week $1,885 per person, double; $2,159, single.
Credit Cards: American Express, MasterCard, VISA
Getting There: From Florence, train or taxi to Chiusi (one hour). By car, Autostrada A–1.
What's Nearby: Siena, Montepulciano.

TERME DI SATURNIA RESORT

Tuscany, Italy

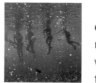

In a grove of plane-top pine trees and cypress, the thermal springs of Saturnia have attracted health-seekers since the Etruscans built temples. Scientific cosmetology and thermal medicine enrich the spa experience at the newly expanded Terme di Saturnia Resort. Harmonizing fire, earth, and water, this is a place of mystical energy.

The rolling hills of the Maremma region in southern Tuscany give little hint of volcanic springs or a modern resort hotel. As you leave the autostrada, about two hours from Rome, the earthy feel of old Toscana makes you breathe a sigh of relaxation.

Hotel guests are received in an ancient stone building. From the lobby bar you can see a lake-size swimming pool and vast lawns where the waters cascade into stone-walled baths and pools.

As you enter the sulfurous water from the canopied doors of the locker rooms, the first thing you notice are blobs of black plankton. Its therapeutic use for skin dis-ease led to the development of Saturnia cosmetics and skin-care treatments. Rising from volcanic springs deep within the pool, this trademarked bio-alga is blended with mineral-rich mud for facials and body wraps. The water bubbles up at a constant 98.6 degrees (37 degrees Celsius)—the same as your body temperature—working its soothing magic on a tired traveler. Getting a Watsu treatment in one of the small outdoor pools is like being in the womb of Mother Nature. Or try the new Thermalion capsule, which combines steam and heat.

The resort can be a busy place on a warm day. Hundreds of day-trippers take up spots on the lawn. Spa appointments have to be made early. (A new building and swimming pools have more than doubled facilities, however.) Programs range from revitalizing an aging complexion to improving the appearance of sensitive skin. Best bet: Day spa package includes your choice of four hydrotherapy treatments, plus free use of pool.

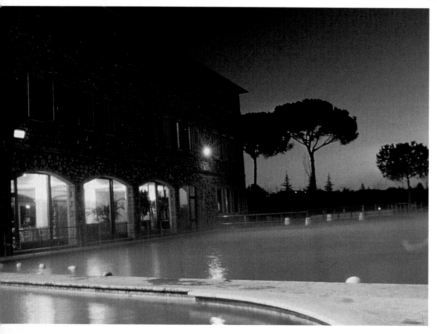

Saturnia doesn't stint on food. Diet, you are informed, means knowing how to live well. A nutritionist is on staff to evaluate your body structure and energy needs, and special diets are served to guests seated as far as possible from the copious buffets. Avoiding wine or alcohol, though, takes self-control. Most of the diners are here to enjoy Tuscany's bounty of fresh produce, game, and pasta. After dinner there is espresso, followed by drinks and dancing in the lounge, where bar manager Umberto has a special menu of nonalcoholic cocktails.

A morning jog with the Italian-American fitness team helps work

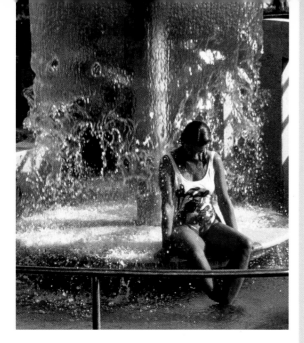

Hotel Terme di Saturnia Resort
58050 Saturnia (GR)
Italy
Phone: 39–0564–601601
Fax: 39–0564–601266
E-mail: info@termedisaturnia.it
Web site: www.termedisaturnia.com

Season: Year-round

General Manager: Glauco San Giovanni

Medical Director: Nicola Angelo Fortunati, M.D.

Fitness Directors: Kirk W. Lemley, Rocco Caloro

Reservations: 800–16–32–50

Accommodations: 140 rooms including ten suites in three buildings, plus nearby lodges with sixty-five rooms. Standard rooms in the original hotel are compact, have modern furniture, full-size bed, bathroom with shower. Luxury junior suites in new wing feature fine wooden furniture, designer fabrics in luminous colors. All are air-conditioned, have satellite TV and VCR, minibar, telephone. Amenities include robe, slippers, and cotton workout clothing.

Meals: Extensive breakfast buffet included with room rate. Villa Montepaldi restaurant table d'hôte fixed-price menu includes pasta, fish, and meat courses, antipasto buffet, and dessert.

Facilities: Institute of Scientific Cosmetology, new well-being center, thermal pools, indoor swimming pools, sauna, steam room, hydromassage, whirlpools, gymnasium with exercise equipment. Golf driving range, all-weather tennis courts (lit at night), bocce, mountain bikes.

Services & Special Programs: Seven-day fitness and anti-stress program. Program includes medical checkup, massage, multijet showers. Treatments booked individually include massage, Watsu, shiatsu, LaStone therapy, fango, reflexology, Vodder manual lymphatic drainage, aerosol inhalations, facial with glycolic acid, dermatology micro-surgery, laser epilation, body gommage, manicure, and pedicure. Fitness classes and personal training, yoga, and postural gymnastics charged per session.

Rates: $$

Best Spa Package: Thermal Week hydrotherapy and fan-gotherapy with exercise includes full board. From $821, double; $946, single.

Credit Cards: Most major

Getting There: From Rome, by car via Civitavecchia on Autostrada to Montalto, Manciano (170 kilometers); scheduled van service from Rome International Airport.

What's Nearby: Perugia, Pitigliano, Tyrrhenian Sea beach resorts, Siena.

off calories and gives you a chance to learn about the area's sports, wineries, olive oil makers, and cultural attractions. The hilltop town of Saturnia is a short distance from the resort. Saturnia Country Club provides horseback riding, fishing, archery, meals, and lodging. But the waters will draw you back.

Healing Waters

Thermal water is extremely relaxing and boosts the immune system, says Saturnia medical director N. A. Fortunati. By increasing resistance to illnesses, Dr. Fortunati explains, thermal water stimulates three functions that link body and mind: the involuntary nervous system, the glands, and the immune system. Saturnia's warm sulfurous waters are enriched with beneficial plant and mineral substances while passing through the volcanic subsoil. The secret of their healing and reinvigorating properties lies in the water's sulfuric-carbonic composition and temperature. Benefits can be experienced on your skin, in your respiratory system, and in enhanced muscular movement.

KEMPINSKI SAN LAWRENZ RESORT & SPA

Gozo, Malta

On an island steeped in history, the elegant Kempinski San Lawrenz Resort & Spa provides the latest in sea-inspired treatments to help you destress and rejuvenate. An exclusive Thalgo marine cure center offers the full range of European body care, facials, and hydrotherapy. Combined with extensive recreational facilities, this is a resort where you can bring children, enjoy hikes and bike rides on unspoiled seaside roads, and simply get back to nature.

Legend has it that the first settlers were a religious cult that worshiped the Earth Mother. Remains of temples predate the pyramids in Egypt. Built of giant boulders in circles similar to Stonehenge, the megalithic temples of Ggantija are a mysterious reminder of nature's power to stir the imagination.

The Knights of Malta, renowned for their hospital on the main island, harvested a healing fungus from rocks near the resort. Known as *fungus gaulitanus,* this rare plant was prized for medical treatments. Set in a deep recess in the rocky coastline, the fungus rock is part of an area called the inland sea of Dwejra, a magnet for scuba divers and sightseers.

Inspired by the architecture of traditional Maltese country estates, the resort is in a picturesque valley that is still being developed with upscale vacation homes. From the marble lobby you walk onto a spacious terrace overlooking eight acres of landscaped gardens and a free-form swimming pool. At garden level, the marine cure center brings the sea indoors, with a pool for relaxation and exercise—only here, springwater has been infused with micronized algae imported from France.

The French cosmetic firm Thalgo teamed up with the resort's developers to create a contemporary healing center that uses products made with seaweed and algae. Body wraps are "rich in minerals, vitamins, and micronutrients." The treatment is said to activate circulation, relieve aches and pains, detoxify, and restore metabolic balance. And it is completely relaxing. Other treatments include a cold marine mask that oxy-

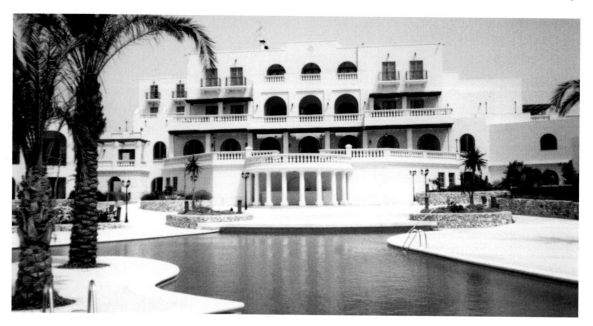

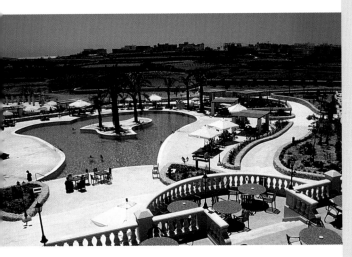

genates the skin, tightening and smoothing stress signs. There are relaxing baths with marine salts, algae, and essential oils, as well as expert massage.

Although there is a well-equipped gym, organized exercise is minimal. The hydrotherapy pool has underwater jets to massage parts of your body and can be used for physical therapy sessions with a local specialist. An indoor swimming pool and whirlpool adjoin the Thalgo center, open to all resort guests. At the outdoor pool (unheated), bar service is available during warm months. Both pools are freshwater; for a swim in the sea, the resort's courtesy bus takes you to nearby sandy and rocky beaches during summer.

Getting a Thalgo treatment here is the next best thing to being in France. And only half as expensive.

Calypso's Cave Lures Lovers

Overlooking the red sands of Gozo's finest beach, Ramla l-Hamra, is the cave assumed to be the home of Calypso, the legendary nymph mentioned in Homer's *Odyssey*. Here the beautiful sea-maiden kept Odysseus as a "prisoner of love" for seven years. Odysseus escaped and returned to his faithful wife, Penelope. Climbing the rocky cliff to see the cave is challenging, and the view is breathtaking.

Mediterranean Marine Cure on a Legendary Island

Kempinski San Lawrenz Resort & Spa
Triq ir-Rokon, San Lawrenz GRB 104
Gozo, Malta
Phone: 356–211–0000
Fax: 356–211–6373
Reservations: 800–426–3135
E-mail: info@sanlawrenz.com
Web site: www.sanlawrenz.com

Season: Year-round

General Manager: Rupert Simoner

Spa Director: Sandy Apap

Accommodations: 106 rooms, virtually all suites, furnished in contemporary style. Rooms have terra-cotta tile floors, separate sitting area with balcony. All have air-conditioning and ceiling fan, coffeemaker, large-screen TV, hair dryer, and ironing board and iron. Bathrooms feature bidet, tub, robes, adapter plug (110v/220v).

Meals: Mediterranean cuisine in the main restaurant, a la carte. Included in room rate is breakfast buffet. Special dinners in the Wine Boutique.

Facilities: Two-floor Thalgo marine cure center with fitness room, hydrotherapy pool, Vichy shower, Blitz shower, pressotherapy, balneo bathtubs. Two private tennis courts, two squash courts, two outdoor swimming pools, indoor pools.

Services & Special Programs: Massage, facials, body and skin care, manicure and pedicure, ayurveda program, marine and herbal cures.

Rates: $$

Best Spa Package: Weekend Rendezvous includes a two-night stay (to include a Saturday night) in the room category of guests' choice, full breakfast in the hotel restaurant or in your room, and a complimentary bottle of wine when you dine in the restaurant.

Credit Cards: Most major

Getting There: From Valletta, Malta International Airport, helicopter transfer to Gozo can be arranged by Air Malta. By car, daily ferry from the main island (thirty minutes). The resort is on the southern shore road.

What's Nearby: Victoria, fortified medieval city, with cathedral, opera house (courtesy bus from resort), Ggantija temples, Calypso's Cave, Comino (by ferry).

LES THERMES MARINS DE MONTE-CARLO

Monte Carlo, Monaco

Overlooking the Mediterranean Sea and Monte Carlo, this lavish, modern seawater spa is lively and happening, at poolside by day, in the casino at night.

Les Thermes Marins is more than a thalassotherapy center; facilities include two beauty salons associated with renowned hairstylists, therapy pools staffed by specialists in restoring equilibrium after childbirth or an accident, a full circuit of LifeFitness exercise equipment, and, of course, a seafood restaurant with dietetic menu. Created in 1995 by Prince Rainier's hotel group, Société des Bains de Mer, this spectacular seaswept aerie is so spacious that a complete vacation can be planned around a day here. And you don't need a princely budget; there are day-spa packages as well as overnight programs with Monaco's four top hotels.

Staying at the Hotel de Paris or Hotel Hermitage gives you direct access to Les Thermes via a marble-walled tunnel. Dip into the largest indoor seawater swimming pool on the Riviera coast. Sea and sky illuminate the shell-shaped pool through tall glass windows, creating the effect of a Botticelli painting. Off to the side are a Turkish steam bath (hammam), cabanas, and the bar. On the terrace, chaise longues fill up quickly, as the lunch crowd arrives early and stays late, cell phones beeping constantly.

Spa package guests get free use of all facilities, plus breakfast in the seaview dining room. Holistic programs are tailored to counteract the stress of modern life and enhance your feeling of well-being. Medical, nutrition, and physiotherapy services can be combined with massage and facials.

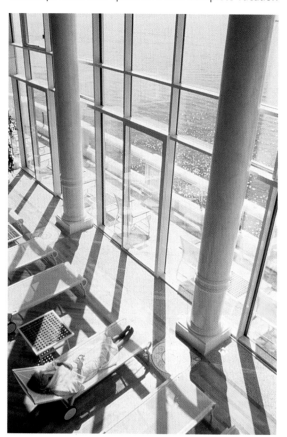

Taking a thalassotherapy cure or course of treatments is considered medical therapy and requires approval from one of the staff doctors. Once past the medical review, a mutilingual hostess guides you to treatments in the four-floor building. Four treatments are scheduled daily, usually a full morning: hydromassage bath, algae or seaweed bath, body wrap, and massage. Exercise sessions in a seawater pool heated to body temperature are led by staff members who pay special attention to physical limitations of participants; sessions last about forty minutes.

Monaco's glamorous entertainment, shopping, dining, museums, and sports are within minutes of Les Thermes Marins. The place to be seen is Hotel de Paris, which faces the historic casino and opera house. The more low-key Hotel Hermitage is ideal as a romantic hideaway, has heated (mosaic-tile) bathroom floors, and a winter garden designed by Eiffel with Tiffany-

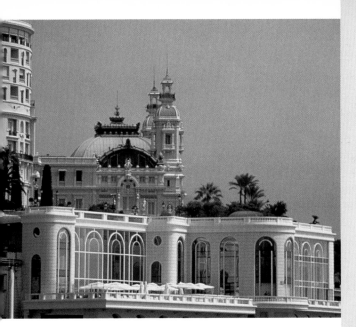

Thalassotherapy Fit for Royalty

Les Thermes Marins de Monte-Carlo
2, Avenue de Monte-Carlo (B.P. 215)
MC 980004 Monaco Cedex
Phone: 377–92–16–40–40
Fax: 377–92–16–49–49
E-mail: thermes@sbm.mc
Web site: www.montecarloresort.com

Season: Year-round

General Manager: Fabienne Guillot-Farneti

Reservations: 800–221–4708

Accommodations: The 227-room Hotel Hermitage and 197-room Hotel de Paris are five-star properties. Rooms with sea view have balcony. All air-conditioned, with TV, full bath, robes, and slippers. Service is formal, dress code to match.

Meals: Dietetic menu available in the spa's restaurant L'Hirondelle. Low-calorie desserts, herbal teas, and mineral water are available throughout the day at the spa pool. In the hotel dining rooms, dietetic selections appear on menus, or you can indulge in Alain Ducasse's cuisine at Le Louis XV. The rooftop restaurant at Hotel de Paris, Le Grill, offers a perfect blend of dining and ambience.

Facilities: Seawater therapy in baths, showers, and pools; marine aerosol inhalations and pressure therapy to stimulate muscles; fitness center with LifeFitness equipment and personal trainers; Turkish steam bath, saunas, beauty salons.

Services & Special Programs: Medical and nutrition consultation, physical rehabilitation in the pool. Weeklong programs for stress control, slimming, anticellulite. Massage, shiatsu, reflexology, aromatherapy, hydrotherapy bath, and affusion massage with seawater, algae, mud.

Rates: $$$

Best Spa Package: The Zen package includes eight "well-being" treatments chosen from a list that includes a facial with floral oil, an Oriental massage, or an underwater jet massage. Also includes daily breakfast, two dietetic luncheons at Les Thermes, and one dinner at a choice of Thai or seafood restaurant. Access to fitness facilities and Gold Card discounts are also included. Rates start at $3,351 for two people staying at The Hermitage (year-round) or the Monte-Carlo Beach Hotel.

Credit Cards: Most major

Getting There: From Nice, frequent express bus schedule at International Airport Côte d'Azur (one hour); helicopter (fifteen minutes); train (forty-five minutes). Limousine and rental car available.

What's Nearby: Eze (artist colony), Matisse and Chagall museums, Fondation Maeght museum, Italian riviera.

style glass ceiling. In addition to free use of the pool and fitness equipment, hotel guests get a VIP "passport" for dining and shopping discounts, and admission to golf and tennis clubs. Take a walk or jog in the casino gardens, down to the yacht-filled harbor, or up to the Grimaldi castle. Monaco is a grande dame who knows how to enjoy life.

Getting the Rhythm for Shape-ups

Seawater workouts at the aqua-fitness center are not only for physical exercise and relaxation; they are prescribed as an indispensable complement for the cures. Lipo-training is a slimming method recently developed by the spa team, tailored to each person's body weight and composition. Workouts in the pool are done at a pleasant rhythm, tuned to the best individual rate for burning fat and boosting metabolism. Before starting sessions in the cardio/strength-training studio, a treadmill test measures your consumption of oxygen. Based on the fitness team's evaluation, your best cardiac working frequency will be the basis for a training program.

MARRIOTT SON ANTEM GOLF RESORT & SPA

Mallorca, Spain

The Holistic Lifestyle Spa at this new golf resort blends ancient and contemporary therapies for beauty and prevention of illness. Designed to serve both resort guests and serious sybarites, the spa facilities are part of a spacious clubhouse set between two golf courses. This combination is ideal for parents with young children, as well as couples who golf and spa.

Verdant greens surround the Andalusian-style Mallorca Marriott Son Antem Golf Resort & Spa. Red-tiled roofs and two-story villas create the feeling of a small village. At its center is the main lodge, more like a hacienda than a hotel. A short walk from your room, the clubhouse is an all-weather attraction: fitness center, cafe, and resort shops upstairs, spa downstairs.

The view of the golf course and outdoor pools enhances both workouts and dining. Equipped with a full line of Technogym cardiovascular and strength-training units, the fitness center stays open late in the evening, as do the steaming thermal pools. It's ideal after a round of golf or to simply relax.

The spa pools are linked for access from outside or inside. Open to all resort guests for a small daily fee or as part of a spa package, the thermal pools are for relaxation rather than swimming. Underwater jets massage your body, and there are places to stretch out and soak. The resort's outdoor swimming pool (unheated) is usable most of the year.

Marriott's spa team worked with designers to create a holistic environment that stimulates all the senses. Revel in thermal water, or seek seclusion in an adult-only area called "Aqua-Zone," where a series of saunas and bubbling bathtubs encourage meditation.

Try the Roman Laconium-Caldarium to steam-clean your skin and respiratory system, the Turkish hammam steam bath for relaxation, and the Finnish sauna. There are fountains for footbaths, floral aromatherapy, and bubbling hot tubs shaped like Cleopatra's casket. Refresh and stimulate blood circulation with crushed ice that spills from the wall.

For total relaxation, book a mood-enhancing session in the oyster-shaped hydromassage capsule. The

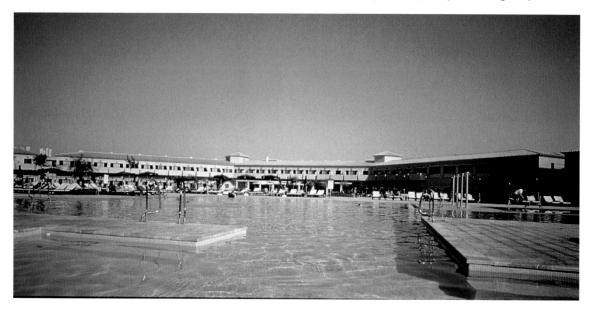

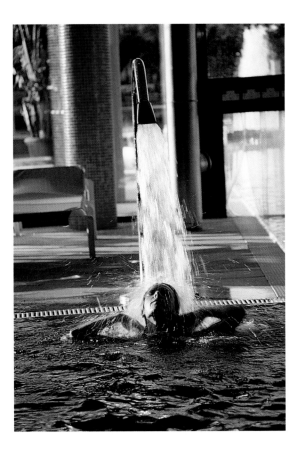

Marriott Son Antem Golf Resort & Spa
07620 Llucmajor
Mallorca, Spain
Phone: 34–971–12–92–10
Fax: 34–971–12–92–11
E-mail: mhrs.pmigs.dir.of.spa@marriott.com
Web site: www.marriotthotels.com/pmigs
Season: Year-round
General Manager: Kurt Strohmayer
Spa Director: Gernot Deutsch
Reservations: Marriott International (USA and Canada, 800–228–9290)
Spa Appointments: 34–971–1292, ext. 4011
Accommodations: 150 rooms including eight suites, with terrace or balcony, desk, reading area, king bed or double queen-size beds, TV, telephones. All have private bathroom, air-conditioning. Amenities include robes, hairdryer, safe.
Meals: Sumptuous buffet breakfast included with room tariff; lunch at clubhouse; dinner menu in main dining rooms; snack bar at swimming pool (summer only).
Facilities: Thermal bath complex with six rooms, whirlpools, dry sauna. Indoor and outdoor swimming pools with thermal water. Private treatment rooms include oyster-capsule bath, shiatsu suite, hydrotherapy tub. Beauty salon for hair and nail care.
Services & Special Programs: Ayurvedic therapies, hydrotherapy, Swedish massage, shiatsu, maternity massage, aromatherapy, facials, mud masque, herbal wrap, body peeling, pedicure, salon services. Consultation and a series of treatments with medical specialists can be arranged. Therapies include magnetic balancing, oxygen enhancement of the immune system, and biofeedback.
Rates: $$
Best Spa Package: Spa/Golf Escape includes room for two persons, breakfast buffet, choice of spa treatment (thirty to forty-five minutes) or round of golf. $231 double occupancy, $216 single, per day, including EVR tax.
Credit Cards: Most major
Getting There: By car from Palma's Airport, follow signs to Playa de Palma, Llucmajor, highway becomes two-lane PM 602, resort entrance on right (fifteen minutes). By plane from Berlin or Frankfurt by Aero Lloyd (two hours); from Barcelona by plane (forty-five minutes) or car ferry (four hours).
What's Nearby: Palma de Mallorca (cathedral, museums, shopping), Llucmajor (bike trails), Es Trenc beach, Costa Nord Cultural Center (Michael Douglas gallery).

spa's medical director, Jose B. Gimmenez Herrero, M.D., adjusts color, music, and aroma inside the space-age capsule as mechanical arms massage your back. Options include a body wrap with fango mud or seaweed to release toxins. To finish, a warm rain showers you within the capsule.

Therapists are highly trained in the latest European and American treatments to enhance your looks and sense of well-being with products by Kanebo, Decleor, and Valmont. Specialties include shiatsu, in a room equipped with tatami mats, and ayurvedic massage. The Salon Estilo provides Epoch hair and scalp care for senoras, caballeros, and kinder.

Active sports abound on the island, from sailing to soccer, biking to hiking. Try the new mountain bike trails at Llucmajor, an ancient village near the resort. Blessed with year-round outdoor recreation, Mallorca offers an ideal combination of sybaritic fun and healthy recreation.

STUREBADET

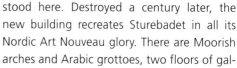

Secret spas are rare, but we've found one in the center of Stockholm that never advertises. The country that brought you ABBA and the Saab keeps Sturebadet to itself. Not exactly a secret—there are 4,000 members—it's the place in Stockholm to work out, get a massage, and enjoy spa cuisine. So here's how to experience Sweden's oldest and grandest spa.

Don't be put off by the location—in a shopping mall called Sturegallerian. The original Sturebadet, opened in 1885 as a communal bathhouse, once stood here. Destroyed a century later, the new building recreates Sturebadet in all its Nordic Art Nouveau glory. There are Moorish arches and Arabic grottoes, two floors of galleries for massage and skin care around the swimming pool, and a well-equipped fitness center for cardio-strength training.

The decor inspires mixed reactions: One member describes it as what a temple to the Vikings might have looked like to an Ottoman sultan. Restoration involved carving antique pine timber for the galleries,

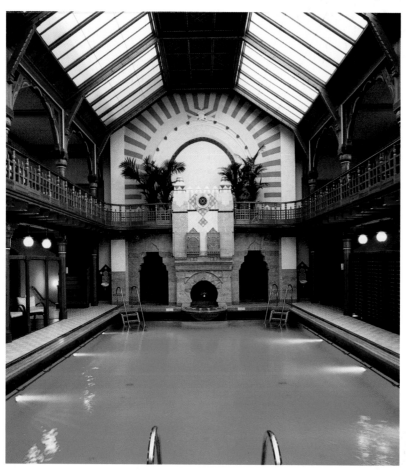

adding warm tones to the granite fountain that fills one end of the pool area. Skylights illuminate the pool, a nice touch in winter when members gather in bathrobes at the cafe/restaurant on the fifth-floor gallery, overlooking the pool.

Busy day and night, the club attracts the young, professional, high-energy, and stressed. Visitors are welcome when space is available for treatments, or you can drop in to swim and exercise by paying for a day pass ($15). Check in at a reception desk on the mall level, collect a robe and locker key, then take the elevator to the locker rooms. An aerobics studio pulses with classes throughout the day, some high-impact, others listed for various levels. In the gymnasium, you may have to wait if your favorite treadmill or Stair-Master is in use, but there are rowing machines, bicycles, and free weights. An instructor is always present; if you don't speak Swedish, the locals are fluent in English and other languages.

With all the high-energy workouts, getting a Swedish massage here is worth taking the next SAS flight. Because therapists are trained for three years at professional schools like the Axellsson Institute, the classic massage strokes are mixed with new techniques that set up a synergy between masseuse and recipient. The spa department also provides facials, body scrubs, manicures and pedicures, and the latest herbal treatments by Kerstin Florian. Treatment cabins surround the pool on all sides, and demand for appointments is so heavy that there is a Web site for members to snag last-minute cancellations.

Two hotels in the area have branches of Sturebadet, where getting treatments may be more convenient. If you stay at the recently built Radisson SAS Royal Park or the historic Grand Hotel opposite the Royal Palace, you can use facilities at all three club spas. But nowhere else can you combine a historic bathhouse with an aromatherapy kur.

Kerstin's Kur

Healthy complexions are a Swedish tradition that's very much alive at Sturebadet. Swedish-born skin-care specialist Kerstin Florian creates some of the spa world's most innovative products for her California-based company, then comes home to Stockholm every summer for workshops and personal training with spa aestheticians. The Kerstin Florian range of products includes Austrian moor mud, Hungarian thermal mineral bath crystals, and German herbal krauter bath oils. Based on the European kur, a centuries-old ritual of renewal and exercise combined with treatment for the face and body, Florian created the kur program to integrate spa treatments at Sturebadet and leading American spas.

Sturebadet
Sturegallerian 36
114 46 Stockholm
Sweden
Phone: 46–8–545–01523
Fax: 46–8–545–01510
E-mail: info@sturebadet.se
Web site: www.sturebadet.se

Season: Year-round

General Manager: Per Rosvall

Accommodations: SAS Royal Park Hotel

Meals: Sturebadet Restaurant offers full-service menu of spa cuisine, breakfast through dinner, every day. Marble-top tables reflect simplicity in food presentation. Fish, vegetable, and pasta dishes change daily.

Facilities: Cardio strength–training fitness center with equipment by Cybex, StairMaster, and free weights; private cabins for spa treatments; hydrotherapy tubs; aerobics studio.

Services & Special Programs: Massage, facials, manicure, pedicure, body scrub, body wraps with aroma oils or moor mud, algae wrap, kur bath, waxing, eye treatments. Chiropractic treatments.

Rates: $

Best Spa Package: Sturebadet half-day kur, $215, includes body scrub, kur bath, twenty-five-minute massage, facial, manicure or pedicure, and full use of club facilities, robes.

Credit Cards: American Express, MasterCard, VISA

Getting There: From center of Stockholm, T-underground train to Ostermalmstorg or Hotorget station, entrance on Stureplan.

What's Nearby: Food halls, Kungsgatan gardens, Vasa museum (1628 royal warship), Old Town.

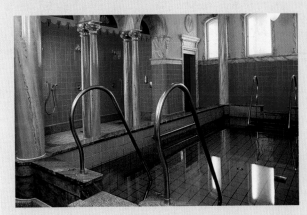

BADRUTT'S PALACE HOTEL AND SPA
St. Moritz, Switzerland

Located on the southern side of the Swiss alps in a sun-drenched corner of the Engadine, St. Moritz has enjoyed a one-hundred-year reputation as a favorite of the jet set, sports enthusiasts, royalty, and spa lovers. Deserving of its reputation as a gathering place for international movers and shakers, this is the nerve center of traditional Swiss hospitality.

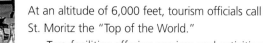

Breathtaking views, crisp alpine air, and a strong tradition of healing waters have made this chic ski resort a coveted word among those who expect the best and can easily afford the cost. Surrounded by twenty-five crystal-clear mountain lakes, majestic glaciers, and deep forests, there are an abundance of outdoor activities available when you stay at Badrutt's Palace, managed since 1999 by the Texas-based Rosewood Hotels & Resorts. The signature tower of this venerable hotel village, with its wooden balconies, stonework, and four-sided green roof, marks its position in the heart of St. Moritz. Gothic arches and hand-carved hardwoods attest to the long history of this landmark hotel, officially opened in 1896.

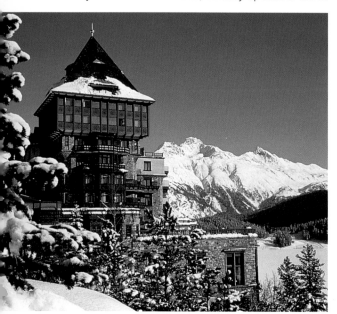

At an altitude of 6,000 feet, tourism officials call St. Moritz the "Top of the World."

Two facilities offering services and activities opened in 2002: Caroli Health Club, named for the Italian judo champion Angelo Caroli (whose motto is "a healthy mind and a healthy body stimulate one another with positive energy"), is where guests check in for their workouts. Daniela Steiner's Beauty Spa is where guests go for all skin-care and body treatments. Enhanced by candlelight and soft music, beauty specialists and body therapists staff ten treatment rooms called care suites. On the spa menu are partial aroma wraps with body massage, classical and luxury facials, and the epitome of luxury bathing—the Cleopatra bath. It's taken in a tub filled to the brim with warm water, milk, honey, and almonds. The spa specializes in beauty treatments for the entire body, using products formulated from the essence of rare botanicals—all laboratory tested for cleansing, healing, and age-defying properties.

Setting this spa apart from others is the Royal Basic Treatment, which can be as short as one day or as long as week. The three-part treatment starts with a personal evaluation and a two-hour First Total Cleansing, which includes a head-to-toe massage and total body exfoliation. Other treatments include an invigorating massage with cypress essences, a crystal bath, a purifying facial mask, and a nourishing hair mask.

Even a regular full-body massage is exquisite. You lay on a heated table in an intimate room filled with indirect lighting. Vapors from a bowl of distilled water infused with drops of neroli oil, lavender oil, and herbs and set below the table help you breathe and relax.

On a strictly personalized basis, a custom-designed wellness program including nutrition and exercise guidelines will leave you feeling on top of the world.

Although the Palace has a wealth of spa opportunities and activities, it does not offer a structured pro-

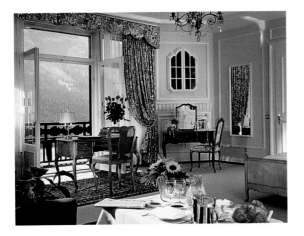

gram with a rigid schedule. Historically, people flocked to St. Moritz for the two- to three-week "cure," a combination of mineral baths, mud baths, drinking the water, alpine walks, and socializing. Today's cure evolved from traditional roots, and it showcases well at the Palace. Everything revolves around guests, and service is as smooth as the snow-capped mountains you see from your guest room.

Arm Yourself against Travel Fatigue

In today's travel-weary world, be prepared for unscheduled delays, long flights, and tight spaces. Prepare and carry with you a spa solution kit, and stow it under your seat in case you need an instant remedy for tired legs, dry eyes, facial dehydration, and dry cuticles. Lip balm, a moisturizer, and a spray of alcohol-free toner will help you pull through. Keep your kit to less than two pounds to save on space and weight. Transfer your favorite remedies to spillproof plastic containers and label each.

When legs feel tired or cramped, try arnica. Apply a leg cream, such as Kneipp's Arnica or EO Revitalizing Lotion, and massage it into your legs from the feet and ankles to midthigh.

Avoid alcoholic beverages, and drink bottled water throughout your flight.

A Champagne Climate for Champagne Tastes

Badrutt's Palace Hotel and Spa
7500 St. Moritz
Switzerland
Phone: 41–81–837–10–00
Fax: 41–81–837–29–99
Web site: www.badruttspalace.com
Season: December 6–April 6, June 27–September 28
General Manager: Roland B. Fasel
Spa Manager: Ulrike Steiner
Reservations: 888–ROSEWOOD (888–767–3966), or e-mail reservations.palace@rosewoodhotels.com
Spa Appointments: 41–81–837–2851
Accommodations: There are 201 guestrooms, including forty-two suites.
Meals: Chesa Veglia, built in 1658 and one of the oldest buildings in St. Moritz, has three restaurants and two bars in a rustic ambience. The Acapulco Snack Bar serves light, healthy cuisine. Le Relais Restaurant offers French bistro cuisine as well as sushi and sashimi. Le Restaurant serves classic French cuisine in a very elegant atmosphere.
Services & Special Programs: Hotel ski school, three outdoor tennis courts, shuttle bus to and from the Corviglia ski lift and Samedan golf course during the summer, bridge hostess, skating instructor, Kids Club Palazino staffed with professional nurses.
Rates: $$$$
Best Spa Package: The four-night Summer Beauty Escape package for two includes accommodations, daily buffet breakfast, fresh fruits and flowers upon arrival, one anti-stress sweet almond and honey wrap, and one luxury facial. Doubles from about $1,653, including taxes.
Credit Cards: Most major
Getting There: British Airways to Zurich. There are daily shuttle flights between Zurich and Samedan airports.
What's Nearby: A Swiss Museum Pass (www. myswitzerland.com) gives you entry to 250 museums throughout the country. St. Moritz offers walking trails, windsurfing, mountain biking, sailing, guided hikes, horseback riding, paragliding, golf, helicopter flights, trips to nearby villages, and treks to glaciers. Municipal swimming pool.

GRAND HOTELS BAD RAGAZ

Bad Ragaz, Switzerland

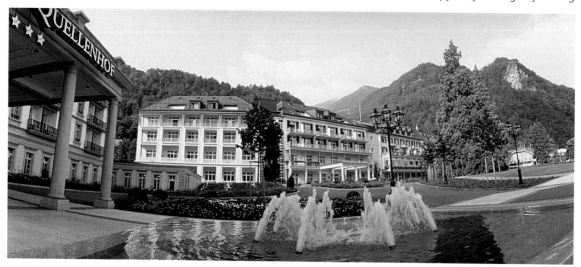

This grande dame of the Swiss spa world is synonymous with "taking the waters." Located in the Alpine foothills in the canton of St. Gallen, the resort has long been a destination for rejuvenation and for relief from rheumatism, arthritis, and other debilitating ills.

The resort consists of two hotels, the chic five-star Grand Hotel Quellenhof and the slightly less expensive, four-star Grand Hotel Hof Ragaz. The elegant Quellenhof underwent a major renovation between 1990 and 1992, transforming itself from a rather stodgy old-world bastion that attracted a rather sickly crowd to an upbeat, trend-setting spa oasis. Although both hotels remain a symbol of the elegant spas of the nineteenth and early twentieth centuries, they have reinvented themselves to reflect today's interest in wellness and preventive health, all the while continuing to maintain their uncompromising standards.

The spa experience Quellenhof-style is a singular one. There are performance diagnostic tests, fitness checkups, massages, and beauty programs. In the well-equipped gym you'll find bicycle ergometers, stepping and rowing machines, Skywalkers, and fourteen training machines. Daily exercise classes include FitBall, stretching, pool workout, and qigong. In some respects the overall program is similar to that found at a traditional American spa, but when it comes to water, the Swiss get serious. The classic water cure has been taken to the next level with some of the most impressive technology in Europe.

The Tamina Gorge, an imposing construction of cliffs and waterfalls, is used for the Kneipp course—a specialized water therapy that originated in Bad Woerishofen, Germany. The Roman influence prevails in the Thermarium (classical steam bath) and the Finnish influence in the coed Sauna Landscape (private saunas are available on request). The cold-water, open-air pool will toughen you up; there are also four individual whirlpools and a large swimming pool. But the heart of this grand European spa is the Helena Bath, the thermal Roman bathing temple adjacent to a Roman-Irish cycle (alternating steam and water baths).

Enhancing the water therapy is the Beauty Oasis for face and body care. A clinic called Prevention of Skin Aging offers the latest therapy—myo-lifting. Myo-lifting

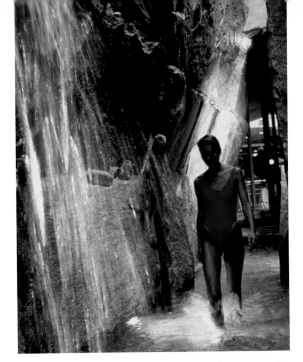

is a non-surgical anti-aging treatment to leave you with younger looking skin. Carita, a French skin-care line, is used for specialized facials. Body treatments using thalassotherapy products are designed to improve circulation, refine, and tone. Slimming and cellulite treatments use partial and whole-body packs, underwater massage, and low-temperature leg treatments.

The Grand Hotels Ragaz represents the new wave of Swiss spas with state-of-the-art technology, a progressive fitness program, a beauty farm, sports, and luxury—all showcasing the efficiency and grace of Swiss hospitality.

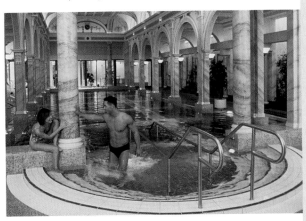

Taking the Waters with Class

Grand Hotels Bad Ragaz
CH-7310 Bad Ragaz
Switzerland
Phone: 41–81–303–30–30
Fax: 41–81–303–30–33
Web site: www.resortragaz.ch

Season: Year-round

General Manager: Hans Geiger

Spa Director: Corrine Denzler

Fitness Director: Brigitte Hallwachs, M.D.

Reservations: (800) 223–6800 (Leading Hotels of the World) or 41–81–303–30–30

Spa Appointments: 41–81–303–20–60

Accommodations: Grand Hotel Quellenhof offers 126 junior suites, eight suites, and a royal suite; all guest accommodations are spacious, decorated in a blue and yellow color scheme, with luxurious baths and balconies with Alpine views. Amenities include remote cable TV, direct-dial telephones, in-room safe, robes, and fresh flowers.

Meals: Restaurant Bel-Air, with sunny terrace, offers popular summer barbecues and spa cuisine; the Dorfbeiz Zollstube serves typical Swiss dishes; the Terrace Cafe Winter Garden offers snacks; and the Golf Club Restaurant has a garden terrace. Gourmet restaurant, Äbtestube.

Facilities: Eighteen-hole golf course with two-story driving range, indoor range, and putting green; six tennis courts (four outdoor, two indoor); two squash courts; two badminton courts; beauty salon; thermal indoor and outdoor pools; complete health club; spa; mountain bikes; shopping arcade; casino; meeting facilities; and hiking trails.

Services & Special Programs: Car rental; laundry/dry cleaning; limousine service; dogs permitted; valet parking; twenty-four-hour room service; business services; children's programs; health and beauty packages; golf packages.

Rates: $$$

Best Spa Package: The His-and-Her Lifestyle Week, with accommodations for six nights, half board (breakfast and dinner), the Fitness & Wellness Experience, daily fitness classes, and the Lifestyle Program (massage, facial, manicure, pedicure, body exfoliation, wave bath, and marine algae gel pack). Price at the Grand Hotel Quellenhof is $1,830 per person double occupancy in winter (January 2 through May 1).

Credit Cards: Most major

Getting There: The resort is one-and-a-half hours from the Zurich-Kloten International Airport and three hours from Munich or Milan. Rail service and limousine transfers are available.

VICTORIA-JUNGFRAU GRAND HOTEL & SPA
Interlaken, Switzerland

The luxury five-star, 220-room Victoria-Jungfrau Grand Hotel, with stunning views of the Jungfrau mountain range in the heart of Interlaken, opened in 1865 and has hosted the

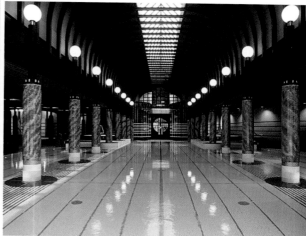

likes of Mark Twain and other visiting dignitaries over the course of its 135-year history. Now the hotel is home to a spa that measures up to its traditional high standards. The ultramodern design of the state-of-the-art Spa Interlaken harmonizes with the venerable hotel, despite the disparity in age. The centerpiece of the spa is a swimming pool meant to evoke the grandeur of a Roman bath.

The spa complex includes a saltwater Jacuzzi, Turkish steam bath, Finnish sauna, bio-saunas with active-light therapy, a solarium, and a relaxation area. The "aqua-fun" water exercises are designed to aid the circulatory system. Foot reflexology, lymphatic drainage, and combined massages are guaranteed to induce relaxation.

Setting this spa apart from the other hotel-based facilities is its medical-fitness program, which was created through the cooperation of physicians and therapists. Each guest is prescribed an exercise regimen based on his or her strength, stamina, speed, mobility, and coordination. The program begins with the Victoria-Jungfrau Fit Test, which takes one hour to administer. Those in the program can use the Cybex 6000 equipment under supervision and can also select electrotherapy, heat and cold treatments, hydrotherapy, and manual therapy. The medical fitness program is combined with an evenly balanced nutritional program of *cuisine minceur* (1,500 calories daily, including a small glass of wine).

At the Victoria-Jungfrau beauty center, an analysis of skin type precedes the selection of a

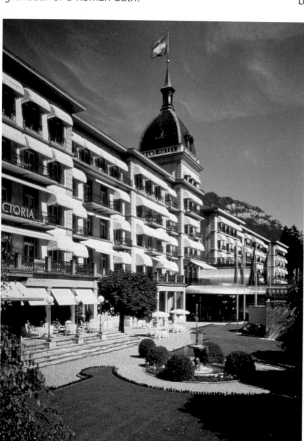

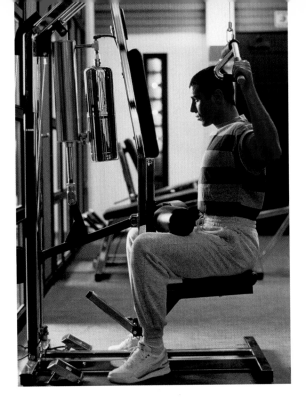

facial. Additional services at the center include anticellulite treatments, personal makeup, and hairstyling.

Hiking, golf, and tennis can be added to your program. There are seven tennis courts (four indoor, three outdoor) and an indoor golf facility. You'll be fit to scale the Jungfrau after this precision-driven Swiss body tune-up.

Few Calories, Lots of Nutrition

The spa's *cuisine minceur* program is very low in calories—just 1,400 to 1,500 per day—but high in nutritional benefits. The aim is to maintain and enhance good health and general well-being, and to prevent nutrition-related illnesses. In addition to breakfast, lunch, and dinner, those following the program enjoy three snacks and a small glass of wine. The theory at Victoria-Jungfrau is that spa cuisine should be a culinary delight rather than a duty; it should satisfy even the most discerning gourmets.

A State-of-the-Art Approach to Alpine Wellness

Victoria-Jungfrau Grand Hotel & Spa
CH-3800 Interlaken
Switzerland
Phone: 41–33–828–28–28
Fax: 41–33–828–28–80
E-mail: interlaken@victoria-jungfrau.ch
Web site: www.victoria-jungfrau.ch

Season: Year-round

General Manager: Emanuel Berger

Reservations: 41–33–828–26–11 or (800) 223–6800, Leading Hotels of the World

Spa Appointments: 41–33–828–28–28

Accommodations: Classic elegance is captured in 212 guest rooms, junior suites, and duplex suites, all with private bath, direct-dial phones, radio, TV, and minibar.

Meals: The hotel has eight distinctive restaurants or bars. Among them: The informal Jungfrau-Stube offers typical Swiss meals and summer barbecues; La Terrasse features elegant dining with piano music; international artists appear at the Cabaret, a private nightclub; Jungfrau Brasserie serves regional specialties; La Pastateca offers southern European favorites; and the Victoria Bar is a good spot for cocktails and dancing.

Facilities: Indoor heated swimming pool; seven tennis courts; fitness center; spa; health and beauty center; indoor golf; billiards; conference rooms; hotel garage parking; boutique.

Services & Special Programs: Sight-seeing excursions, hiking weeks, adventure packages; various spa packages; numerous family and children's events and programs; complimentary hotel kindergarten.

Rates: $$$

Best Spa Package: The Spa Deluxe six-night package includes a spa fitness test, private training with a qualified instructor, massage, and nutritional counseling. $1,340 per person, double occupancy.

Credit Cards: Most major

Getting There: Two-hour drive from Zurich and Geneva airports and one-half hour from Bern airport. Direct train connections are available; limousine service can be arranged through the hotel.

What's Nearby: Shopping; 18-hole golf course; horseback riding; wide range of sports from downhill and cross-country skiing to hiking and mountain biking; William Tell Open-Air Theatre.

CHAMPNEYS HEALTH RESORT & SPA
Tring, Hertfordshire, England

A destination spa providing more than twenty daily activities, more than one hundred treatments, holistic health services, and gourmet meals, Champneys is England's version of California's Golden Door. Founded more than sixty years ago by a naturopath, the resort has evolved with the times and currently emphasizes organic food, a balanced regimen of exercise and stress management, state-of-the-art treatments, and the simple pleasures of country walks. Recently given a facelift, new restaurant, and additional guest rooms, the resort attracts a lively mix of fitness-oriented and stressed-out men and women.

Arriving at the mansion, about an hour from London, you are welcomed and escorted to the registration desk. The mansion's Victorian elegance and sunny

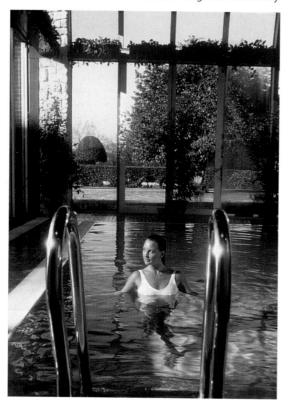

garden terraces immediately create an air of relaxation. Beyond an oaken door to the drawing room is a bar that serves herbal teas, mineral water, and after-dinner coffee. There's also a quiet music room, a game room with a snooker (pool) table, and a smoking room. In the west wing are exercise studios equipped for strength training and cardiovascular workouts.

Champneys is on the cutting edge of preventive medicine, holistic health, and stress management. At the spa, skin care and hair treatments feature products by Clarins, Decleor, Guinot, Aromatherapy Associates, Jessica, Lamour, and O-Lys. The staff outnumber guests by two to one, and it doesn't take them long to make a visitor from abroad feel at home. On arrival, you meet a nurse (called "sister" in England) to go over any health problems and plan a personal program. Appointments can be made for the bath or wrap and massage, which are included in the daily fee. Beyond that, treatments are a la carte or part of packages for two to five nights, and you are free to join scheduled group exercise or simply relax.

Dieting here has an elegant edge: Meals are served on Wedgwood china, and dinner can include wine in crystal goblets. Selections are rated by fat and fiber content, and you can chose from the fixed light diet menu or an elaborate salad bar and hot buffet of local game, trout, sea bass, salmon, and vegetarian pasta. In warm weather you can dine on the terrace. Meet people at the Champneys table reserved for single guests.

Set on 170 acres of sweeping lawns and colorful flower beds, the mansion, which was once owned by the British branch of the Rothschilds, is an ideal getaway spa. Country house informality encourages dressing down during the day (jogging suits are fine; some guests wear a dressing gown or the robe and slippers supplied in your room). Sturdy walking shoes or boots are advised for exploring the Chiltern hills,

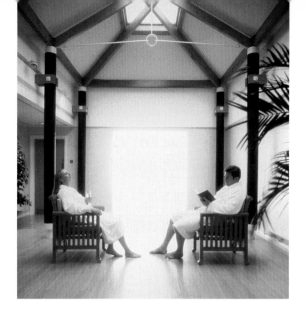

Country Pleasures for Mind, Body, and Soul

Champneys Health Resort & Spa
Wigginton, Tring, Hertfordshire HP23 6HY
England
Phone: 44–144–2291000
Fax: 44–144–2291001
E-mail: resort@champneys.co.uk
Web site: www.champneys.com

Season: All year, except Christmas week

General Manager: Robert Nipper

Spa Manager: Mette Haxthausen

Accommodations: Seventy-eight rooms, including eight suites in mansion. All with en-suite bathroom, except fourteen budget rooms in west wing. Modern rooms facing gardens have traditional pine furniture, chintz fabrics. Spacious suites Nos. 17–19 on second floor of mansion consist of a living-dining area, elaborately draped king-size bed facing bay window overlooking garden, marble-walled bathroom with whirlpool tub. Centrally heated and air-conditioned, with phones.

Meals: Included in daily tariff. Choice of menu in dining room: light diet or gourmet cuisine a la carte, with vegetarian option.

Facilities: Fitness center with advanced cardiovascular equipment, StairMaster, VersaClimber, stationary bikes. Separate spa baths for men and women, forty-four treatment rooms. Indoor swimming pool and squash court; whirlpool indoors and outside, croquet lawn, three tennis courts, mountain bikes, snooker table, volleyball and badminton, darts; art studio, aerobics gym.

Services & Special Programs: More than one hundred treatments offered a la carte, including acupuncture, shiatsu, LaStone massage, aura-soma, homeopathy. Nutrition consultation, cooking demonstrations; holistic health programs; breast examination. Art instruction and craft workshops.

Rates: $$$

Best Spa Package: Two-night package with daily massage and heat treatment, three meals daily, choice of group exercise. $784–$1,200 per person.

Credit Cards: Most major

Getting There: Train to Berkhamsted from London Euston Station; taxi or limousine meets trains and planes, on request. By car, the M–1 from London, exit 8, follow A–4147 to A–41.

What's Nearby: Windsor Castle, Stratford-upon-Avon, Oxford, Henley, Woburn Abbey, Dunstable Downs Gliding Club, Tring Museum.

where horseback riding, golf, and guided walks are offered daily. Bring rain gear; the concierge supplies Wellies (high rubber boots).

This twenty-first century wellness center, which can be traced back to 1307 when the estate was owned by the Champneys family, brings together the best of Europe and America.

Shedding Light on Facials

Exposure to light treatments using O-Lys equipment and products is said to increase your body's production of vitamin D, thus aiding the natural absorption of calcium, phosphorus, and magnesium. Focused by a specially trained aesthetician, the equipment concentrates light with no laser burn. Other modes improve muscle function (including that of the heart), lower blood pressure, and help those suffering sleep disorders or jet lag. Try it in conjunction with reflexology for a head-to-toe rejuvenating experience. Another blend of light and color therapy, called aura-soma, stimulates natural healing and self-discovery based on your selection of bottled herbal extracts, essential oils, gems, and crystals that reveal energy auras.

CHEWTON GLEN HOTEL, HEALTH & COUNTRY CLUB

Hampshire, England

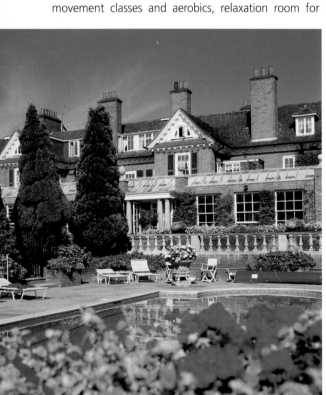

Traditional country-house hospitality has been honed to a fine art at Chewton Glen. Not content with winning every award in the United Kingdom, owners Martin and Brigitte Skan unveiled an expanded health club in 2002. Larger than most resort spas, the club's airy, light-filled spaces include a vast indoor swimming pool, separate changing rooms for men and women, each with steam rooms and saunas, and a hydrotherapy pool. Exercise equipment is arranged so that you enjoy views of the woodlands, croquet lawn, and golf course.

Contrasting with the chintz and dark wooden furniture of country houses, the new health club is sleek and modern. The range of facilities includes a studio for movement classes and aerobics, relaxation room for "after treatments," and a large gym with air-resistance equipment. New treatment rooms offer skin care based on natural ingredients and aromatherapy straight from English gardens.

Time moves in measured paces here, so don't expect lots of activity. Aside from scheduled sessions in the studio, you may want to work with a personal trainer. Advance consultation with the spa director also assures appointment times for treatments, especially on weekends and during holidays when there is a full house.

Privacy is paramount, and formal dress is required in the dining room. From the moment you are greeted in the courtyard, tradition is carefully observed. Wellies, the rubber boots beloved of country gents, are lined up at the door so that guests can borrow a pair before taking off on walks. Floral arrangements are in every room, and teatime is a social ritual. Each suite and bedroom is decorated with individual flair, mixing heirlooms, antique furniture, and the refined taste of the owners. Dating from the early 1700s, the main house had Palladian additions in the 1890s, faithfully preserved in recent renovation.

Attention to detail is a hallmark. Nothing goes unnoticed. That can be intimidating for newcomers, but the gracious staff make it all seem natural. Especially in the dining room—Chef Pierre Chevillard and many staff members have been here for years and cater to your personal pleasure.

Set in a tranquil landscape, the resort is close to the English Channel as well as nature preserves, 90 miles southwest of London. Take long walks on the beach or perhaps a badgerwatch trek in the New Forest. But with a private 9-hole golf course on site, indoor and outdoor tennis, culinary celebrations and musical galas, most guests simply settle in and enjoy being at this quintessential country retreat.

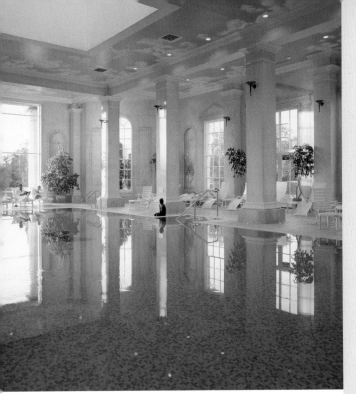

Chewton Glen Hotel, Health & Country Club
Chewton Farm Road
New Milton, Hampshire BH25 6QS
England
Phone: 44–1425–275341; U.S. toll free (800) 344–5087
Fax: 44–1425–272310; U.S. toll free (800) 398–4534
E-mail: reservations@chewtonglen.com
Web site: www.chewtonglen.com
Season: Year-round
Owners/directors: Martin and Brigitte Skan
General Manager: Peter Crome
Spa Manager: Clive McNish
Reservations: U.S. toll free (800) 344–5087; UK 44–1425–275341
Accommodations: Fifty-nine rooms, many with sitting area; nineteen suites. Country casual means lots of floral chintz, pinch-pleated drapery, solid wooden furniture. All guest rooms have private bath, Frette bathrobes and slippers, telephone, TV, trouser press, hair dryer, Molton Brown toiletries. Complimentary sherry, shortbread, and mineral water.
Meals: Full English breakfast and dinner included in daily tariff. Balanced nutrition and fresh seafood are features of the new Conservatory restaurant. Marryat restaurant (Michelin star) offers a varied menu. Extensive wine list available.
Facilities: Full-service health club with gym, aerobics studio, computerized air-resistance equipment, eleven private treatment rooms. Swimming pool indoors (ozonated) and in garden, whirlpool, eucalyptus-scented steam rooms, and saunas. Tennis courts (two indoor with Marka-Grain surface, two outdoor), 9-hole golf course, golf club loan, bikes. Nearby horse riding, sailing, ten golf courses.
Services & Special Programs: Massage, reflexology, Indian scalp massage, facials, Thai massage, reiki, shiatsu; Pilates; hypnotherapy; skin care by ESPA, Guinot, and Clarins. Fitness evaluation, personal trainers, sports rehabilitation program; massage workshop, tennis clinics, flower-arranging class.
Rates: $$$
Best Spa Package: Three-night Getaway Break, from $1,118 per person, double, includes breakfast and dinner daily, spa treatments.
Credit Cards: Most major
Getting There: From London by car, M3 to M27 westbound, after Bournemouth becomes A31, right on A35 at the Swan pub toward Walkford (two hours). By train from Waterloo Station (two hours); helipad on site.
What's Nearby: Southampton, New Forest, Beaulieu (estate with car museum), Portsmouth, Cowes (sailing), Stonehenge (druids).

Stressbuster British-Style

Balanced by a hearty dose of exercise and relaxation, stress loosens its hold. Add a healthy diet, and you've got it beat. Chewton Glen gets it together, indoors and out. The Greco-Roman design of the spa immediately relaxes you: honey-colored stone walls, leafy green trees, and the pool's silky-crystal ozone-treated water. Windows rise floor to ceiling, flooding the pool with natural light. The ceiling is painted a scenic sky blue with puffy white clouds conjuring memories of childhood. There's even a specially designed couch for pregnant ladies.

After a damp steam in the hammam, swim laps in the pool, relax in the bubbling whirlpool. "We avoid faddy here-today-gone-tomorrow therapies," says club manager/sports therapist Clive McNish. Indulge in treatments like Indian scalp massage that send you into a state of utter relaxation.

FOREST MERE HEALTH FARM

Liphook, Hampshire, England

The English countryside is a perfect counterpoint to the luxuries of Forest Mere. Natural beauty surrounds this classic country manor set amid farms on 120 acres of tranquil woodland about an hour south of London. But the beauty within comes from treatments with top European brands of skin care and cosmetic products.

New Age energy meets old English charm in the spa department. Reservationists check you into comfortably appointed lounge areas; then it's up to you to plan a program or simply relax. With two aerobics studios offering unlimited free group workouts and a gymnasium full of LifeFitness equipment and free weights, the ambience is much like that at an American resort. Then you discover the pools: a glass-walled ozonated 25-meter (half–Olympic length) indoor swimming pool, a

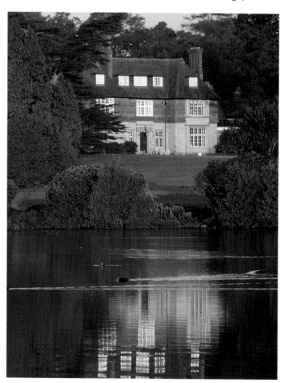

whirlpool, and a saltwater hydrotherapy pool. And there are seventy treatment rooms, more than most destination spas. Between serious pampering and workouts, your choices can be the most difficult exercise.

In addition to traditional treatments, alternative medicine specialists offer Chinese herbal care, hypnotherapy, and osteopathy. In the hands of therapists who are credentialed and caring, you are quickly lulled into a state of serenity.

How about trying something exotic? Aromatherapy is practically a necessity for the stressed young executives who make up a large portion of Forest Mere regulars. Try a full-body massage with essential oils on the acupuncture points for relaxation or stimulation. Then there are seaweed and mud wraps, and a dry flotation bed where you relax cocooned in the seaweed wrap. For sensual luxury, there is a Cleopatra milk float, and an evening primrose oil float. Plus the pièce de résistance: a mud treatment in the Serail-Bad, an Oriental steam room with brightly tiled walls, a fountain that puffs herbal mist, and a selection of muds for gentle exfoliation.

British-style thalassotherapy starts with group exercise in a huge saltwater hydrotherapy pool. Led by a staffer and supported by the saltwater (the pool has a mix of springwater and sea salts—a first for the United Kingdom), you move through a series of underwater jets and overhead cascades that add a watery massage to the experience.

Just outside the grounds are two championship golf courses. Nearby is the Pilgrims' Way, a 100-mile path that traces the route believed to have been taken in the fourteenth century by pilgrims headed for Canterbury, immortalized by Geoffrey Chaucer in *The Canterbury Tales*. Join a guided hike or cycling group to explore the peaceful byways and vast green fields populated with fluffy white sheep. Sometimes a gentle mist provides nature's facial. And there's always a pub at the next crossroad.

Meals add another dimension to this British version of healthy living. With an executive chef who trained at some of London's trendy new restaurants, health farm cooking is based on organic, fresh, locally grown British produce. Simple cooking, basic ingredients, and favorites like pasta and fish make each meal a showcase for healthy options.

The informality of a country house quickly sets you at ease. Robes can be worn in the dining room for breakfast and lunch. Afternoon tea is a good time for socializing. A hostess or concierge is on hand to arrange transport for sight-seeing or to help you catch the train for London. Created by the owners of Henlow Grange and Springs Health Farm, Forest Mere, with its innovative combination of destination spa and lifestyle programs, was honored as Spa of the Year by the British Beauty Awards in 1999.

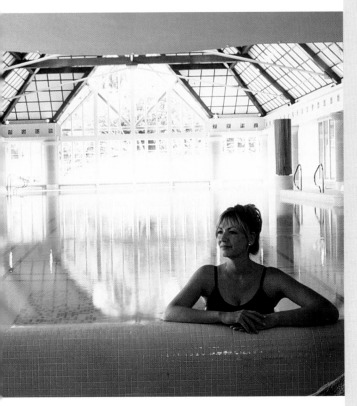

Health Farm Harvest of Well-Being

Forest Mere Health Farm
Liphook, Hampshire GU30 7JQ
England
Phone: 44–1428–726000
Fax: 44–1428–723501
Web site: www.healthfarms.co.uk

General Manager: Stephen Purdew
Spa Director: Haley Neech

Accommodations: Seventy-seven rooms done in country-style wooden furniture, flowered chintz, and fluffy pillows, private (en suite) bathroom. Most rooms are in garden-level wings that connect to the main house and dining rooms. Suites have French doors that open to a terrace. All are air-conditioned and have TV and phone.

Meals: Three meals included in daily tariff. Extensive breakfast and lunch buffets. Cooked vegetarian breakfast available for supplementary charge. Dinner menu includes gravlax, wild mushroom soup, sole with mock hollandaise sauce, chargrilled marinated vegetables. Vegan, kosher, and detox diets available. Wine by bottle or glass, mineral water, soft drinks.

Facilities: Beauty farm with seventy treatment rooms, aerobics studios with sprung floors, gymnasium with computerized cardiovascular and strength-training equipment, Pilates studio, indoor and outdoor swimming pools, men's and women's locker rooms with sauna, steam room, cold plunge pool; outdoor tennis court, bicycles. Smoking lounge. Robe hire.

Services & Special Programs: Comprehensive range of traditional and alternative therapies, skin care, bodywork, and exercise. Saltwater hydrotherapy pool. Hair salon. Programs for stress management, weight loss. Personal training in Pilates, tai chi, and healing circles.

Rates: $$

Best Spa Package: Four-night Break package includes two massages, facial, algae wraps, thalassotherapy pool session, unlimited use of facilities and exercise classes, all meals, evening talks. Single: $781–$923; double per person, $704–$767, plus tax. Package includes two massages, facial, head-shoulder massage, thalasso pool session; all meals, and scheduled program daily. Upgrade to premier service includes robe, treatments in private area.

Credit Cards: Most major

Getting There: By train from London Waterloo station to Liphook (one hour) on Portsmouth line; by car, A–3 southbound toward Portsmouth, exit after Hindhead on B–2131 to B–2070.

What's Nearby: Chichester, Guildford, Portsmouth.

MANDARIN ORIENTAL HOTEL, HYDE PARK
London, England

Reflecting the sophisticated international style of London, the spa at Mandarin Oriental Hotel is a dramatic fusion of East and West. Setting the mood are slabs of jet-black Zimbabwean granite, furniture made of black American walnut, and elaborate Asian art. Water is the central element: Relax in a soaking pool, steam away stress in the amethyst crystal chamber, and let the therapist soothe you with a ritual welcoming footbath of herbal oils and flower petals. Cocooned, intimate—it's hard to believe this fantasy is minutes away from busy Knightsbridge shops.

Treatments designed by ESPA meld traditional therapies with the latest mind/body concepts of holistic medicine. Perhaps the best example is the jet lag reviver massage. Plan to arrive early; the meditative mood of the soaking pool is yours to enjoy at no extra cost. The steam room is home to a large amethyst crystal, said to have serenity-inducing properties.

As you pad along halls paved in granite or pause in the tea lounge, calm colors backlight arrange-ments of orchid sprays. Whether you've just arrived from far away or need an escape from London's hectic pace, the treatments here restore balance and renew energy.

The Total Luxury Experience extends to three hours of rituals created for you by therapists trained in exotic treatments and philosophies. Other mind-and-body packages include blissful back, face, and scalp treatments. Exercise equipment is available in the adjoining fitness club; there is no hydrotherapy or swimming pool.

Finding this haven of tranquility in the center of London is a bonus reserved for hotel guests, but appointments can be made without overnight stay. The stately hotel overlooking Royal Park has long been a landmark of hospitality. After a shopping foray, porters will collect your packages while you head for the spa. Later, join fashionable Londoners at the Mandarin Bar, then stay for dinner at The Park restaurant as the Royal Horse Guard pass en route to Buckingham Palace.

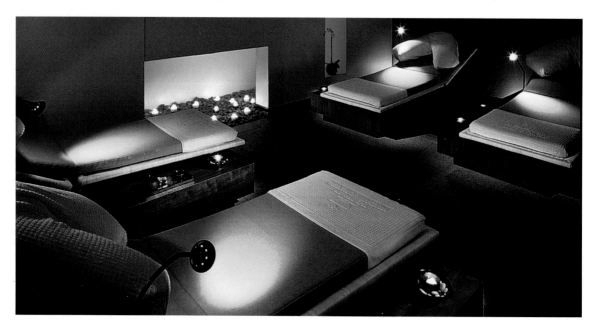

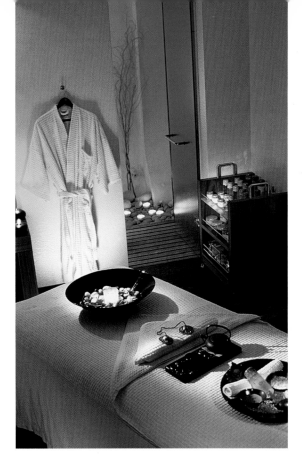

Mandarin Oriental Hotel, Hyde Park
66 Knightsbridge
London SW1X 7LA
England
Phone: 44–20–7235–2000
Fax: 44–20–7235–2001
E-mail: reserve-molon@mohg.com
Web site: www.mandarinoriental.com
Season: Year-round
General Manager: Liam Lambert
Spa Director: Claire Raynor
Reservations: (866) 888–6780
Accommodations: Two hundred rooms and suites, individually decorated with traditional English style. Many rooms overlook Hyde Park; those facing front may be affected by traffic noise. Completely air-conditioned, rooms have full bathroom tiled in marble, king-size or double beds. Amenities include robe and slippers, hair dryer, daily mineral water, fruit, and newspaper. Rooms are equipped for high-speed Internet, have CD player and disks, TV, phones. This five-star hotel opened in 1899 and is now part of Mandarin Oriental Hotel Group based in Hong Kong.
Meals: Traditional English breakfast, daily buffet. Menu features spa cuisine at The Park restaurant and Foliage restaurant for lunch and dinner.
Facilities: Relaxation pool, steam room, lounges for men and women offer daybeds, shower. Private treatment rooms on two floors; adjoining fitness club. Locker, slippers, and robe provided.
Services & Special Programs: Massage, reflexology, facial, ayurvedic scalp treatment, men's facial, Oriental body glow.
Rates: $$$
Best Spa Package: The Total Luxury Experience includes three hours of sheer indulgence at the spa, overnight accommodation, and fitness breakfast. Your Total Luxury spa program has been created to ensure that you leave feeling radiant and relaxed. Float back to your room where fresh fruit and exotic fruit juices await you, and the following morning indulge in Mandarin Oriental's legendary Fitness Breakfast. Rates start from $938.
Credit Cards: All major
Getting There: London Underground's Knightsbridge Station is directly in front of the hotel.
What's Nearby: Victoria & Albert Museum, Harrod's, Buckingham Palace, Picadilly Circus, Chelsea.

London Bespoke Spas

Tailor your spa experience: men- or women-only or mixed gender. London has spas to suit every style. Trendsetting spas include the Refinery in Mayfair, for the male executive seeking privacy and pampering; services range from hair styling to hydrotherapy. On a court-yard off Old Bond Street, the Elemis Spa blends Eastern and Western philosophies of beauty and relaxation. In Covent Garden, women work out at the Sanctuary. Champneys at Picadilly Circus has the best swimming pool and social scene. Agua at the Sanderson Hotel attracts celebrities. From posh retreats in exclusive hotels to trendy leisure clubs, London spas have gone mainstream.

THERMAE BATH SPA
Bath, England

The ancient thermal springs of Bath, once considered holy by the Romans, now flow in England's most unusual spa. Completed in 2003, the new, modernist bathhouse at Bath revives a centuries-old bathing tradition. Bath, a Georgian city straight out of *Masterpiece Theatre,* is the ultimate twenty-first century spa town.

Sheathed in glass, the new spa building reflects the past. Surrounded by Georgian colonnades dating from the eighteenth century, the five-story spa features a Roman sauna, a caldarium of steam rooms, cold pool, and mist showers. Treatments range from Kneipp herbal wraps to Watsu, Italian fango mud packs, hydrotherapy tubs, massage, and reflexology. The rooftop swimming pool has views of ancient hills and farms, plus a restaurant. Essentially

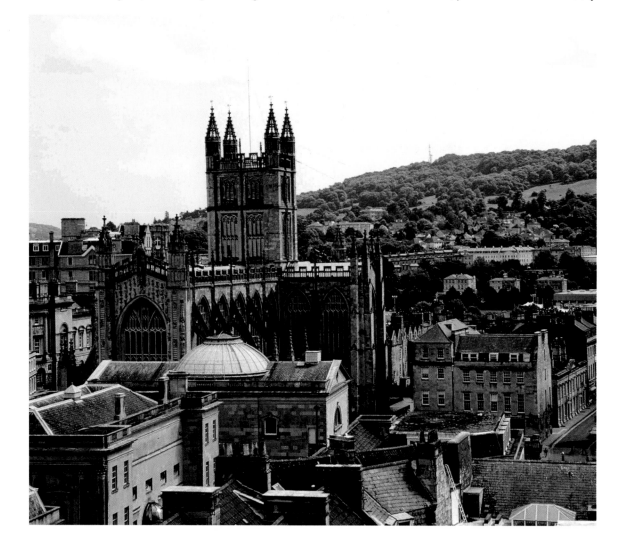

a day spa with admission fees based on two-hour increments, treatments are booked a la carte. Overnight packages are available at nearby hotels and B&Bs.

The Bath experience is a pleasurable mix of history, culture, and country rambles. Learn about ancient bathing rituals at the Roman Bath Museum. The Romans built a temple here honoring the goddess Minerva in A.D. 43. Excavated and partially rebuilt, the large complex of pools and heated relaxariums can be traced back to the water cults of the Celts and their deity Sul. By the eighteenth century the hub of Bath's social life was the Pump Room, where visitors still line up for a cup of the sulferous mineral water.

An easy excursion from London, Bath can be reached by direct trains from Paddington Station. Stay at one of the Georgian townhouses that offer B&B accommodations or at the upscale Duke's Hotel. For Regency luxury, book a suite at the Royal Crescent Hotel and take treatments at its luxurious, intimate Bathhouse Spa. Jane Austen's legacy lives on in a small townhouse devoted to mementos of her times in Bath. Throughout the year there are literary festivals, professional shows on stage at the Theatre Royal, and cricket matches.

A Royal Crescent Retreat

Privacy and a taste of Georgian elegance come with a spa retreat at the Royal Crescent Hotel. Set in a crescent-shaped residential block built just before the American Revolution, when classical architecture set the style under King George III, the hotel occupies three stately townhouses and has a private garden in the back, where the restaurant and spa are located. The Bathhouse spa resembles a Japanese onsen: a lap pool embedded in black slate, soaking pools sheathed in teak, stone floors. Above a tiny sauna and steam room, private cabins offer massage, aromatherapy facials, body wraps, nail care, and hair styling.

Bathing in Georgian Bath

Thermae Bath Spa
9-10 Bath Street
Bath BA1 1SN
England
Phone: 44–1225–477710
Fax: 44–1225–477110
E-mail: info@tdcbath.com
Web site: www.bathspa.co.uk
Season: Year-round
Director: Henk Verschuur
Spa Manager: David Rowlands
Reservations: info@tdcbath.com
Accommodations: The Royal Crescent Hotel, 16 Royal Crescent, has forty-five bedrooms, plus suites, decorated with Georgian antiques, all with private bath. Reservations: 44–800–9800987 (U.K.); (888) 295–4710 (U.S.); phone: 44–1225–823333; e-mail: reservations@royalcrescent.co.uk. The Duke's Hotel & Fitzroy's Restaurant, Great Pulteney Street, offers eighteen recently renovated rooms in a four-story Palladian townhouse with no elevator. All have private bath, heated towel rack. Reservations: 44–1225–787960; e-mail: info@dukesbath.co.uk, www.dukesbath.co.uk.
Meals: Full English breakfast included with room at hotels; Restaurant at Bath Spa offers light menu daily; the Roman Bath Museum Pump Room (no reservations) has traditional menu for breakfast, lunch, and dinner.
Facilities: Thermae Bath Spa includes indoor and outdoor thermal baths, steamrooms, and treatment rooms. Featuring naturally hot mineral water, the rooftop swimming pool is included with admission to the spa. A medical center in the restored eighteenth-century bathhouse offers treatments plus central thermal pool.
Services & Special Programs: Hydrotherapy, physiotherapy, massage, acupuncture, herbal wrap, Kneipp bath, Watsu, fango mud pack. Visitor Centre provides introduction to spa complex.
Rates: Spa Sessions (two hours) from $27; all day $55. Hotels $–$$$.
Best Spa Package: Royal Crescent Hotel two-day retreat, from $1,140 per person, double.
Credit Cards: Most major
Getting There: By express Thames train from London (Paddington Station) eighty minutes; driving from London, M4 (exit 18) take A46 to Bath, two hours; by air, Heathrow Airport, two hours, London Gatwick, three hours.
What's Nearby: Stratford-upon-Avon (Shakespeare Theater), Oxford, Cotswolds walks, the American Museum, Roman York, Bristol, Kennet & Avon Canal cruise, golf.

THE SHERATON GRAND HOTEL AND SPA
Edinburgh, Scotland

Kilts and clans aside, Scotland is marching into the spa world with flair and finesse. And it's all due to a hotel-based spa that is attracting worldwide attention.

The Sheraton Grand Hotel, located in the center of Edinburgh, is linked via a covered glass bridge to an amazing new spa, One Spa, which opened in 2001. As you walk through this glass bridge, blue neon lights illuminate the passageway, and you begin to think you are in a spaceship. You see a stunning structure before you. As you open the beautiful wooden door to One Spa, you enter a space so different that you think indeed you have arrived on a different planet. There is an immediate feeling of openness and calm. Because each floor is a split-level, the space radiates with a positive energy. This new building with three split-levels of spa services is the first of its kind in the United Kingdom. The spa is a jewel designed to rejuvenate locals and tourists alike. The building is destined to become a landmark. Adjacent to the hotel is Edinburgh's Conference Square and nearby are theaters, restaurants, and numerous attractions, including the foreboding Edinburgh Castle, lurking high above.

The building is designed to allow ease of movement and makes maximum use of natural daylight.

There are three restaurants that boast everything from fine Italian dining to healthy bistro food.

The exclusive consultant for One Spa is ESPA, an international company. It offers unique treatments, heat and wet experiences, fitness activities, and relaxation methods carefully blended to encourage well-being. There is a fully equipped fitness studio, a 60-foot ozone-friendly swimming pool, eleven multipurpose treatment rooms, an Oriental massage room, a hydrotherapy room, and a carefully designed thermal suite with a range of hot and cooling therapies to cleanse the body and aid in relaxation. Unique to the spa is the outdoor hydropool, a stainless steel pool cut into the building with a cedar-plank curved rear wall; it is accessed by swimming from the indoor hydropool. It has an infinity edge with glass panels to protect it from the wind and offers spectacular views of Edinburgh. Dramatically lit at night, the 95-degree salt water, which lets off steam into the cool air, is quite a sensation.

Sophisticated technology services the building with computerized lighting programmed to change throughout the day to create changing moods. Each spa visitor gets their own watch containing a microchip that is individually programmed to allow access to different zones in the spa.

The fitness studio has the most advanced Technogym equipment. Fine Italian leather is among some of the materials used in the Technogym. And the pièce de résistance is the thermal suite which offers a range of hot and cooling therapies to cleanse the body and aid in relaxation. These include:

- Hammam: A Turkish concept, with beautifully tiled white floors and blue tile walls lined with seven ice-filled sinks. The entire room is swathed in shades of purple and violet light.

- Aroma grotto: A room infused with aromatherapy scents and oils from herbal extracts to enhance complexions and hair.

- Rock sauna: A classic Finnish sauna with a temperature of more than 144 degrees, which has a purifying effect on the body.

- Bio sauna: A room with a temperature of 165 degrees infused with a measure of humidity to create a more gentle experience, enhanced with colored fiberoptic lights.

- Tepidarium: An area with several curved concrete benches heated to release toxins.

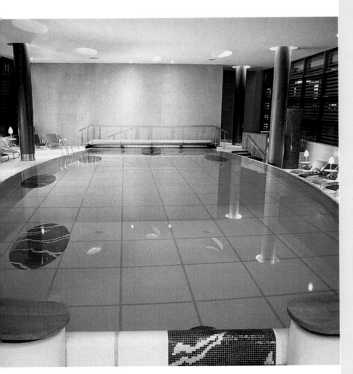

Intense Pulse Light (IPL)

There is a promising solution for rosacea, a troublesome skin problem that can make your complexion look red as a beet, according to Renato Calabria, M.D., a Beverly Hills, California, plastic surgeon.

"There is no permanent cure," says Dr. Calabria, "but there are ways to improve the skin."

Dr. Calabria recommends intense pulsed light laser as a solution. Pulsed light laser requires five treatments under a local anesthetic, in a physician's office, one month apart. IPL also reduces the size of pores, smoothes the skin, and reduces pigmentation.

Dr. Calabria said there is a predominance of rosacea of women in their thirties. Heat, stress, and a poor diet are triggers for it. The National Rosacea Society says that eliminating these factors will help those prone to this problem.

The Sheraton Grand Hotel and Spa
1 Festival Square
Edinburgh EH3 9SR
Scotland
Phone: 44–131–229–9131
Fax: 44–131–228–4510
Web site: www.one-spa.com
Season: Year round
General Manager: Peter Murphy
Spa General Manager: Brian Hunter
Spa Treatments Manager: Jane Ross
Fitness Manager: Graham Hunter
Reservations: 44–131–221–7780 or (800) 325–3535
Spa appointments: 44–131–221–7777
Accommodations: 260 rooms, including seventeen elegantly appointed suites.
Meals: Broad range of international flavors at Terrace Room for breakfast, lunch, and dinner; the Rosettes Grill for fine dining; and Santini for Italian cuisine.
Facilities: Fitness studio has Technogym key-system cardio and resistance equipment, 19-meter swimming pool, outdoor and indoor hydropool, eleven treatment rooms, Thai massage room. Heat experiences include hammam, aroma grotto, rock sauna, bio sauna, laconium, and tepidarium.
Services and Special Programs: There are eleven treatment rooms offering a remarkable range of treatments from around the world, including ayurvedic, Chinese, and Thai. Within the spa is a Thermal Suite, beauty salon, gymnasium, and a relaxation lounge. Santini, a chic Italian Restaurant, is one of the city's trendiest.
Rates: $$
Best Spa Package: Relax and Revitalize, a three-day residential program that includes lifestyle programs, hydrotherapy bath, salt and oil scrub, face and scalp treatment with hot stone therapy. Breakfast, lunch, and dinner. $395 daily.
Credit Cards: Most major
Getting There: Eight miles to Edinburgh International Airport.
What's Nearby: The gardens and shops of Princes Street, Edinburgh International Conference Center and theaters, pubs and narrow streets of Old Town; Turnberry and St. Andrew's golf courses, Holyrood Palace, and Balmoral Castle.

WESTIN TURNBERRY RESORT AND SPA
Ayrshire, Scotland

World-class golf meets a world-class spa at the hallowed grounds of Turnberry, an Edwardian-style country house dating back to 1906, now a Westin resort. The opening of the Turnberry Health Spa in 1991 symbolized a new era for this landmark golf resort. The legendary Ailsa course has hosted the British Open three times. The spa is located in a long complex adjoining the main hotel. The natural coastline and wild countryside now has a civilized spa where golfers and spa-goers alike may enjoy it all, from a challenging aerobics class to squash to an aromatherapy massage.

The weather in this corner of Scotland is famous for mild temperatures and sunshine. That, plus exclusive spa treatments, championship golf on two courses, and the highly touted cuisine of Chef Stewart Cameron makes Turnberry a popular destination. The Westin resort is rated five stars by both the Scottish Tourist Board and the Royal Automobile Club.

Sue Harmsworth launched her successul product line ESPA here, with the goal of promoting guests' well-being. As with the golf, the spa here is already a legend, with an outstanding range of treatments for both men and women. Aromatherapy is the spa's specialty, with treatments such as the aromatherapy total body. The spa's centerpiece is a magnificent 20-meter pool with breathtaking views across the Irish Sea to the island of Ailsa Craig.

The spa has its own restaurant with Mediterranean-inspired dishes; there are two other fine restaurants as well. The bright and airy guest rooms are all individually decorated and extend the feel of a fine old country estate.

As you approach, Turnberry is like a vision from a vintage etching. The two-level white edifice with red tile roof cries out to be photographed. In the evening,

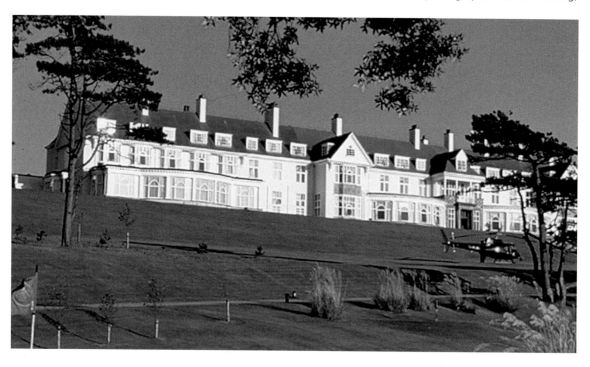

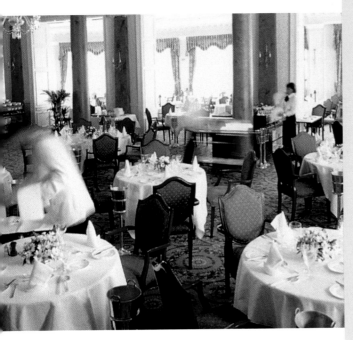

Westin Turnberry Resort and Spa
Ayrshire KA26 9LT
Scotland
Phone: 44–1655–331–000
Fax: 44–1655–331–706
E-mail: turnberry@westin.com
Web site: www.turnberry.co.uk or www.westin.com

Season: Year-round

General Manager: Stuart Selbie

Spa Director: Suzy Pieroni

Fitness Director: Peter Conlan

Reservations: 44–1655–331–000 or (800) 325–3535 or (800) WESTIN–1

Spa Appointments: 44–1655–331–000

Accommodations: 221 guest rooms, all individually decorated.

Meals: The resort offers three restaurants. The Turnberry Restaurant, the main dining room, features local produce and fish as well as French delicacies. The Clubhouse restaurant strides off the eighteenth green of the Ailsa course. The Spa restaurant serves health-conscious, low-fat entrees.

Facilities: Full-service, 50,000-square-foot spa with six treatment rooms and spa-side Jacuzzi; 65-foot pool with views across the Irish Sea to Ailsa Craig; two hydrotherapy rooms; fully equipped gym; beauty salon; two squash courts; saunas; two championship golf courses; private landing strip; helicopter pad.

Services & Special Programs: Chauffeur-driven car service; business services; golf clinics; one-on-one personal fitness training.

Rates: $$$

Best Spa Package: The three-day Spa Revitalizer Package includes two nights' accommodation, two breakfasts and dinners, personal profile with therapist, hydrotherapy treatment, body polish, aromatherapy facial, Kanebo makeover, and aromatherapy massage, as well as full use of the spa's facilities, including pool, sauna, steam room, and gym. $490–$780, depending on season.

Credit Cards: Most major

Getting There: Glasgow Airport is forty-five minutes away by car; a private landing strip and helicopter pad are located on the premises.

What's Nearby: Culzean Castle; Burns Country (poet Robert); Castle Kennedy ruins and gardens, 35 miles away; Bargany Gardens, 9 miles from the resort; and Dunure Castle, 8 miles away.

as the sun sets over the heather, a lone bagpiper dressed in full tartan plays his bagpipes. Another idyllic day has passed at Turnberry.

Skin as Smooth as a Scottish Morn

The Turnberry Spa's approach to healthy skin is a holistic one—your skin reflects your inner well-being. Treatment at the spa begins with a lifestyle consultation to detect such underlying problems as stress, hormonal changes, or erratic sleep patterns. This is followed by a purity program, based on the belief that the key to body balance is regular purifying. The program includes a jet blitz to increase circulation and improve skin tone; a hydrotherapy bath using an infusion of detoxifying mineral sea salts, seaweed, and essential aromatherapy oils; an aromatherapy massage for relaxation of mind and body; and home care advice on products to ensure that the benefits of purification last well after the trip to the spa is over.

THE CELTIC MANOR RESORT—FORUM HEALTH CLUB AND SPA

Newport, Wales

Opened in 1999 on a 1,400-acre estate rich with scenery and history, the Forum Health Club and Spa capped development of the most complete resort in Wales. Combining exceptional golf, leisure, and convention facilities, the Celtic Manor Resort includes a 400-room hotel and three championship golf courses.

Crossing the Severn estuary on a dramatic new bridge, you can't miss the Manor. An in-your-face newly built megalith dominating the M–4 motorway, the resort is all about thinking big. Canadian telecommunications tycoon Terry Matthews invited golf course designer Robert Trent Jones Sr.—both were born in Wales—to launch the project in 1995. At the resort's center is a refurbished nineteenth-century manor house. Set into a hillside, the hotel's soaring central atrium links three wings of bedrooms to the spa and leisure club, and to a high-tech convention center.

The Forum Health Club and Spa surpasses many European resorts. Taking up most of the hotel's lower floor are a 20-meter swimming pool, fifty-person whirlpool with underwater sound and light beneath a constellation of fiber-optic stars, and luxurious changing rooms with sauna and steam room, plunge pool, and whirlpool. The sixteen therapy rooms are spacious and well-equipped for a range of treatments by Clarins, Elemis, and Guinot, including sports massage and skin care for men. Perhaps the most interesting feature is the spa's rasul chamber, where mud-caked guests socialize as they steam out impurities under a star-studded dome.

Spacious and elegantly appointed, the Forum's wide corridors, high ceilings, and light-filled exercise studios are a pleasant environment, even when the weather isn't. The fifty-four-station gym allows you to watch TV or enjoy music while you work out on cross-trainers, steppers, bikes, rowers, free weights, and treadmills. Personal trainers are on hand, and scheduled sessions of yoga and aerobics are held in a wood-floored studio. The gym also offers fitness assessment and counseling packages from Fitech. Kids up to age fifteen have their own Hideaway Club, with gym,

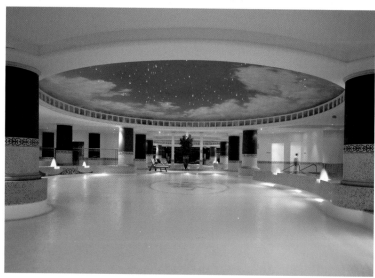

swimming pool, whirlpool, computer, and cinema. Taking care of the entire family are an Aveda concept hair salon, run by local-TV celeb Philip Mungeam, and a spa cafe.

At the golf clubhouse, open to the public as well as members, a second health club called Dylans offers an aerobics studio, gym, indoor swimming pool, and treatment rooms. The focus here is on sports medicine, osteopathy, and physiotherapy. Shape up your game at the golf academy and its twenty-four bay driving range, floodlit for evening use.

Secluded amid woodlands and

valleys, the resort has views of nearby Cardiff and industrial developments. Tennis, mountain biking, riding, walks, and hiking are on offer, as well as pony trekking, clay pigeon shooting, archery, and off-road driving. Elegant restaurants offer Welsh fusion cuisine and Mediterranean classics. Legendary Wales has a new star.

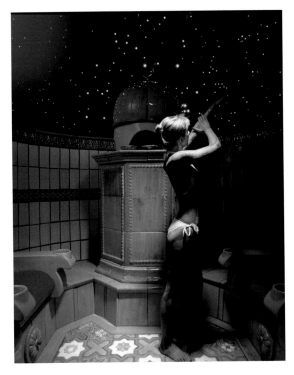

Detox Dome Is Muddy Marvelous

Rasul, an ancient cleansing ceremony originated by Eastern healers, debuts here in a lushly tiled chamber. Seated under a blue dome twinkling with fiber-optic stars, you apply mud mixed for your skin type. Steam rises through herbs in a central pillar, gradually increasing the humidity and temperature of the chamber. After showering off the mud you are coated with nourishing oils by a therapist. Four friends can share the experience, au naturel, or borrow disposable knickers. Cost: $30 per person.

The Celtic Manor Resort—Forum Health Club and Spa
Coldra Woods, Newport
Gwent NP18 1HQ
Wales
Phone: 44–633–410349
Fax: 44–633–410229
E-mail: postbox@celtic-manor.com
Web site: www.celtic-manor.com

Season: Year-round

General Manager: Robert Church

Sports and Leisure Manager: Ian Phillips

Reservations: (800) 223–6800

Accommodations: 400 luxury rooms, thirty-two suites in contemporary hotel, most with balcony. All have private bath and shower, air-conditioning, speaker phone with voice mail, desk with fax modem and dual voltage power, CD player, TV. Amenities include hair dryer, trouser press, iron and board, tea- and coffeemakers, robe, toiletries. Library lounge.

Meals: A la carte menu in two restaurants and spa cafe. Also available at golf clubhouse, conservatory and terrace, games room and library, and piano bar.

Facilities: Two indoor swimming pools and whirlpools, sixteen treatment rooms including hydrotherapy, dry flotation bed, rasul chamber, two fitness centers with cardiovascular and strength equipment, aerobics/dance studios, men's and women's changing rooms with sauna/steam rooms, plunge pool. Hideaway Club for kids. Admission is free to hotel guests.

Services & Special Programs: Skin care, facials, massage, G5 machine massage, body wrap, aromatherapy, Cathiodermie, hair and nail care; jet shower, hydrotherapy tubs. Fitness evaluation, personal trainers.

Rates: $$$

Best Spa Package: Elemis aromatherapy, top-to-toe, two-hour treatment for $80, plus gratuity. Spa Energizer package with room, treatments, meals for two, $416–$603 daily (three-night minimum).

Credit Cards: Most major

Getting There: By train to Cardiff/Newport from London Paddington Station on Great Western (two hours); by car, M–4 to Severn Bridge, junction 24 (approximately two hours).

What's Nearby: Cardiff Bay, Wentwood Forest, Caernarfon Castle, Tintern Abbey.

INDIA & AFRICA

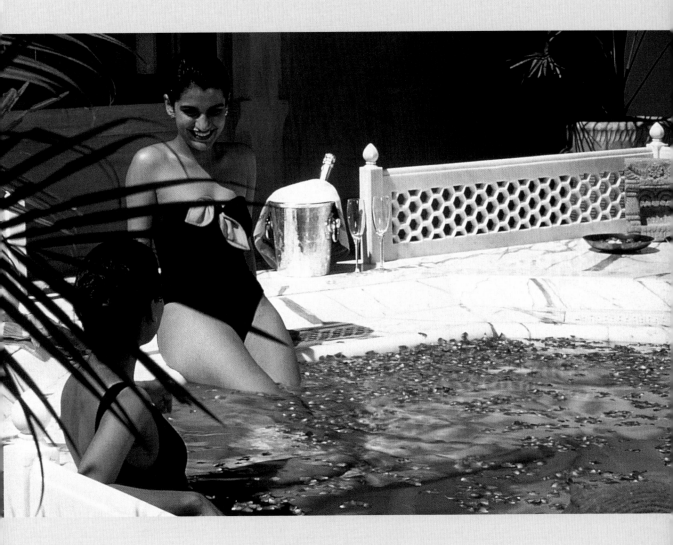

RAJVILAS

Jaipur, India

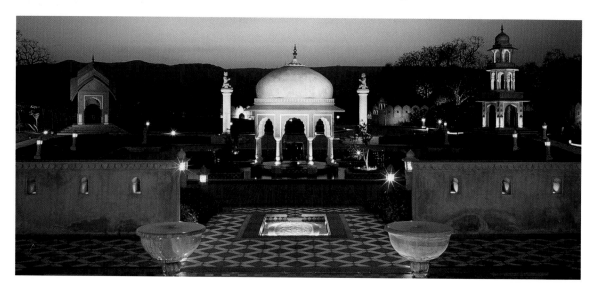

In the perfumed gardens of a maharaja's palace, a cool retreat blends Eastern and Western wellness treatments. At Rajvilas, ritual purification, a centuries-old tradition in India, is reinterpreted through herbal body care, aromatherapy massage, and deep-cleansing facials.

The location says it all: Jaipur. A city of storybook forts and palaces, of polo-playing maharajas and colorful desert people, and the source of ayurveda—traditional natural healing for purity of body and mind.

This sumptuous palace was built in 1727, amid parched, pale desert. Restored in 1995 as the jewel in the crown of the Oberoi Hotel Group, the stunning public rooms and guest suites are nothing less than regal. Rajvilas brings past and present together in a glorious fusion of styles.

Water gardens that would have delighted royal princesses now harbor a lavish spa complex devoted to soothing body and soul. The spa is a private hideaway for hotel guests. The setting is graced by a 250-year-old Shiva temple surrounded by a lotus pond, fragrant herb garden, and 25-meter lap pool. Managed by the international Banyan Tree Group, the spa is housed in the original building on the site, a classic Rajasthani mansion called a *haveli*. The ornate interior features treatment rooms for both holistic Western and ayurvedic relaxation and pampering, a whirlpool in an open-to-the-sky courtyard, shaded terraces for meditation, and an air-conditioned gymnasium outfitted with the very latest exercise equipment.

Enhancing your enjoyment of the spa are ready supplies of cold towels, fresh juices, herbal teas, and a light cuisine. There are massage suites with private lounge and recreation areas, individual Finnish saunas, steam rooms, separate hot and cold plunge pools, and showers for men and women.

Guest rooms are an architectural amalgam of traditional Rajasthani flat-roofed houses and *havelis*. Clustered around courtyards, each building is hand-decorated with colorful frescoes depicting tropical birds and flowers. The rooms are an eclectic blend of colonial and Indian influences, furnished with four-posters, dhurrie rugs, and wicker. Sunken marble baths

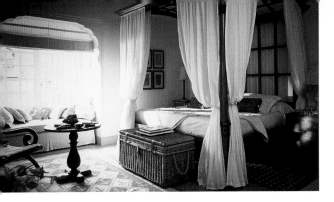

look onto secluded gardens. Dramatically lit at night by flaming torches, the fort's central courtyard has a dais where traditional dances are performed while you dine in an open-air section of the restaurant.

For a touch of desert living, you can stay in a tent that a prince might have used while on safari. Appointed with teak floors and campaign chests, as well as cool white and beige block-print fabrics, these cloistered tents are perhaps the most distinctive accommodations in Oberoi hotels, which can be found from Bali to Lombok, London to Hong Kong.

Rajvilas offers an exotic retreat, complete with elephant ride at the Amber Fort. Located thirty minutes from the Jaipur airport, it is another world.

Ayurvedic Rejuvenation

Ayurvedic methods of relaxation, massage, and herbal treatments are the core of the Rajvilas experience. With treatments based on ayurvedic principles to relax the mind and promote well-being, the spa uses therapeutic essential oils developed in Asia by Banyan Tree Spas. Experiences include such traditional treatments as massage, shirodhara, and katibasti. Using local ingredients, a shirodhara therapist drizzles a fine stream of warm sesame oil or buttermilk onto your "third eye" (the center of your forehead) to help calm and clear the mind. Or a therapist may prepare you for massage with an herbal "ubtan"—a body polish using sandalwood and rose powder to slough off dead cells that leaves your skin soft, smooth, and glowing.

Ayurvedic Rejuvenation in a Maharaja's Palace

Rajvilas
Goner Road, Jaipur 303 012
India
Phone: 91–141–680–101
Fax: 91–141–680202
E-mail: rchopra@oberoidel.com
Web site: www.oberoihotels.com

Season: Year-round

General Manager: Huvida Marshall

Reservations: (800) 223–6800

Accommodations: Sixty-eight rooms in small clusters of traditional houses and tents. Private villas (three) have swimming pool. All are air-conditioned, with marble bathroom, sunken tub.

Meals: Gourmet European and Indian cuisine served in the Surya Mahal Restaurant. Spa menu available a la carte.

Facilities: Separate wings for men and women, each containing changing and rest rooms, sauna, steam room, plunge pool, therapy rooms. Gymnasium with Cybex and LifeFitness equipment. Salon for hair and nail care. Tennis on two floodlit courts, heated swimming pool.

Services & Special Programs: Yoga, meditation, massage, ayurvedic full-body massage, body wrap, facial, shirodhara (head massage), Swedish massage, aromatherapy, eye treatments.

Rates: $$$

Best Spa Package: The Unforgettable Experience includes two nights and three days' accommodation in a deluxe room, spa breakfast and dinners for two, daily spa treatment, guided yoga and meditation. Chauffeur-driven limousine transfers on arrival and departure. $900 for two people, $750 single occupancy, including tax and service charge.

Credit Cards: American Express, Diners Club, MasterCard, VISA

Getting There: Jaipur can be accessed either by rail, air, or road from Delhi. Complimentary transfers to hotel from airport or railway station. A helipad is on the grounds.

What's Nearby: The Amber Fort, Jagarth Fort, the "Pink City" of Jaipur, Ramgarth, Jantar Mantar Observatory.

WESTERN CAPE HOTEL & SPA: ACQUABELLA WELLNESS CENTER

Hermanus, South Africa

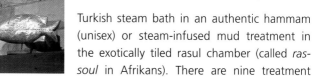

Cradled in the heart of the Arabella country estate, the new Western Cape Hotel & Spa incorporates both modern and ancient concepts of wellness for a unique South African spa experience. The integration of a well-designed spa complex with an 18-hole championship golf course, full-service hotel, and recreation on a large country estate provides a relaxing and affordable vacation.

Plan a holistic program of physical, mental, emotional, social, and spiritual components. To achieve this objective, the Acquabella Wellness Centre offers a wide range of internal arts, such as meditation and yoga, to better integrate mind and body. Therapies incorporate the healing power of touch, which facilitates relaxation, disease prevention, and general health. This is the only place in Africa equipped with a space-age capsule for thermal baths, a rasul chamber for herbal mud skin treatments, and an indoor saltwater pool for relaxing soaks with underwater music.

Entering the spa complex you have a choice of Turkish steam bath in an authentic hammam (unisex) or steam-infused mud treatment in the exotically tiled rasul chamber (called *rassoul* in Afrikans). There are nine treatment rooms, plus a winter garden where you can relax and sip herbal tea between treatments. The hydropool area offers an indoor lap pool and whirlpool. Treatments feature Phytomer marine products from France and Dermalogica skin care.

Group exercise sessions are scheduled four times per day, from 6:00 A.M. to 6:00 P.M. Each session lasts four hours and is free to hotel guests and Acquabella members. Personal trainers are on hand for wellness evaluations and a program designed to meet your goals or physical limitations.

Overlooking a vast lagoon, the resort offers a wide range of outdoor recreation, from bird-watching to mountain biking to trail rides on horseback. Nearby is the vibrant city of Cape Town, with ocean beaches, vineyards, and museums of world-class quality.

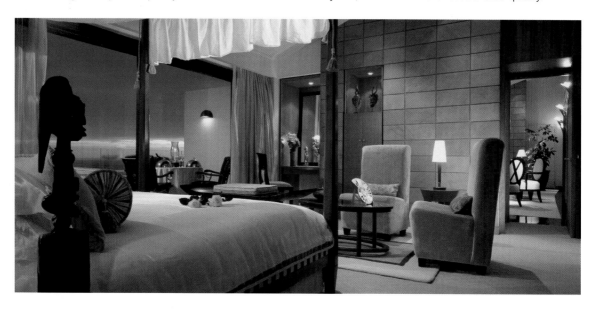

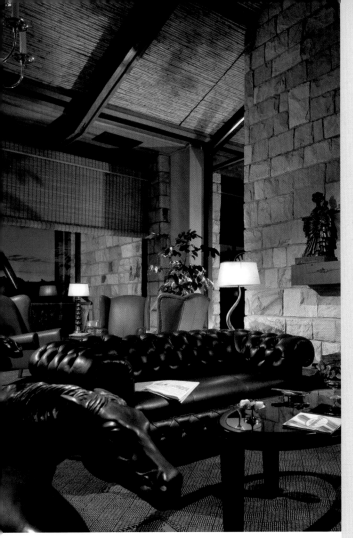

Western Cape Hotel & Spa
P.O. Box 593
Kleinmond 7195
South Africa
Phone: 27–28–284–0000
Fax: 27–28–284–0011
E-mail: reservations@w-capehotel.co.za
Web site: www.arabellasheraton.co.za
Season: Year-round
General Manager: Sebastian Berinato
Spa & Wellness Director: Rob Cowling
Reservations: (800) 325–3535 (Sheraton Worldwide)
Spa Appointments: cowlingr@w-capehotel.co.za
Accommodations: 145 spacious, terraced rooms and suites, done in sandstone, timber, and glass. Completely air-conditioned, with TV, telephone. All have private bathroom with bidet and a wall that folds back to let you soak while enjoying the view. Deceptively low key, the hotel's architecture enhances the wraparound views of mountain and lagoon.
Meals: Jamani's Restaurant has an international menu as well as spa cuisine prepared in consultation with the resident dietician; service is informal. The Premier offers fine dining.
Facilities: The spa building houses nine treatments rooms, hydropool complex, indoor lap pool, and steam treatment rooms (rasul, hammam), Swiss shower, Hydrotone thermal capsule. Sports facilities include tennis courts and an 18-hole, par-72 golf course. On the estate are walking trails, mountain bikes, and horseback rides.
Services & Special Programs: Hydrotherapy bath, Swedish massage, sports massage, reflexology, aromatherapy, body wraps and peels, sea mud pack. Personal consultation on nutrition and diet, physical fitness evaluation, and personal training.
Rates: $
Best Spa Package: Three-night Wellness Break includes hotel accommodation and breakfast daily, one buffet dinner, three wellness treatments, pregolf massage. $213 for two persons, plus tax.
Credit Cards: MasterCard, VISA, Diners Club, American Express
Getting There: From Cape Town by car, coastal route R44 via Gordon's Bay (one hour).
What's Nearby: Cape Wine Route, Hermanus (whale refuge).

Nature Safari

Take a walk on the wild side of Arabella estate. Acquabella Spa is set on a lagoon bordered by Kogelberg Nature Reserve. There are beautiful birds, wild horses, and a penguin colony. Nearby Hermanus is a haven for dolphin and whales at certain times of the year. Seaweed harvested here is used in spa treatments. Inland, trek mountains and valleys of the wine-growing district around Stellenbosch, and visit one of the wineries for a free tasting of outstanding vintages.

THE RESIDENCE—PHYTOMER SPA

La Marsa, Carthage, Tunisia

Tunisia is forging ahead with an ambitious master plan to attract tourists, and the fabulous Phytomer Spa at the luxurious Residence resort is destined to put this North African country on every spa-lover's map. And plan a few days before or after your visit to explore this legendary country sandwiched between Algeria and Libya.

The spa, with its spectacular dome-covered pool, offers massage, lymphatic drainage, skin care, hydromassage, bubbling seawater massage, circular showers with affusion, and seaweed therapy—all in a luxurious setting of arches, columns, balustrades, cupolas, arcades, fountains, urns, and sculptures. There are thirty treatment rooms, and the staff is expertly trained.

The thalasso-based spa complies with the French standards of thalassotherapy, but goes well beyond them. Water from the Mediterranean, highly charged with sodium chloride and magnesium, is pumped into the spa for all thalassotherapy treatments. The bubbling seawater is kept at a cool temperature. Sessions last from fifteen to twenty minutes, depending on the spa doctor's recommendations.

Speaking French is helpful here, but not necessary. The multilingual spa director can arrange your appointments. The beauty salon has limited hours. There is a lovely spa restaurant with an excellent luncheon buffet and juice bar.

Guest rooms are brochure-perfect, with private balconies overlooking the sea and all of the amenities imaginable, from satellite TV to minibar refrigerators. The elegant, oversized bathrooms are decorated in red and black marble and feature dressing tables, telephones, bathrobes, and slippers.

The Residence is ideal for the spa-goer who seeks a world-class spa in one of the most exotic settings in the world.

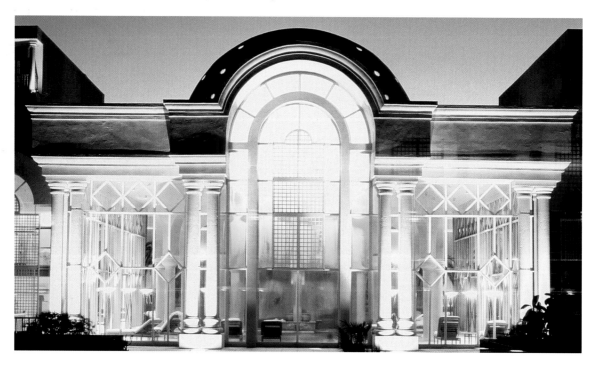

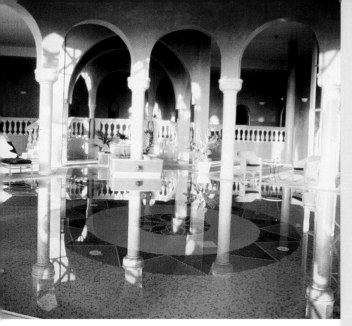

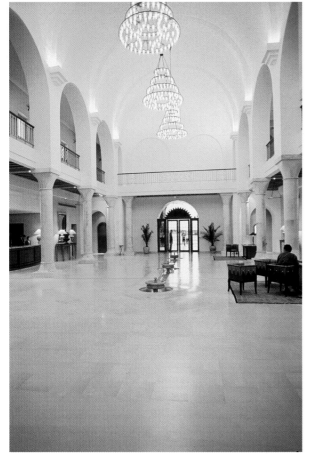

The Residence—Phytomer Spa
Les Cotes de Carthage
Boîte Postale 697
2070 La Marsa
Tunisia
Phone: 216–71–910–101
Fax: 216–71–910–144
E-mail: residence.tun@gnet.tn

Season: Year-round

General Manager: M. Jean-Pierre Auriol

Spa Director: Emna Bouchoucha

Reservations: (800) 223–6800 (Leading Hotels of the World); (800) SICILY–1 (Amelia Tours).

Accommodations: 161 rooms and nine suites, most suites with sea views. All accommodations are double, furnished with king-size beds or two double beds. All contain minibars; satellite TV; private terrace; marble bathrooms.

Meals: The Juice Bar offers a light spa luncheon buffet and freshly pressed juices. Mediterranean dining is offered in L'Olivier; Li Bai serves Chinese cuisine. All dining is a la carte.

Facilities: 37,650-square-foot spa with German hydrotherapy equipment; six massage rooms; four jet showers; two affusion showers; two facial rooms; four rooms for body wraps; steam; sauna; Turkish hammam; gym and fitness room; pool with aquatic circuit.

Services & Special Programs: A personal program is created for each guest after consulting with a spa doctor. Treatments range from those dealing with getting in shape to back care to a special antistress marine cure for men.

Rates: $$

Best Spa Package: The seven-night, six-day Thalassotherapy Cure starts at approximately $1,280 per person, based on double occupancy in the low season (November–March). This includes four thalassotherapy treatments daily, a superior category of room, and breakfast and lunch or dinner daily.

Credit Cards: Most major

Getting There: Flights from London, Paris, Amsterdam, and Zurich to Tunis. British Airways flies four times a week from Gatwick; Tunisair has four flights a week from London's Heathrow. The hotel concierge can arrange airport transfers, or you can use a taxi.

What's Nearby: Bardo Museum (famous mosaics); the Tunis medina (twenty minutes away); archeological tours to Thuburbo Majus.

MIDDLE EAST

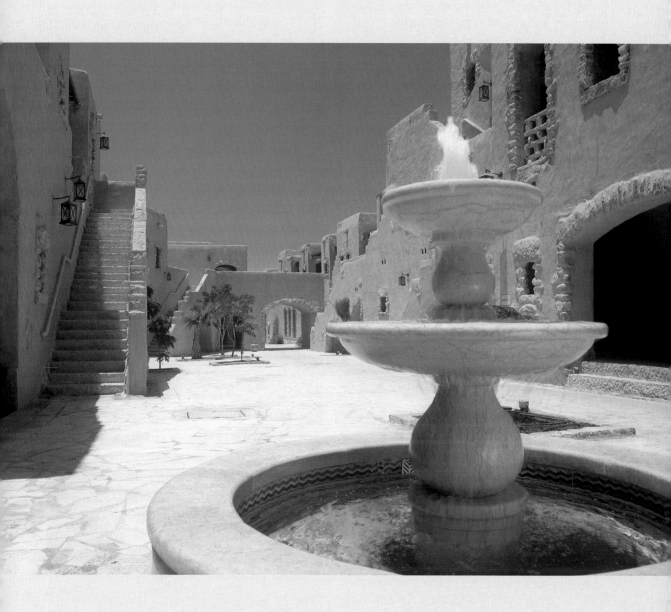

CARMEL FOREST SPA RESORT

Haifa, Israel

The Carmel Forest Spa Resort is set into a hillside in the forests of the Carmel Mountains. The hotel is hardly visible until you round the driveway. Dedicated to renewal and relaxation, this is Israel's top destination spa. With views stretching to the Mediterranean and acres of manicured lawns, the resort draws inspiration from nature and the Bible. According to the ancient sage Maimonides, "The wholeness of the body preceded the wholeness of the soul." Today's mantra is relaxation and pampering.

An extensive menu of facials, skin care, and bodywork distinguishes the spa. Treatments feature mud from the Dead Sea, seaweed, and aromatic oils made for the resort from flowers and herbs used since biblical times. Ayurvedic massage appears here for the first time in Israel, as do Parisian facials by Decleor.

Surrounded by a nature preserve, the spa offers unique peace and quiet. Signs posted on the grounds call for quiet, and, astonishingly, the guests generally comply. Guests range from Tel Aviv fashion models and stressed-out software executives to television news presenters and immaculately coifed forty-something women wearing lots of jewelry. Children younger than

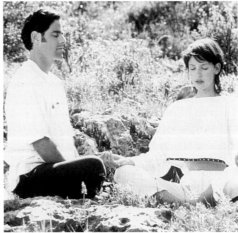

sixteen are not welcome. There is no bar, but you can order wine with dinner. The restaurant gets noisy, but most of the talk is about politics. As one woman explained, Israeli parents worry about their kids doing military service. Men and women on duty actually get special rates to come here for a few days of R&R, adding a young element not often found at Israeli spas.

Lavishly decorated, inside and out, the building belies its origin as a sanatorium constructed with German reparation money for Holocaust survivors. Converted to a world-class resort by Ben Yakar's Isrotel Hotel Group, the hotel rooms and spa facilities are topnotch. Among unique features: an indoor swimming pool with views down the mountain, adjoining reading and music rooms with fireplaces, and an imported Turkish steam room (hammam) for body scrubs. Interiors have lots of glass, tile, and polished wood floors. Native stone walkways lead to trails through the forest.

Borrow a mountain bike or join the daily guided fitness walk. Activities are scheduled every hour, from body shaping in the morning to a predinner stretch. Choices include yoga, qigong, tai chi, aquaerobics, and FitBall sessions. Resort guests have free access to

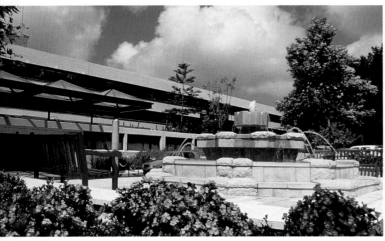

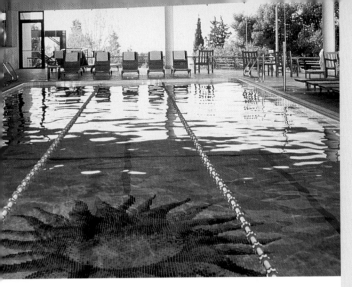

all scheduled programs, including lifestyle lectures in English and guided meditation. At night there are movies, concerts, and guest speakers (in Hebrew) on subjects like sexuality and women's health. The all-inclusive tariff covers three meals daily, even barbecue nights. The menu may be low fat, but the buffets are extensive, with cooked-to-order steak and seafood, and there's no limit on seconds.

Staffed by experts from Israel and abroad, the resort offers spa services a la carte or in packages. Day spa only arrangements can be prescheduled, and you may want to take advantage of discounts offered on Saturdays, when scheduled activities are limited.

Controlling Stress

In a country where stress is daily news, Carmel Forest Spa Resort is an island of peace and tranquillity. Revitalizing programs include weight loss and meditation, guided hikes and tai chi. Being surrounded by a forest adds to the spa's serenity, and spa treatments are designed with natural products derived from local plants and herbs. Antistress workshops focus on tools to prioritize your daily life. At day's end, relax on the terrace and drink in the view of forest and sea, a natural tranquilizer.

Carmel Forest Spa Resort
PO Box 9000
Haifa 31900
Israel
Phone: 972–4–8307888
Fax: 972–4–8323988
E-mail: carmelf@isrotel.co.il
Web site: www.isrotel.co.il

Season: Year-round

General Manager: Stephen W. Ayers

Spa Director: Guy Nadler

Accommodations: Destination spa with 126 rooms, including sixteen suites, facing the Mediterranean. All with private bath, balcony, or wooden terrace. Amenities include robes, slippers, air-conditioning.

Meals: Buffet breakfast and lunch, dinner menu served. Salad bar and extensive selections of yogurt, grains, vegetables, and fruits complement cooked-to-order eggs, fish, and steak. No strict kosher rules, just fresh, low-fat meals. Herbal teas, coffee available.

Facilities: Comprehensive physiotherapy and pampering in a focused environment. Aerobics studio, indoor and outdoor swimming pools, gymnasium. Turkish hammam, private hydrotherapy baths.

Services & Special Programs: Massages range from Swedish to Hawaiian lomi lomi, Thai, shiatsu, four-hand ayurveda, and sports. Reiki, reflexology, craniosacral balancing, mud and seaweed wraps, facials, aromatherapy. Guided walks, exercise classes. Nutrition counseling and structured weight-loss program. Stress-management program.

Rates: $$$

Best Spa Package: Three-day antistress program (Sunday to Thursday) teaches positive, practical steps for managing stress. On arrival, the resort nurse checks your medical record and gets a body composition report. Individually tailored exercise and meal plan, plus daily selection of treatments, are included in this $210 package, per person, plus room.

Credit Cards: MasterCard, VISA

Getting There: From the Haifa–Tel Aviv Old Road outside of Haifa, follow signs for Carmel Forest on Beit Oren Road, Route 70 (twenty minutes).

What's Nearby: Vered Hagalil dude ranch, Hammat Gader hot springs, Safed artist colony, Biblical sites of the Galilee and Nazareth, Druze village, Tiberias hot springs, Caesarea beaches, golf.

THE DEAD SEA: SPA TOWN

Dead Sea, Israel

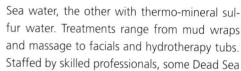

Life-enhancing waters and mud are the main attractions at Dead Sea resorts. Lying an astonishing 400 meters (1,312 feet) below sea level, the Dead Sea has a unique, healing environment, one that has been documented since biblical times. It attracts vacationers as well as persons seeking relief from rheumatism and skin problems, and taking a cure here today is a combination of age-old natural elements and high-tech therapy.

The drive from Jerusalem to the Dead Sea takes less than an hour and passes through 2,000 years of civilization. Arid desert suddenly gives way to a silver-colored sea as the road turns toward a flowering oasis at Ein Gedi, the massive fortress of Masada, and the Ein Bokek hotel area. Set against the bleached hills of the Judean Desert, the region is a vast nature reserve, where wildlife like the Nubian ibex can be spotted among ruins of ancient cultures.

Strung along the shore, the modest kibbutz and glamorous high-rise hotels all boast in-house spas. Standard facilities include two pools, one with Dead Sea water, the other with thermo-mineral sulfur water. Treatments range from mud wraps and massage to facials and hydrotherapy tubs.

Staffed by skilled professionals, some Dead Sea spas specialize in medical treatments for which the seaside microclimate, mineral-laden water, and mud have achieved recognition, although not universal acceptance. But for vacationers, there are state-of-the-art oases at the **Hyatt Regency Hotel, Golden Tulip Resort, Crowne Plaza,** and other members of the Dead Sea Hotel Association.

Along with water sports, these destinations offer freshwater swimming pools and a variety of restaurants, from kosher to Oriental, steak house to Italian.

Exploring the region starts at Masada, a mountain-top fortress that King Herod transformed in 35 B.C. as his winter palace. Hikers brave the heat and dust to follow a serpentine Roman path to the summit, but a quick cable car ride allows you to enjoy panoramic views of the sea and desert. The ruins tell a story of heroism by Jews who defied the might of the Roman empire.

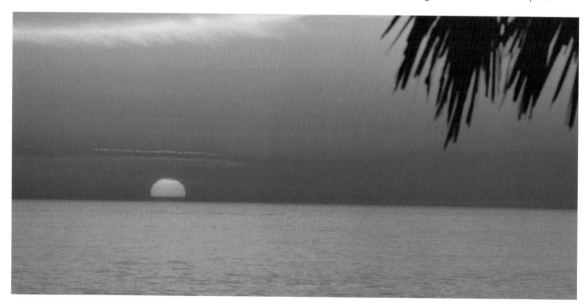

Plan a day trip, or stay a week; packages are offered at all the resorts. Hiking trails at **Kibbutz Ein Gedi** take you past bird sanctuaries, waterfalls, springs, caves, canyons, and an early Bronze Age temple. A thriving health resort where modest accommodations come with access to hot springs and mud treatments, this hillside kibbutz also operates a day spa on the shore road. Here you can purchase cosmetics and bath products made with Dead Sea minerals, water, and mud.

At the top-rated **Hyatt Regency Dead Sea** in bustling Ein Bokek, the Mineralia Spa rests on a hill commanding views of the Judean Mountains. Palm trees and lush gardens shelter the glass-walled Roman pool, providing a respite from the sun. There are six mud therapy rooms and seventeen private rooms for skin care, massage, and beauty treatments. Aerobics and group exercise are scheduled in a well-equipped fitness center where workouts come with a view of the water. A private medical clinic provides dermatology care and postsurgery recovery, plus natural health and complementary medicine programs.

Awesome as the Dead Sea looks, there is a calming effect in the pristine air. Sunlight's harmful rays are filtered by this oxygen-heavy, salt-laden atmosphere. Floating effortlessly in the warm, mineral-rich saltwater is better than a water bed, and it gives your skin a tingling, healthy glow.

Taking Natural Healing to a Higher Dimension

Dead Sea Hotel Association
P.O. Box 25056
Tel Aviv 61250
Israel
Phone: 972–5–363–5510
Fax: 972–3–571–2611
E-mail: info@deadsea.co.il
Web site: www.deadsea.co.il

Season: Year-round

Rates: $–$$$

Credit Cards: Most major

Accommodations: Ein Bokek on the southwestern shore has 2,800 hotel rooms, mostly in high-rise resorts close to a shopping mall. Kibbutz Ein Gedi offers motel-style rooms for 200 guests, a freshwater swimming pool, and central dining hall.

Getting There: From Jerusalem and Tel Aviv, scheduled motor coach service operates daily, except Saturday. Rental car or taxi available at Tel Aviv Ben-Gurion International Airport (150 kilometers).

Balneotherapy

Balneotherapy is a European term for therapeutic bathing. The role of balneotherapy in the treatment of rheumatism is a subject of much debate in medical circles. Although the therapeutic value of bathing in the Dead Sea has been reported for at least 2,000 years, systematic study of the effects of balneotherapy has started here only recently. The sea's concentration of minerals (about 30 percent) and its composition (there are large amounts of magnesium and bromide, rather than sodium chloride, which is the predominant salt in most European spa waters) are said to account for its healing properties. According to recent research, while bathing in the sea, your relative weight is practically nil, so moving sore joints and muscles becomes easier. Definitive studies are still lacking, but bathers who coat themselves in mud and frolic in the Dead Sea waters emerge with a healthy glow.

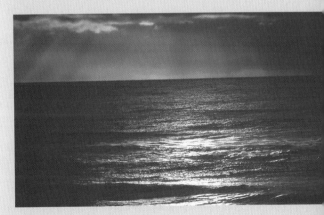

HERODS VITALIS

Eilat, Israel

Inspired by legendary kingdoms, Herods Sheraton Resort Eilat rises on the shore of the Red Sea like a vertical village. This complex consists of the family-oriented Palace, where Middle Eastern traditions meet high-tech fun and games, and the Vitalis tower, which shelters a self-contained spa with lifestyle programs.

The magnificent Vitalis spa is a total experience. Everything is geared toward your physical, emotional, and spiritual well-being. From the time you awaken in your luxury spa guest room or suite till the end of your day, there is a sense of timelessness. Set against a panorama of sea and mountains, the desert climate engulfs you in a relaxing, tension-free experience.

Getting away from it all doesn't mean you can't have fun. The namesake of this vast resort, King Herod, was a Roman ruler of Judaea who enjoyed taking the waters and having nightly orgies. Managed by Sheraton, this is a family resort for Israelis who can burst into a hora at the drop of a matzo ball. Activities range from water sports to theme restaurants. So you can enjoy the Vitalis spa, then dip into the action at the Palace pool.

Herods Vitalis is an adults-only stand-alone tower with sixty-four rooms and three floors of spa facilities devoted to making you look and feel your best. Indoor and outdoor treatment rooms take advantage of the seafront location, offering the most extensive selection of bodywork, skin care, and hydrotherapy in the Middle East. Waterview weight training in an air-conditioned gym, and both indoor and outdoor exercise pools and aerobics studios, keep fitness buffs busy. Special emphasis on exercise in the pools includes body toning and aqua stretch classes. Relax in a thermal mineral salt pool, hydromassage pool, or under cascading waterfalls.

Dining on the outdoor terraces at Vitalis is another perk for spa guests. There is a special daily menu for your personal nutrition program, as well as gourmet spa cuisine. Many activities are held in small groups, enabling single persons and couples to make new friends. Structured programs (three, five, or seven days) called Lifemasters are all about learning to stay well. Participants share the excitement and fun of exercise and recreation. A personal focus can be included, such as weight reduction, body toning, sports training,

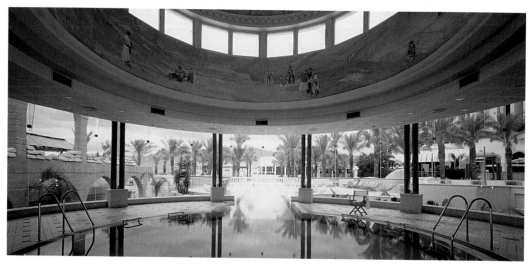

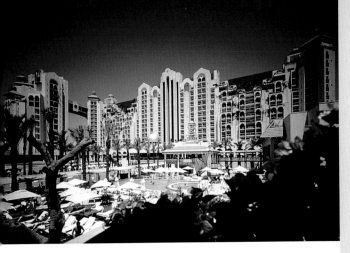

Red Sea Rejuvenation at Vitalis Spa

Herods Sheraton Resort Eilat
North Beach, Eilat 88000
Israel
Phone: 972–8–638–0000
Fax: 972–8–638–0060
E-mail: dana_alter@sheraton.com
Web site: www.herods.co.il

Season: Year-round

General Manager: Jean-Patrick Thiry

Spa Director: Moti Zingboim

Fitness Director: Zur Sofer

Reservations: (800) 325–3535

Accommodations: Herods Vitalis has sixty-four nonsmoking rooms, including four suites, fourteen single rooms, and forty-six double rooms, all with balcony and sea view. Bathroom has Jacuzzi, hair dryer, robe and slippers. Herods Palace offers 300 rooms, themed to historical periods of the region, with kitchenette and minibar. All the rooms are air-conditioned, have color TV, radio, and personal safe.

Meals: Herods Vitalis has gourmet spa cuisine in the Seven Spices Spa Restaurant, which features seafood and Middle Eastern specialties. There is a special daily menu of low-calorie selections.

Facilities: Twenty-seven body treatment rooms, ten massage rooms, seven skin care rooms, three hydrojet massage rooms, exercise pools, soaking pool, dry and wet saunas, gym with full line of exercise equipment, roof garden with mud treatments, jet showers and cascades, beauty salon with cosmetic treatments.

Services & Special Programs: Bodywork and skin care a la carte; Lifemasters all-inclusive programs designed to effect a positive change in lifestyle.

Rates: $$$

Best Spa Package: Three-Day Lifemasters, per person, double occupancy $675–$975, including accommodations, meals, treatments.

Credit Cards: Most major

Getting There: By car from Jerusalem, four hours. Road #1 south to Road #90 via Dead Sea, Aravaa Valley. Scheduled flights to Eilat from Tel Aviv airports on Arkia Airline or Israir, one hour. Free shuttle bus to Herods.

What's Nearby: Eilat Mountain Nature Reserve, bird-watching sanctuary, King Solomon's Pillars, underwater observatory.

or relaxation. Each program includes face and body treatments, fitness classes, workshops, lectures, and meditation. Eastern philosophies mix with the latest in stress management techniques to help you manage a personal program of well-being.

Located on the shores of the Red Sea, the southernmost point of Israel, Vitalis offers guided walks and excursions for a variety of fitness levels. Borrow a mountain bike to enjoy cycling trails through the wild desert landscape or sunrise in the mountain nature reserve. Kayaking in the sea strengthens muscles of the upper body as you explore this fabled part of the ancient world.

Beauty from the Sea Comes Naturally

Ancient springs on the site of the Herods Resort were thought to bring youth and rejuvenation. Much visited by spice caravans centuries ago, today the Vitalis springs' mineral-rich water is combined with modern technology in treatments designed for relaxation. Combinations of seawater, sea algae, and bath products by Repechage and Yon-Ka are featured. An innovative hydrotherapy experience combines underwater massage with color and light, aromatic oils, and therapeutic minerals. Your body and soul experience a unique sensation of floating in a sea of color selected to lift your spirits.

PACIFIC RIM

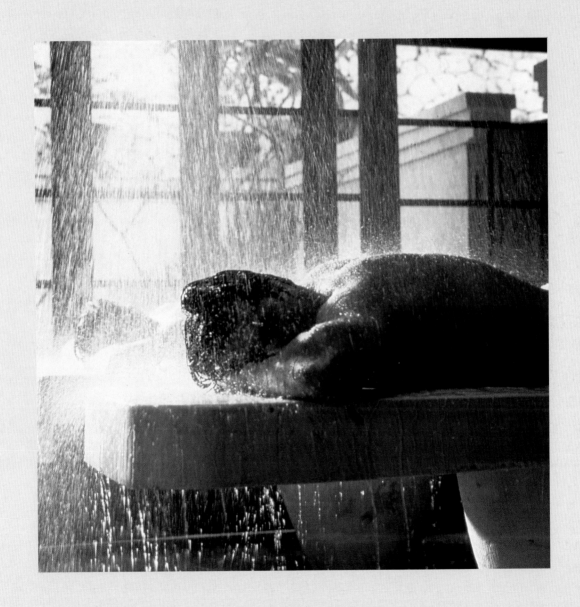

FOUR SEASONS RESORT BALI AT JIMBARAN BAY
Jimbaran, Bali, Indonesia

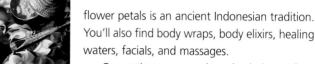

If you have ever harbored thoughts of a spa hideaway with tempting treatments, flower-filled bathtubs, and moonlit massages, this is the place to hang your straw hat. Celebrities such as Cindy Crawford, Whitney Houston, and Sylvester Stallone flock to the Four Seasons Resort Bali at Jimbaran Bay, enticed by the privacy and treatments so captivating that *USA Today* named it one of the "Ten Great Spas for Him and Her." The innovative treatments differ from traditional American treatments in technique, ingredients, and orientation.

This low-rise resort on thirty-five lush acres has spacious one- and two-bedroom villas that are intimately arranged, with twenty villas clustered around seven village squares.

The 10,000-square-foot spa with nine treatment rooms features treatments and products—potions as well as lotions—indigenous to the island. In any language, they are an exotic experience, designed for those who seek the unconventional. Try the lulur Jimbaran, which uses ginger root, spices, ground turmeric, and a fresh yogurt splash. Soaking in a warm bath filled with flower petals is an ancient Indonesian tradition. You'll also find body wraps, body elixirs, healing waters, facials, and massages.

One unique approach to body beautification is called the "coconilla." A body scrub that combines fresh shreds of young coconut, vanilla beans, and coconut milk polishes the skin while naturally adding moisture and luster. The process is completed with a rub of coconut lotion. Graceful and gentle Balinese therapists guide you through the treatments. You may have to be awakened when the procedure ends.

The spa bar serves healthy cuisine and can revitalize you with refreshing tonics and elixirs. Other dining choices range from gourmet cuisine to casual munching. Warung Mie, the newest dining spot, presents exotic and traditional noodle dishes from Japan, China, Vietnam, Thailand, and Indonesia. Guests dine at large, antique communal dining tables while the chefs cook right before their eyes. The resort also offers a cooking class that celebrates the island's culinary traditions and preparations.

Various honeymoon packages are offered at the Four

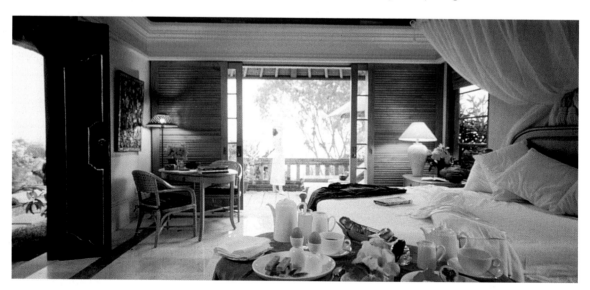

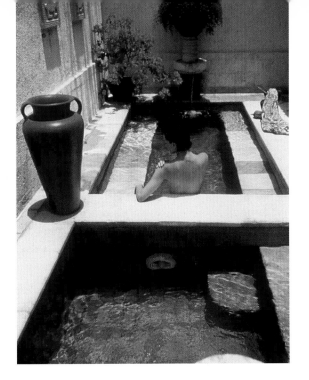

Four Seasons Resort Bali at Jimbaran Bay
Jimbaran, Denpasar 80361
Bali
Indonesia
Phone: 62–361–701010
Fax: 62–361–701020
E-mail: worldreservations@fourseasons.com
Web site: www.fourseasons.com

Season: Year-round (less rainfall April through October)

General Manager: Chris Norton

Spa Director: Belinda Shepard

Reservations: 62–361–701010 or (800) 332–3442

Accommodations: 139 one-bedroom villas; six two-bedroom villas; and two royal villas; CD and cassette sound system; TV and VCR (video and CD library in lounge); telephone; deluxe bathrooms; robes and slippers; in-room safe; air-conditioning and fans.

Meals: Five main restaurants: the Warung Mie (exotic and traditional noodle dishes); the Pool Terrace Cafe; the Taman Wantilan Restaurant (bayview dining with contemporary and spa cuisine); the Terrace Bar and Lounge; and the Pantai Jimaran (alfresco beachside cafe).

Facilities: 10,000-square-foot spa with nine treatment rooms, fitness facility, salon; 112-foot swimming pool with waterfall into free-form soaking pool; two tennis courts; library and lounge; art gallery; meeting facilities.

Services & Special Programs: Beach activities center with complimentary windsurfing, sailing, and snorkeling equipment and instruction; twenty-four-hour villa meal service; private tennis lessons; wedding coordination and receptions; cooking classes; arranged tours to arts and crafts centers and cultural events.

Rates: $$$

Best Spa Package: The four-night Romance in Bali includes round-trip transfers, fruit and flowers, breakfast daily, candlelight dinner in your villa, and a lulur Jimbaran spa treatment for each partner. The cost is $2,350 plus tax and service charge.

Credit Cards: Most major

Getting There: Many international airlines offer routes to Denpasar's Ngurah Rai International Airport. The resort is only a fifteen-minute limousine ride from the airport.

What's Nearby: The Bali Golf and Country Club's 18-hole course; scuba diving; white-water rafting; bicycling and trekking tours; art galleries; cultural events.

Seasons Bali, where idyllic weddings take place daily thanks to the resort's wedding consultants who shepherd couples through the process from permits to reception.

The Jimbaran experience is definitely a "Bali high."

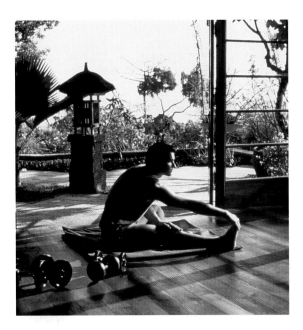

LE MERIDIEN NIRWANA GOLF & SPA RESORT
Tanah Lot, Bali, Indonesia

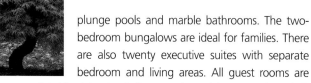

Breathtaking vistas accentuated by volcanic mountain backdrops, rice terraces, and views of the Indian Ocean greet guests as they enter the five-star Le Meridien Nirwana Golf & Spa Resort. Opened in 1997, this sprawling, 278-room resort is a world unto itself, with lush gardens and deep-blue pools enhanced by views of the crashing surf. It is no wonder that the Pacific Asia Travel Agents Association awarded Le Meridien "The Best New Resort Hotel in Asia" in 1998.

The resort complex is made up of low-lying buildings and laid out in an ecofriendly way. Rice terraces alternate with belts of forest, broad fairways, streams, and tropical flora. At least 70 percent of the resort is dedicated to landscaping and open green spaces.

Guests choose from a variety of accommodations, including twelve Balinese-style bungalows, all with private

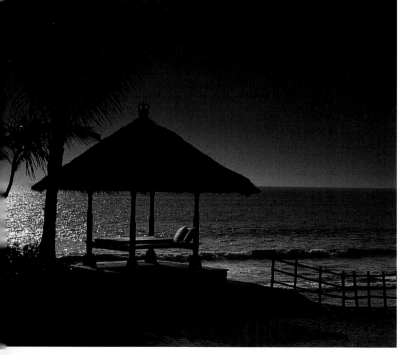

plunge pools and marble bathrooms. The two-bedroom bungalows are ideal for families. There are also twenty executive suites with separate bedroom and living areas. All guest rooms are furnished in the Balinese style and have spacious balconies, perfect for watching the orange-hued sky at dusk.

Three Balinese-designed bungalows are devoted to the spa, which features a variety of Balinese treatments. A recently added treatment, *nyuh gading sreed,* is wonderfully exotic. A body scrub made from the pulp of a young yellow coconut and turmeric seeds is used to cleanse and exfoliate the skin. The treatment, used historically for religious ceremonies, is followed by a traditional Balinese massage. Also new to the spa is *singgul beraban,* or beraban scrub. A mixture of ground coffee beans, volcanic rock, pumice stone, and red rice flour is formed into a paste used to cleanse the pores and exfoliate dead skin. This is also followed by a Balinese massage using soothing moisturizers. The highlight of the Balinese mud treatment is when cool jasmine-scented water is poured all over the body. The spa menu also includes a variety of massages, such as Swedish, French, lomi lomi, and Balinese, in addition to facials. Treatments may also be taken in the privacy of your room or in one of the outdoor huts, which have spectacular ocean views.

The hotel has three Balinese swimming pools, a waterslide, and a swimming lagoon with a man-made, white-sand beach and waterfall. A Greg Norman–designed 18-hole, par-71 golf course is uniquely landscaped with rice fields serving as roughs and hazards. The Indian Ocean backdrop makes this course one of the most beautiful in the world.

This traditional Balinese spa set in paradise promises a memorable stay.

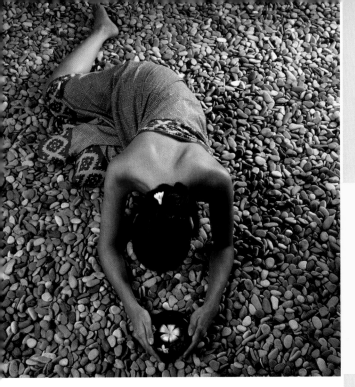

A Fantasy Spa Nestled in the Balinese Countryside

Le Meridien Nirwana Golf & Spa Resort
P.O. Box 158
Kediri, Tabanan 82171
Bali
Indonesia
Phone: 62–361–815–900
Fax: 62–361–815–901
E-mail: info@balimeridien.com
~~~~~~~~~~~~~~.com

~~~~~~~~~~~~~~~~ Griffiths
~~~~~~~~~~~~~~ tajaya
~~~~~~~ 15–900 or (800) 543–4300
~~~~~~~ ooms, including one- and two-
~~~~~~~ ve suites. Rooms offer marble
~~~~~~~ showers, in-room safes, and fully

~~~~~~~ nt is the resort's signature restau-
~~~~~~~ nese specialties. The resort also
~~~~~~~ dana Restaurant for all-day din-
ing, and the Nautilus Pub. The lobby lounge, overlooking pools, gardens, and ocean, serves an elaborate high tea. There is no spa menu, but the French culinary staff can accommodate special requests.

Facilities: Full-service spa with authentic Balinese body treatments; beauty salon; three swimming pools; waterslide; swimming lagoon; 18-hole golf course; conference facilities; fitness center; two tennis courts; gift shops.

Services & Special Programs: The Pirates Club for children, with supervised games, pool, and playhouse; guest services center arranges daily activities; daily complimentary shuttle alternate days to Ubud, an arts colony.

Rates: $$

Best Spa Package: The three-night Spa and Life Style Package offers deluxe accommodations in a one-bedroom villa with its own private plunge pool, an open-air and indoor shower, daily breakfasts for two; airport transfers; complimentary spa consultation; six health and beauty treatments per person; unlimited squash, tennis, gym use; and complimentary shuttles to shopping and Ubud. The package costs approximately $1,205 for two, double occupancy.

Credit Cards: Most major

Getting There: The Ngurah Rai Airport in Denpasar is thirty minutes away by car. Airport transfers can be arranged by the hotel.

What's Nearby: Tanah Lot Sea Temple; Ubud, a flourishing art colony; art colonies of Mas and Celuk; Sangeh Monkey Forest; Mengwi Temple.

A Spa Treatment Good Enough to Eat

The young yellow coconut and turmeric seed scrub, once reserved for religious ceremonies, has been adapted for use in the spa here. All of the ingredients used for the exfoliation and cleansing process are natural and free from commercial processing. Because the ingredients used in the scrub are all edible foods with vitamins and minerals, the body does not need to reprocess them, according to the spa therapist. As a result the beneficial effects of the forty-five minute treatment are felt sooner. The full-body treatment at Nirwana has three phases: The body scrub ensures that the skin is exfoliated; the body mask allows the newly opened pores to absorb the vitamins and minerals; and the full-body massage relaxes the body and improves circulation. The total 120-minute process, known as *nyuh gading sreed*, simply stated is a coconut/turmeric scrub, a carrot/seaweed/lime body mask, and a Balinese massage. Yum!

INN SEIRYUSO
Shimoda, Japan

Simplicity and silence so luxurious that all you want to do is sit for hours, watching the light, listening to rippling water. This silence is the first thing you notice at a *ryokan,* or traditional Japanese inn, like Seiryuso. Stepping into the reception area, you enter a realm of shadows and screens, tatami mats and polished stone.

Always a country where tradition melds with First World living, Japan has raised the ritual of bathing to an art form in the onsen. These hot-spring bathhouses are everywhere, in isolated forests, on beaches, and at mountain resorts. Staying at a *ryokan* is a different way of seeing the world, where space, time, and self are in harmony. Seiryuso has all the classic amenities, plus outside and inside baths *(onsen)* fed by hot springs.

The bath ritual is observed in exquisite detail. Don a light cotton robe provided in the room, slip into wooden clogs, and follow the maid to a private soaking pool. First you wash your body by dipping water from a pail. Then you climb into the tub. By the time you have soaked to a lobster-pink shade, the table has

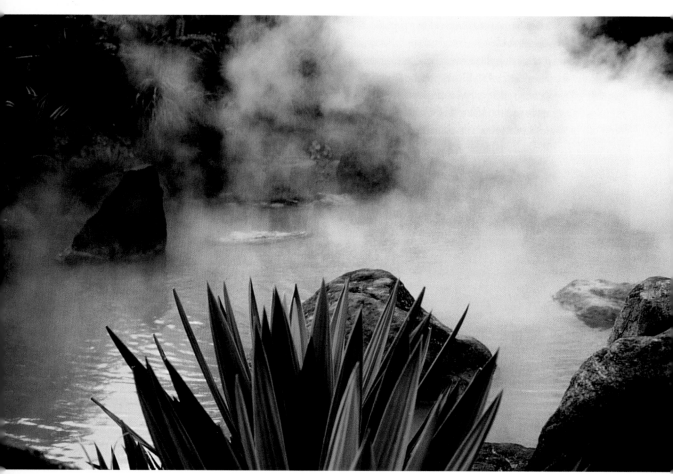

been set in your room for dinner. Prepare for a two-hour ceremony of culinary art. Each of the courses (usually ten) is served like miniature artwork. Maids shuffle in and out amid a flurry of bows and smiles, bringing in one course after another. This traditional tasting dinner may account for half the price of your room.

Massage and body treatment services distinguish Seiryuso from older inns. Spa services are separate from the baths, are performed in your room, and should be requested in advance of your arrival. Guest rooms, in six pavilions set in beautiful gardens, capture the enchanting Pacific light and air.

There are outdoor garden baths, beloved by both visitors and Japanese alike. From an indoor enclosure, where one washes up with modern bathing apparatus, a door leads to the heightened pleasure of bathing in the garden. These baths are sculptural masterpieces in green slate rock, basic angles, and curves. Protected from the wind and opening onto scenic views and cooling fresh air misted by steam from the water, they are favorite places for after-dinner soaks.

Seiryuso, built about one hundred years ago, resolutely clings to tradition. Aesthetically pleasing, the interior garden has stone-paved walkways amid century-old trees. *Ryokan* etiquette is followed precisely, but you'll see many people strolling around town in their robes. Following a bath, it's considered beneficial to your skin not to shower, as thermal water leaves a natural moisturizer on your body.

Spa Haiku

The Japanese speak of *wabi* and *sabi*, terms that connote loneliness, simplicity, and rustic purity; think of a haiku (or poem) in which the spaces between words convey as much as the words themselves. The overall effect is to screen you from the world, making you free to meditate. Time stops. A deep sense of relaxation, a cedar tub in your bathroom, and the sweet smell of the garden are your reward.

Inn Seiryuso
2-2 Kochi
Shimoda-shi
Shizuoka-ken 415-0011
Japan
Phone: 81–558–22–13–61
Fax: 81–558–23–20–66
E-mail: ubpi@seiryuso.co.jp
Web site: relaischateaux.com/seiryuso

Season: Year-round

General Managers: Kenichi and Hideo Tanaka

Reservations: (800) 735–2478 or www.relaischateaux.com

Accommodations: Thirty spacious traditional rooms equipped with modern amenities are in six pavilions. All have private bathroom with cedar tub.

Meals: Kaiseki menu of small plates featuring seafood, vegetables, miso soup, steak filet wrapped in bacon, tofu with caviar, sashimi, lobster or large shrimp, fruit, green tea, sake, and beer. Dinner and breakfast, afternoon tea, included in room rate. Gratuity not expected; 8 percent tax added to bill. Fine dining at Casa Vino features fish and wines.

Facilities: Hot baths (*rotenburo*) in garden, tubs inside, in-room massage and body treatments.

Services & Special Programs: Massage, shiatsu, reflexology.

Rates: $$$

Credit Cards: MasterCard, VISA

Getting There: From Tokyo by train, take the shinkansen (bullet train) to Shimoda, taxi 3.5 kilometers from station. By car, Tomei Highway to Route 135 (250 kilometers from Narita Airport).

What's Nearby: Gulf of Japan, Naoshima Cultural Village, Mount Fuji.

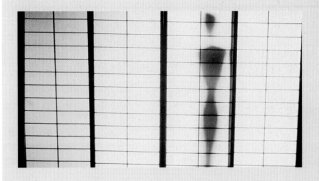

THE DATAI—MANDARA SPA

Kedah Darul Aman, Malaysia

On a faraway island surrounded by deep-blue water, almost at the Earth's edge, is The Datai. This five-star retreat is a piece of paradise where the stars shine so brightly at night you can almost reach out and touch them. Surrounded by an unspoiled rain forest, this tropical resort resonates with the sounds of birds. The air is tempered by soft breezes from the Andaman Sea. This startlingly beautiful resort on the northwestern tip of Langkawi has one of the most private and hard-to-find spas in the world.

You'll find the Mandara Spa along a wooded stream in four free-standing villas designed to blend harmoniously with the lush jungle. (The word *mandara* stems from an ancient Sanskrit legend concerning the gods' quest for a natural elixir of eternal youth and immortality.) The treatments at Mandara, which have such exotic names as Andaman Ecstasy and Langkawi Luxury, have been inspired and influenced by Bali. One two-and-one-half-hour specialty is called the Ultimate Indulgence. The

treatment uses two therapists per guest, starts with a refreshing footbath (using salt from the Andaman Sea), and includes a natural pumice, peppermint conditioners, a natural body scrub, and a warm aromatherapy flower bath while you overlook the rain forest. Follow this with the Mandara massage and conclude with a soothing facial and reflexology treatment for your feet. More traditional treatments at the spa include lulur, boreh, coconut scrub, a Bali coffee scrub, and a rain-forest herbal scrub.

The fifty-four deluxe guest rooms and eighteen suites are housed in forty free-standing villas scattered throughout the rain forest and connected by a series of pathways. All have steam showers, outside bathtubs, and private balconies that jut out over a stream. The decor and furnishings are stunning in their straightforward, natural style.

The Pavilion, an authentic Thai restaurant, provides open-air dining among the treetops, while the Dining

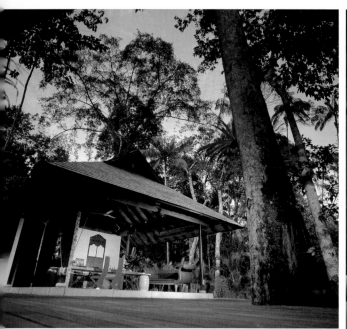

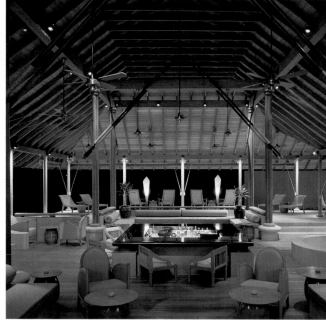

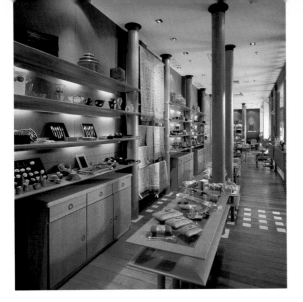

Room serves Malaysian and Western cuisine.

Adjacent to the resort is the 18-hole Datai Bay Golf Course, carefully landscaped to blend with the surrounding natural beauty. The Datai, submerged within this mystical island of jungle-covered mountains, lakes, caves, and waterfalls, is a perfect oasis from which to explore all there is to uncover in the realm of self-discovery.

Jet Lag Antidote

Jet lag does not have to ruin the start of your holiday. With a bit of forethought and on-arrival care, you can avoid feeling tired and stressed and begin to enjoy your holiday refreshed and relaxed. While on the plane, wipe your face and neck regularly throughout the flight with a warm, damp washcloth sprinkled with two drops of lavender and one drop of ylang-ylang essential oil. After eating, rub the washcloth over pulse points to soothe, calm, and promote sleep. Always drink plenty of water during a flight and avoid alcohol. Once you arrive at the Datai, use the spa's tranquillity massage oil blend for a prebath massage, then from the spa's new bath menu, choose the special bath aimed at relieving jet lag. You will feel as if your holiday has truly begun.

Mandara Spa at The Datai
Jalan Teluk Datai
07000 Pulau Langkawi
Kedah Darul Aman
Malaysia
Phone: 60–4–959–2500
Fax: 60–4–959–2600
E-mail: datai@ghmhotels.com
Web site: www.ghmhotels.com

Season: Year-round

General Manager: Jamie Case

Spa Director: Pat Choa

Reservations: 60–4–959–2500 or (800) 223–6800 (U.S.), Leading Hotels of the World

Spa Appointments: 60–4–959–2500 or (800) 223–6800

Accommodations: Ninety-eight rooms and twelve suites. All villas and suites have private terrace, elevated dining area, and CD player. All accommodations have veranda views of jungle or Andaman Sea. Suites feature a bedroom with separate living area and dining table.

Meals: Authentic Thai cuisine at the Pavilion in an open-air, treetop setting; Malaysian and Western dishes at the Dining Room; alfresco dining at the Beach Club.

Facilities: The Mandara Spa located in four individual villas; the 18-hole Datai Bay Golf Course; gymnasium; boutique; library; two tennis courts; beauty salon; and two swimming pools.

Services & Special Programs: Concierge; car hire and chauffeur-driven island tours; nature walks led by resident naturalist; shopping tours, including one to the night market; complimentary nonmotorized water sports.

Rates: $$$

Best Spa Package: Rates for a deluxe room start around $325 per night double occupancy. Tax and service charges are included.

Credit Cards: Most major

Getting There: Guests fly into Kuala Lumpur and then take a fifty-five-minute connecting flight to Langkawi on Malaysian Airlines.

What's Nearby: Temurun Waterfall; Kok Beach; Datai Bay; Tengkorak Beach; Cenang Beach; the Budaya Craft Centre; the Langkawi Crystal Factory; mountain biking.

BANYAN TREE MALDIVES

Vabbinfaru, The Republic of Maldives

The journey to this spa on a coral atoll is an experience in separation. Being here for a few days brings new meaning to the term "island hideaway." The resort is the sole occupant of this private island, and indeed, it is privy to registered guests only. Those intrepid enough to buy a ticket to Male, the Republic's gateway, are in for a spa journey like no other. After traveling halfway around the world, you'll feel like you're in a dream when you slip away for an aromatic massage in a thatched villa without walls.

Guests are met at the airport and make their way to a speedboat, which takes off for the twenty-minute ride to the resort: a cluster of forty-eight villas, some with a private outdoor Jacuzzi and sundeck by the beach. The fine white-sand beach is at your front door, and guests spend most of their time comfortably barefoot.

If privacy is your goal, this is the place to make it happen. With no traffic or other intrusions of today's techno-lifestyle, tranquillity is guaranteed. An essential component of the spa experience is thirty minutes of relaxation time for each guest, which includes a cooling mint footbath, an energy-boosting shower, and, as a finale, a soothing herbal drink and refreshments. The magic of the Maldivian lifestyle erases memories of stress and tension, and having several spa treatments daily under the capable hands of a Thai therapist is about as close as you can come to spa bliss. This is no surprise—the spa menu was developed at the Banyan Tree Spa Academy in Phuket, a school in Thailand where therapists undergo a 430-hour training program.

If you really want to take your mind, body, and spirit to where they have never been before, there are two choices. Both are three-hour treatments. The Harmony Banyan is a synchronized massage performed by two therapists. The Royal Banyan is based on massage techniques used in past centuries and features an oil-free

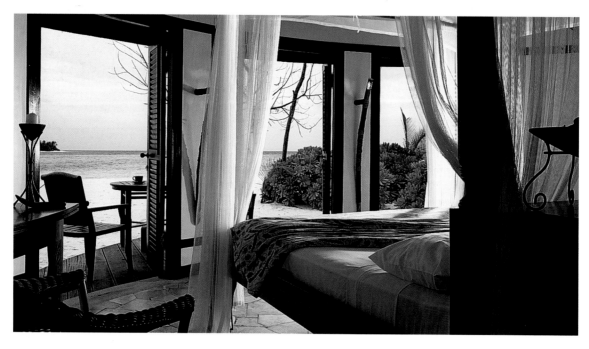

Royal Thia acupressure massage. The signature Banyan massage is performed with warm herbal pouches.

For those who want to explore the breadth of Thai-inspired treatments, the Thai Healer is extraordinary. This three-hour treatment features a traditional Thai yoga massage based on ancient ayurvedic principles. You will emerge from this inimitable spa experience with a radiant glow and a new lease on life.

What you won't find here is a structured program, a state-of-the-art gym, and lifestyle/wellness programs. This is an island-based spa, where the soft waves lap against the pristine beach and stars shine so bright at night you need sunglasses. Leave your cares and cell phone behind; this is a golden opportunity to enjoy the delights of a sunshine-blessed spa that most people still have trouble finding on the map.

The Lure of the Baths

A visit to the public baths in Roman times was an "irreplaceable part of the day's routine," an opportunity for personal regeneration, and a deeply rooted social and cultural habit, according to Fikret Yegul, history of architecture professor at the University of California at Santa Barbara. Yegul is the author of *Baths and Bathing in Classical Antiquity*, an uncommon resource that diagrams spas in ancient Greece, Rome, North Africa, and Asia Minor.

He notes that the Hippocratic School advocated that the "patient should not attempt to wash himself, but let others do it for him." This bathing prescription is followed today at such spas as the Sanctuary in Scottsdale, Arizona. Spa guests steep in aromatic marine water combined with sage, lavender, and essential oils, which are thought to increase circulation, regenerate cells, and act as anti-inflammatories. The evolution of bathing is a worldwide phenomenon.

As bathing rituals flourish at spas around the world, they echo ancient cultures and our enduring need to revitalize, rejuvenate, and relax.

Banyan Tree Maldives
North Male Atoll
Republic of Maldives
Phone: 960–443–147
Fax: 960–443–843
E-mail: maldives@banyantree.com
Web site: www.banyantree.com
Season: Year-round
General Manager: Maximillian Lennkh
Spa Director: Jeannie Sng
Reservations: (800) 525–4800 (Small Luxury Hotels) or reservations@banyantree.com.mv
Spa Appointments: Can be made upon arrival with guest services.
Accommodations: Each of the forty-eight villas has a four-poster king-size bed, step-down shower, fully stocked mini-bar, recessed sitting area, hair dryer, and telephone. Villa categories are garden, Jacuzzi garden, beachfront, Jacuzzi ocean view, Jacuzzi beachfront, and the presidential.
Meals: Buffet breakfast, lunch, and dinner included.
Facilities: Banyan Tree Gallery, which showcases indigenous arts and crafts; volleyball, table tennis, snooker, and badminton; TV room, reading area, and board games.
Services & Special Programs: Snorkeling, PADI Dive Center, deep-sea fishing, night fishing, water skiing, windsurfing, catamaran, sea-plane excursions, glass-bottom boat rental. On-site cooking school.
Rates: $$$$
Best Spa Package: Garden villas start at $440 per couple, nightly. Full board is an additional $100 per person, per day. Half board is $65 per person. Add to this $6.00 city tax and 10 percent service charge. Spa treatments are additional. April through September is the low season.
Credits Cards: Most major
Getting There: British Airways operates daily flights between London and Dubai. From Dubai, Emirates operates daily flights to Male.
What's Nearby: Male sight-seeing, island hopping, private yacht charters.

BANYAN TREE PHUKET

Amphur Phuket, Thailand

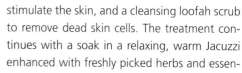

Banyan Tree Phuket is one of Asia's most luxurious spas and was voted "World's Best Spa Resort" in 1999 by *Condé Nast Traveler*. But you won't find sophisticated equipment or cutting-edge technology here. The drive to rev up in the gym is not part of the picture. Nor are doctors. You decide what is best for you.

The theory behind the treatments at Banyan Tree Phuket is not technology but touch. The absence of gimmicks and gadgets is evident in the treatment areas, many of which are outdoors, surrounded by lush gardens and a panoply of gorgeous flowers. The ambitious and comprehensive spa menu includes several exclusive treatments, such as one called the Honey Release Massage, which uses fresh orange juice mixed with pure honey to release muscle tension, increase blood circulation, and moisturize the skin.

Then there is the one called Oasis of Enlightenment—fifty minutes of sheer joy that begins with a choice of wet steam or dry sauna, a cold shower to stimulate the skin, and a cleansing loofah scrub to remove dead skin cells. The treatment continues with a soak in a relaxing, warm Jacuzzi enhanced with freshly picked herbs and essential oils; after this revitalizing ritual, you are "anointed" with a body moisturizer. Spa guests emerge from these rarefied treatments with a blissful smile.

The gardens of the resort flow into and around the guest villas, which are among the most spacious in Asia, each with its own garden, raised king-size bed, and sunken open-air bath. For ultimate luxury, choose one of the villas with its own private swimming pool.

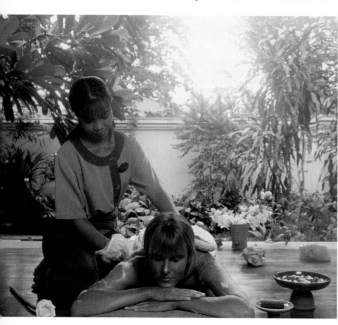

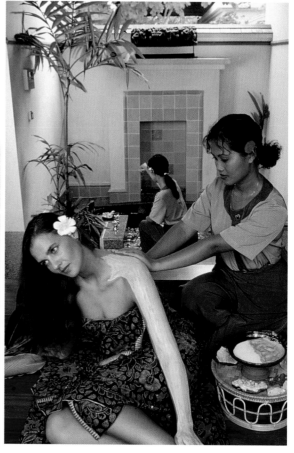

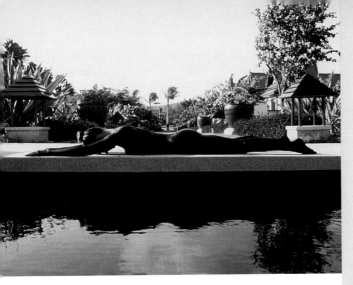

Banyan Tree Phuket Resort
33 Moo 4 Srisoonthorn Road
Cherngtalay, Amphur Phuket 83110
Thailand
Phone: 66–76–324374
Fax: 66–76–32375
E-mail: phuket@banyantree.com
Web site: www.banyantree.com

Season: Year-round

General Manager: Kamal Chaoui

Reservations: 66–76–324374 or (800) 525–4800 (Small Luxury Hotels)

Spa Appointments: 66–76–324374

Accommodations: 108 spa pool villas and two-bedroom pool villas, plus fifty-eight two-bedroom villas with private swimming pools. All have king-size beds and open-air baths.

Meals: Tamarind Restaurant offers light fusion cuisine with a range of culinary styles that includes Thai, Mediterranean, Indian, and Japanese. The cuisine is high in fiber and vitamins, low in fat and cholesterol, and has no added sugar and salt. The juice bar offers a large selection of fresh vegetables and health juices, smoothies, assorted teas, and wines.

Facilities: Full-service spa; golf club; outdoor swimming pool; two tennis courts (one floodlit); gallery of indigenous arts and crafts; a free-form pool with bubble mats and a rapid-water canal.

Services & Special Programs: Horseback riding; fishing; daily tours; bungee jumping.

Rates: $$$

Best Spa Package: The four-day, three-night Banyan Spa Sampler features daily breakfast; a ninety-minute massage or body wrap treatment; discount on a la carte spa treatments; use of all water-sport facilities, including wind surfing, canoeing, and sailing; and use of fitness pavilion. Rates are $750–$1,280 per person.

Credit Cards: Most major

Getting There: Take British Airways to Bangkok. There is a one-and-one-half-hour flight to Phuket Airport. The resort is twenty minutes by car from the airport. Transfers can be arranged in advance.

What's Nearby: Phang Na Bay for sea canoeing and scuba diving.

The spa's setting is spectacular, from the lap pool set in a fragrant garden to the outdoor treatment areas. Once your senses have been awakened here, you will understand why most spas in Asia are compared with the Banyan Tree.

The Joy of Ginger Tea

Kim and Cary Collier, an American couple considered by many to be the pioneer spa consultants in Asia, recommend ginger (*jahe*) tea as an antidote for jet lag. They lived in Indonesia for seven years, devoting their energy toward the study of traditional spa therapy. The Colliers find this recipe for ginger tea effective in relieving indigestion and in improving systemic blood circulation. Boil a cup of hot water; cut and peel a fresh ginger root. Boil this in the water for two minutes. After it is boiled and before you turn off the stove, crush the ginger root in the water. Add a tablespoon of unrefined sugar (*gulah merah*). Allow the water, crushed ginger, and unrefined sugar to steep for five minutes before straining and serving. Relax and slowly sip the tea. Ginger tea should be sipped during and after your flight. You will find ginger tea at various spas using Jamu treatments. It is often served iced.

CHIVA-SOM INTERNATIONAL HEALTH RESORT
Hua Hin, Thailand

This destination health resort, set on seven acres of beachside gardens near the king's summer palace, accommodates those seeking a rare blend of fitness, spa cuisine, skin care, and rejuvenating treatments. The resort, which offers fifty-seven private units in Thai-style pavilions, was the brainchild of Boonchu Rojanastien, Thailand's former deputy prime minister. With the help of private investors, his dream has become a reality. Together they set high standards, so expect a serious wellness program and a well-qualified staff. Chiva-Som was named "Second Best Overseas Spa" by *Condé Nast Traveler* magazine in 1998 and 1999. In 2000, the resort was named number one in the destination spa category by *Conde Nast Traveler*'s readers.

The fifteen treatment rooms have separate heat treatment suites for men and women. Treatments range from aromatherapy and face and body massages to body reshaping. There are also a music therapy room, a flotation chamber for destressing, and outdoor massage pavilions for special pampering. The spa program was developed by an international staff and is managed by an international team. As a result, you will meet an international clientele in your classes and at meals.

The belief at Chiva-Som ("haven of life") is that mind, body, and spirit should work in unison and that putting them in balance will prevent or help cure many age-related illnesses. All guests receive a private medical consultation. Physicians, nurses, and dietitians are on staff. Recommended programs may include such alternative methods as equilibropathy—a combination of acupuncture techniques, exercises, and spinal correction. Iridology, an analysis of markings in the iris, is used to reveal information about the digestion, circulation, and other body systems.

A typical spa day could start with a power walk along the beach or an exercise class in the air-conditioned gym. Yoga is presented in pavilions designed especially for the purpose. The bathing pavilion features

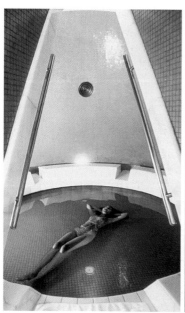

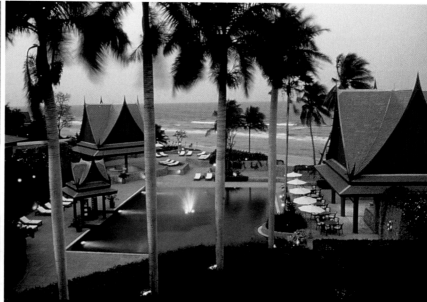

an indoor pool for aqua aerobics, a plunge pool, a Kneipp bath with pebbles for massaging the feet, and a large hydropool.

The spa cuisine is a harmonious blend of Asian and Western specialties. It is gourmet in preparation and presentation while being both low calorie and highly nutritious. Herbs, vegetables, and fruit are grown in the resort's private organic garden. Wine and champagne are the only alcoholic beverages served. For those seeking weight loss, a dietitian will provide a

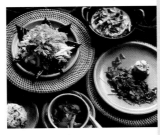

sensible program. Meals are served in an emerald-green dining room with air-conditioning or on an outdoor terrace. Those on an unrestricted diet may dine at the Waves seafront restaurant, which serves healthy snacks and beverages. The Orchid Lounge serves coffee and tea throughout the day.

Exotic Chiva-Som meets its goal of integrating mind, body, and spirit in its personalized training, enlightenment exercises, luxurious body treatments, and healthy cuisine. This realistic wellness program, carried out with a staff-to-guest ratio of four to one in a beautiful natural setting by the sea, is fit for a king or queen.

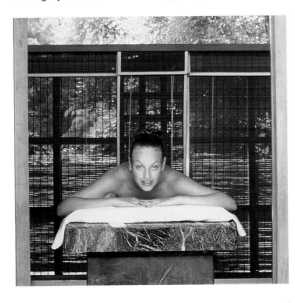

A Harmonious Spa Haven for Mind, Body, and Spirit

Chiva-Som International Health Resort
73/4 Petchkasem Road
Hua Hin, Prachuab Khiri Khan 77110
Thailand
Phone: 66–32–536–536
Fax: 66–32–511–154
E-mail: mktg@chivasom.com
Web site: www.chivasom.com

Season: Year-round
Managing Director: Joy Menzies
Health & Wellness Director: Sarah Noble
Reservations: 66–32–536–536 or (800) 525–4800 (Small Luxury Hotels of the World)
Accommodations: Fifty-seven guest accommodations are located along the beachfront in either private Thai-style pavilions or oceanview rooms or suites. Guest room interiors were designed by international and Thai designers.
Meals: Rates include three spa cuisine meals a day in the dining room with Asian and western specialties. During the day, the Waves Restaurant serves healthy snacks and beverages. The Orchid Lounge offers fruit juices, coffee, and tea.
Facilities: Conference room; spa with fifteen treatment rooms, beauty bar with hairdressing and manicure and pedicure services, outdoor massage pavilions; air-conditioned gym; bathing pavilion with indoor pool, multilevel unisex steam room, plunge pool, Kneipp bath, and large hydropool; outdoor seaside pool.
Services & Special Programs: Lectures; board games in library; arts and crafts at boutique; water sports, from windsurfing to sailing; private medical consultations and nutritional counseling.
Rates: $$$
Best Spa Package: The seven-night package (ranging from $2,734 to $5,859 plus taxes) includes accommodations, three Chiva-Som spa cuisine meals daily, individual health and beauty consultations, and choice of a daily massage, fitness class, and leisure activity. Add to this a spa bath, loofah scrub, and Oriental foot massage.
Credit Cards: Most major
Getting There: Guests can fly on British Airways to Bangkok and then on to Hua Hin Airport. The resort is fifteen minutes from the airport. The resort can also arrange ground transportation from Bangkok International Airport or Bangkok City, a three-hour drive.
What's Nearby: The Summer Palace; Floating Market; Sam Roi National Park; Pala'u Waterfall.

THE ORIENTAL HOTEL BANGKOK—
THE ORIENTAL SPA

Bangkok, Thailand

This is a city spa, a Thai-style house sublime in its simplicity and grace that has been recognized as "Best Spa in the World" by *Travel and Leisure* magazine. Appropriately referring to itself as a "temple of well-being," the spa is housed in a 120-year-old residence across the Chao Phraya River from the Oriental Hotel Bangkok.

The hotel is another story. It's legendary as a favored haunt of past literary masters Graham Greene, Somerset Maugham, and Joseph Conrad. And it's been rated as the "Number One Business Hotel Worldwide" by the British publication *Business Traveler*.

The 1,000-meter Oriental Spa is a haven of tranquillity. The Thai-style house is made from beautifully carved golden teak wood. Soothing aromas fill the air. The myriad beauty and relaxation treatments are performed in the privacy of your own luxurious suite—many of the suites have been frequented by movie greats, such as Elizabeth Taylor and Goldie Hawn, and by VIPs, such as former President George Bush.

Spa services are for a full day or half day. The six full-day programs include such offerings as the Oriental herbal wrap, a marine balneotherm treatment, an Orien-

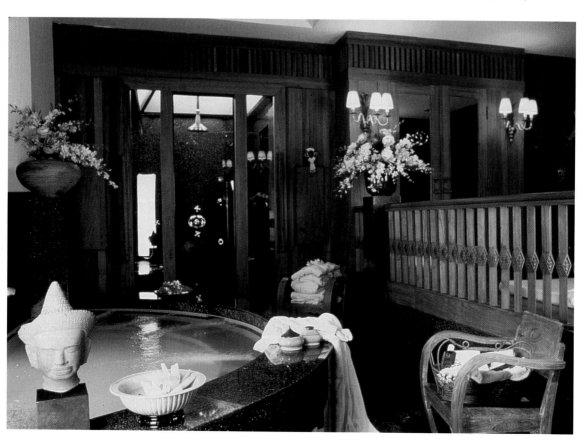

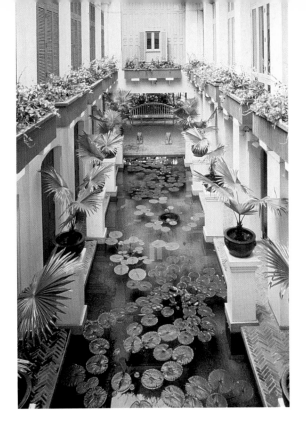

The Oriental Hotel Bangkok—The Oriental Spa
48 Oriental Avenue
Bangkok 10500
Thailand
Phone: 66–2–659–9000
Fax: 66–2–659–0000
E-mail: orbkk-reservations@mohg.com
Web site: www.mandarinoriental.com/bangkok

Season: Year-round

General Manager: Kurt Wachtveitl

Spa Director: Orawan Choeysawat

Reservations: (800) 223–6800 or 66–2–439–7613 (Leading Hotels of the World); or (800) 526–6566 (Mandarin Oriental Hotel Group).

Spa Appointments: 66–2–439–7613

Accommodations: 395 guest rooms and thirty-five suites; rooms in garden wing rooms are split-level; all rooms offer air-conditioning, color satellite TV, refrigerators, minibars, dual phone lines, and river views.

Meals: Ciao (Bangkok's only outdoor Italian restaurant); the Normandie (French cuisine); the Sala Rim Naam restaurant (spicy Thai fare).

Facilities: Oriental Spa; two outdoor swimming pools; sports center with high-tech gym, tennis courts, squash courts, and sauna; barbershop and beauty shop; flower shop; shopping arcade; fully equipped business center.

Services & Special Programs: Thai cooking school; Thai cultural program; Oriental river cruises to the old capital and the summer palace; boat rides to River City shopping mall; golf arrangements and transportation; helicopter service to airport; medical service; twenty-four-hour room service; laundry and valet service.

Rates: $$$

Best Spa Package: The Oriental Spa Day gives you the ideal way to experience the spa. This five-and-one-half-hour program is $250 per person. To this add the cost of accommodations at the Oriental Hotel, which range from $280 to $340 for River Wing rooms, and from $430 for the suites, per night, double occupancy. Add 10 percent service charge and taxes.

Credit Cards: Most major

Getting There: The hotel is close to Bangkok's new skytrain station and within easy access to Bangkok International Airport by expressway.

What's Nearby: River City (antiques shopping); New Rod (arts, crafts, and silverware); championship golf courses; Ayudhaya, the ancient capital.

tal massage, a European stress recovery treatment, a manicure or pedicure, a spa cuisine lunch or dinner, and a variety of herbal teas, fruit juices, or mineral water throughout the day. The spa also offers a special ninety-minute jet-lag recovery treatment.

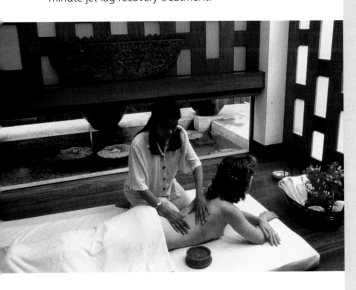

THE REGENT RESORT CHIANG MAI—
LANNA SPA
Chiang Mai, Thailand

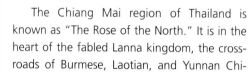

This handsome, secluded resort, with its twenty acres of gardens studded with lakes, streams, waterfalls, and countless varieties of plants and trees, is sure to put you in the mood for some of the most luxurious spa treatments in Asia.

You'll find them in the three-level, 9,000-square-foot Lanna Spa, nestled amid tropical gardens, with views of the surrounding rice fields. Inspired by a northern Thai temple and graced with sculpture and artwork, the spa has seven stunning and spacious suites. The Laan Chiang penthouse treatment suite occupies the entire third floor. Here you can experience a rice and spice skin rub (an aromatic massage) along with an aloe and lavender hydrating body wrap. The lavish suite also has Thai and Western massage beds, an outdoor soaking tub in a private *sala* (outdoor terrace), an herbal steam room, and a double semi-outdoor shower—not to mention a breathtaking view of the Doi Suthep Di Pui mountain range.

You may choose from Thai-inspired treatments, such as a honey seed rub or a lemon grass body wrap, or indulge in garden baths, massages, and facials—all presented in spa suites with individual soaking tubs on semi-enclosed private terraces. Five suites are equipped with private herbal aromatherapy steam rooms, and two spa treatment suites have double rain-shower massage beds. The relaxation lounge is the perfect sanctuary for repose between treatments. There is also a full-service beauty salon on the premises.

Guest pavilion suites are designed with rich gold teak timber, handmade local ceramic tiles, and bright accent colors. Teak also predominates in the Sala Mae Rim Restaurant; the natural upholstery is accented by Lanna-style tapestries. The restaurant features fine Thai cuisine, including both northern and vegetarian specialties. The restaurant has its own organic garden.

The Chiang Mai region of Thailand is known as "The Rose of the North." It is in the heart of the fabled Lanna kingdom, the crossroads of Burmese, Laotian, and Yunnan Chinese cultures. Combining your spa experience with this fascinating region of the world will make for an unforgettable spa journey.

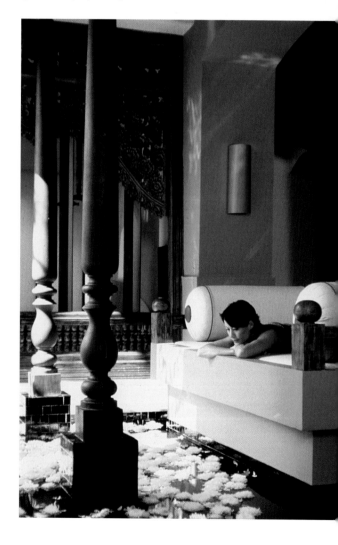

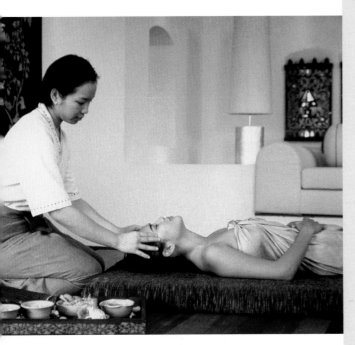

The Regent Resort Chiang Mai—Lanna Spa
Samoeng Old Road
Mae Rim Valley
Chiang Mai 50180
Thailand
Phone: 66–53–298–181
Fax: 66–53–298–189
E-mail: rcm.reservations@fourseasons.com
Web site: www.regenthotels.com

Season: Year-round

General Manager: Michael J. Kemp

Spa Director: Rungratree Kong Kwanyuen

Fitness Director: Joel Johnson

Reservations: (800) 332–3442 or 66–53–298–181

Accommodations: Seventy-two suites with in-room safes, sound system, CD player, satellite TV.

Meals: The Sala Mae Rim and Lanna restaurants serve Thai cuisine; the Elephant Bar is an open pavilion lounge with afternoon tea, cocktails, and after-dinner drinks; the Pool Terrace and Bar offers poolside dining and weekly barbecues.

Facilities: Lanna Spa with seven treatment rooms, outdoor showers, private herbal steam rooms, outdoor soaking tubs, and tropical rain-shower massage tables; hair salon; conference and banquet facilities; library; tennis and health club, with two courts and fitness/exercise studio.

Services & Special Programs: Lanna Cooking School, "Art of Thai Cuisine"; six-day program (Monday–Saturday).

Rates: $$$

Best Spa Package: Lanna Spa Discovery (four nights/five days) includes private airport transfers, welcome drink and jasmine garland on arrival, daily American breakfast, daily fresh fruit bowl and newspaper, daily dinner for two, ten hours of spa treatments (four two-hour sessions for two people). The cost is $2,356 double occupancy, plus tax and service. Rates change seasonally.

Credit Cards: Most major

Getting There: Take British Airways to Bangkok. Thai Airways operates daily flights between Bangkok and Chiang Mai (ten in summer, fourteen in winter). Limousines are available for airport transfers and local transportation.

What's Nearby: Chiang Mai's temples; Chiang Dao Elephant Training Camp; Wat Phra That Suthep, a holy fourteenth-century shrine on a 5,000-foot mountain; Wat Suan Dok, home to a 500-year-old Buddha.

The Cold-Water Cure for Jet Lag

Just getting to one of these tropical but remote spa resorts can take up to twenty hours—even more if you meet up with unscheduled delays. So when you finally arrive after so many hours cooped up in a plane, you're probably pretty uncomfortable, and your biological clock is pretty out of whack. But there is an unusual way to bounce back. Try cold-water bathing! A cold-water bath can revive your sluggish senses, and some people swear by it. It is said to improve circulation, increase muscle tone, assist in preventing premature aging, build up resistance against colds and infections, and enhance glandular functioning. Spraying the soles of the feet with cold water draws excess blood from the brain and helps relieve cranial congestion, so say believers. After a spray of cold water, massage your neck and shoulders. Then rest in bed for twenty minutes.

CARIBBEAN ISLANDS &
THE BAHAMAS

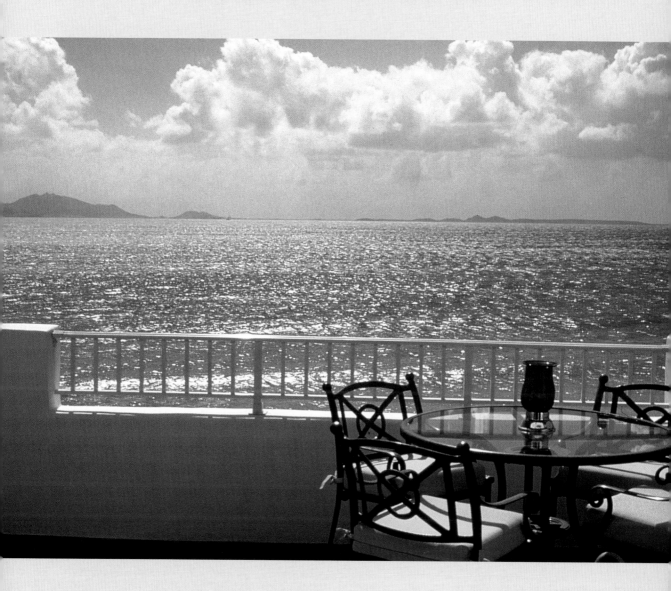

CUISINART RESORT & SPA
Anguilla, British West Indies

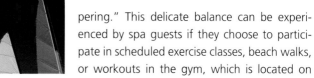

The elongated island of Anguilla in the British West Indies measures merely 16 miles long by 3 miles wide. But within its limited borders is a destination that for spa-lovers that is well worth seeking: CuisinArt, a stylish ninety-three-room resort tucked away on the white-sand beach of Rendezvous Bay. The startling blue-green water of the bay meets with the white-washed villas, designed to resemble the Greek island of Mykonos. This sets the idyllic stage for the intimate, three-level, 7,500-square-foot spa. The gardens surrounding the resort are lush with 37,000 plants, representing 150 species, such as tamarind, guava, citrus, and banana.

The resort's goal is to offer "the best in healthful living, gourmet cuisine, fitness, relaxation, and pampering." This delicate balance can be experienced by spa guests if they choose to participate in scheduled exercise classes, beach walks, or workouts in the gym, which is located on the first level of the spa. The second level of the spa is reached by a winding staircase that leads to five treatment rooms and a full-service beauty salon. Hair and skin-care products from the Rusk line are left in your room daily, along with a generous selection of seashell soaps and bath salts.

The spa program is unstructured, but the spa director will happily help you schedule classes and treatments. Repêchage skin-care products, a French line, are used exclusively for body treatments, facials, and body scrubs. A schedule of activities is posted daily; an evening pro-

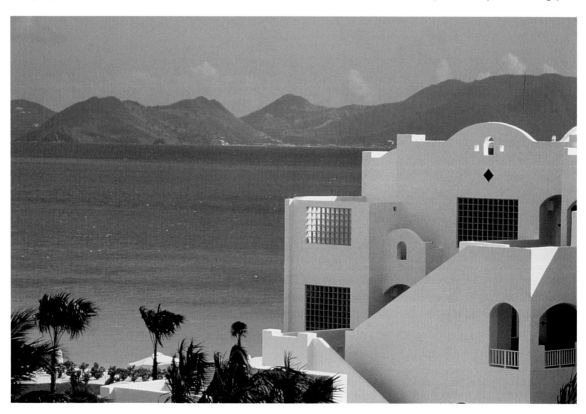

gram might be a half-hour informal talk by the fitness director on the quickest route to fitness success.

Those who enjoy healthful dining also usually enjoy the tour of the resort's hydroponic farm, a huge air-conditioned greenhouse that is totally free of soil. Hydroponic farming cultivates plants in nutrient-enriched water without soil. The resulting pesticide-free vegetables—bright red tomatoes, yellow and red peppers, and butter lettuce—are served in the resort restaurants (Santorini offers gourmet dining; the Mediterrano is poolside). You can also have a lunch that is both healthful and educational at the Hydroponic Cafe, tucked away in the greenhouse, where a colorful buffet of salads is served daily and irresistible tropical fruit smoothies are made to order.

One of the best places to sunbathe (or stargaze) during your free moments is on your own guest room patio with its views of neighboring Saint Martin and Rendezvous Bay. Bathrooms are outfitted with Italian marble, and you'll find monogrammed robes there too.

The beach, one of the most perfect in the Caribbean (if not the world), offers plenty to do, but you can just plain relax if that's your pleasure. Comfortable lounges for beach-lovers dot the sand. During the day, guests are treated to homemade sorbet and cool towels. Paradise is sunning and spa-going at CuisinArt.

Sea Salt for Smooth Skin

CuisinArt Resort & Spa uses the island's natural resources in its roster of treatments, from sea salts to stones to the soothing sounds of the sea. One skin treatment uses salt harvested from local salt ponds, which is combined with pure essential oils to cleanse, detoxify, and exfoliate the skin, while at the same time stimulating and smoothing it. After the skin is renewed, an application of self-tanning lotion is applied in preparation for a holiday in the sun.

A Spa with Gourmet Cuisine on a Caribbean Beach

CuisinArt Resort & Spa
P.O. Box 2000
Rendezvous Bay, Anguilla
British West Indies
Phone: (264) 498–2000
Fax: (264) 498–2010
E-mail: reservations@cuisinart.com
Web site: www.cuisinartresort.com

Season: Year-round

General Manager: Rabin Ortiz

Spa Director: Kathy Eggleston

Fitness Director: Peter Vasilis

Reservations: (212) 972–0880 or (800) 943–3210

Spa Appointments: (800) 937–9356

Accommodations: Ninety-three rooms and suites surrounded by lush, tropical foliage. Accommodations range from superior rooms to luxury, to junior suites to one- and two-bedroom suites with solariums. Guest rooms include such features as private patios, marble bathrooms, some oceanfront views, and Italian furnishings.

Meals: Gourmet dining in Santorini; poolside dining in the Mediterrano; lunch in the Hydroponic Cafe, tucked away in the greenhouse.

Facilities: Three-level spa; gym; billiards room; tennis courts; hair salon; boutique; tennis pro shop; children's playground; library; swimming pool; croquet field; bocce court.

Services & Special Programs: Daily continental breakfast on guest-room patio; satellite TV, and VCRs on request; equipment for snorkeling; windsurfing; horticultural tours; boat charters; beach beverage service; laundry services; baby-sitting; day trips; and cooking classes.

Rates: $$$

Best Spa Package: Five-Night Indulgence (available April 15–December 16): accommodations in junior suite, continental breakfast, one massage and one facial (each for one person), one dinner for two, complimentary water sports, use of fitness facilities. Cost is $2,355.

Credit Cards: American Express, MasterCard, VISA

Getting There: Flights are available to Wallblake Airport from neighboring islands served by international carriers. Nearest international airports are on Saint Maarten and Puerto Rico. Ferry service is available from Marigot Bay, French Saint Martin, to Blowing Point, Anguilla.

What's Nearby: The islands of Saint Barthélemy (St. Barts), Nevis, and Saint Martin are all day-trip destinations.

MANDARA SPA AT THE OCEAN CLUB
Paradise Island, Nassau, The Bahamas

East meets West at this new Bahamian spa. Clustered under palm trees in tropical gardens, eight luxurious Oriental villas provide an exotic retreat for body and mind. Mandara Spa is ideal for romance or for simply getting away from it all.

Step into your private garden, complete with whirlpool bath. Relax on an open-air Balinese daybed, cushioned and comfortable enough for two; feel the stress fall away as your Bahamian therapist offers herbal tea and washes your feet. Breathe sea air perfumed by tropical flowers, cooled by bamboo fans. Two treatment tables and individual wardrobes are in the air-conditioned suite where you change into robes, shower, and start the ritual.

Mandara spa rituals combine many elements for stress release. The Caribbean coffee body scrub exfoliates and refines your skin with finely ground coffee beans, which adds a rich aroma to the experience! Forget steam cleaning; Mandara scrubs and creams open pores and smooth skin. An ideal antidote to jet lag and dehydration, the Elemis Japanese silk facial masque delivers nourishment deep into the skin.

Pamper your palate in two restaurants. Open throughout the day and evening, Dune overlooks the beach, with alfresco and indoor seating. More formal dinner in the Courtyard Terrace reaches gourmet heights (and prices) inspired by New York Master Chef Jean-Georges Vongerichten.

Cocooned in comfort, no sounds intrude other than the ocean. The beach is never crowded, and you can walk or jog for miles. From the days when this was an exclusive hideaway for the rich and famous, the resort's terraced gardens, tennis complex, and mansion house have been completely refurbished, although the place retains the ambience of a private club. New accommodations reflect the stately British Colonial look of the original and feature a Roman bath and entertainment center. Nearby developments are changing the island's seclusion, but paradise doesn't get much better than this.

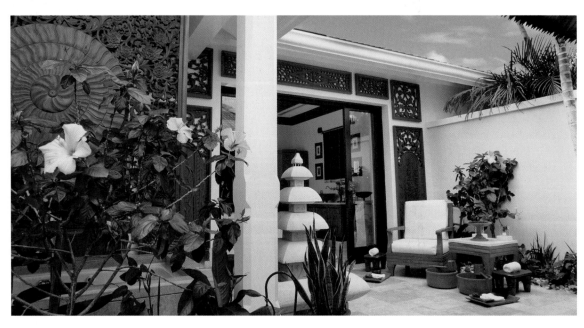

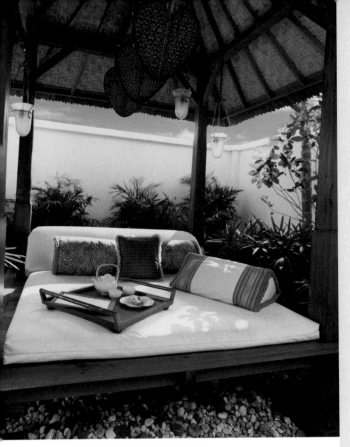

Mandara Spa at the Ocean Club
P.O. Box N-477
Nassau, The Bahamas
Phone: (242) 363–2501, ext. 64808
Fax: (242) 363–5901
E-mail: bahamas@mandaraspa.com
Web site: www.OceanClub.com
Season: Year-round
General Manager: Youlanda Deveaux
Spa Director: Shian Wing
Reservations: (242) 363–3000 or in U.S. (800) 321–3000
Accommodations: The Ocean Club has 107 rooms and suites in two-story beach lodges, plus two-bedroom villas near the tennis courts and pool. All are air-conditioned, with balcony or terrace. Rooms in the new Crescent Wing are spacious, with ocean view, mosaic-tile bath with separate shower and toilet, two commodes, TV, DVD, CD, phone, modem, clothes press, robes.
Meals: Daily a la carte menu at Dune restaurant featuring seafood, Thai specialties; dinner alfresco at the romantic Courtyard Terrace starts with conch chowder, lobster bisque, or roasted garlic soup.
Facilities: Eight private Mandara Spa suites with two treatment tables, whirlpool bath, shower, garden pavilion; two-room salon for hair and nail treatments. On the thirty-five-acre property: Nine Har-Tru tennis courts (lit for night play); lap pool; ocean beach; 18-hole, par-72 golf course.
Services and Special Programs: Floral aromatherapy bath, footwash, reflexology, massage (Swedish, Thai, Balinese, warm stone), Elemis facials and wraps, Balinese boreh herbal body scrub, Caribbean coffee scrub, salt glow, ayurvedic shirodhara, mother-to-be skin care and massage, men's facial. Salon for hair and nail care, makeup lesson, waxing.
Rates: $$$
Credit Cards: All major
Best Spa Package: Global Fusion three-hour ritual for two persons ($820) or solo ($460) includes foot treatment, massage, wrap, facial, tea ceremony, whirlpool bath, eye zone therapy. Service charge 15 percent.
Getting There: Located 13 miles from the international airport, Paradise Island is reached by two causeways from Nassau's main road, Bay Street. Limousine transfers available; also taxi, helicopter pad, yacht marina. Airlines serving The Bahamas include American, Delta, USAir. Valid passport required.
What's Nearby: Sivananda yoga ashram, Atlantis Resort and casino, marina, Eleuthera, and neighbor islands.

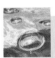

On the Wild Side

Staying at the Ocean Club gets you access to Kerzner Resorts' awesome Atlantis Resort, including that resort's twenty-four-room Mandara Spa, with King and Queen treatment suites, a seawater whirlpool, a Cybex fitness center, a lap pool, and a tennis complex. While you spa, kids (age four to twelve) can learn about sea creatures at day camp, and teenagers can surf the Internet and indulge in PlayStation challenges at Club Rush (no adults allowed). Atlantis has a casino with 1,000 slot machines and 78 gaming tables, designer boutiques, restaurants overlooking big yachts in the sixty-three-slip marina, kayaking, and water sports. The only thing free is a shuttle bus that connects resort properties.

SANDY LANE HOTEL
Barbados, West Indies

Greeted at the airport by a chauffeur-driven Bentley, you are ushered into a world of privilege and pricey services at the Sandy Lane Hotel. From the airy coralstone and Italian marble lobby to your suite (where the butler demonstrates electronic controls), the look of luxury is impressive. So are prices: Room rates start at $600 a night; $165 for a round of golf; $350 for synchronized massage with two therapists. But the well-heeled crowd, largely British and German, doesn't seem to mind. Sandy Lane has been cosseting celebrities, royalty, and the rich for forty years, and its recent $200 million reconstruction keeps it at the forefront of luxury resorts.

Although the hotel's stretch of public beach is pretty, there is constant distraction from people hawking Jet Ski rides and souvenirs. Escape to the cool, quiet spa, palatial in marble and limestone, with cascading waterfalls. It feels like a cross between a Roman emperor's baths and the Starship Enterprise. The 47,000-square-foot guests-only spa features a steam room centered on a huge chunk of agate, which is said to produce healing effects.

As you descend a grand staircase, your view takes in four swimming pools. Set in tropical gardens, the spa provides a separate area for teenagers and a playroom and restaurant for young children. Adult sybarites head for the hydropool, which features lounges below the water's surface that are made of steel rods from which bubbles escape to create a comfortable cushion. Landscaping shuts out the rest of the resort and isolates you from the beach.

After-sun therapy and sports massage for golfers are house specialties. Offering a wide range of skin care and bodywork, the spa features ESPA products. Inspired by the example of the ancients, the spa rituals can encompass a full day and blend traditional therapies from the Caribbean, the Far East, and Europe with a modern philosophy of health and well-being. These are treatments of rare quality and exceedingly high standards, delivered by a team of well-grounded professional therapists. Ask for one of the garden suites, and enjoy your island oasis.

For a unique experience, steam first in a unisex

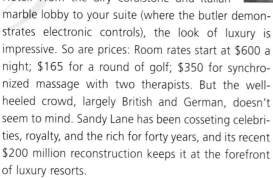

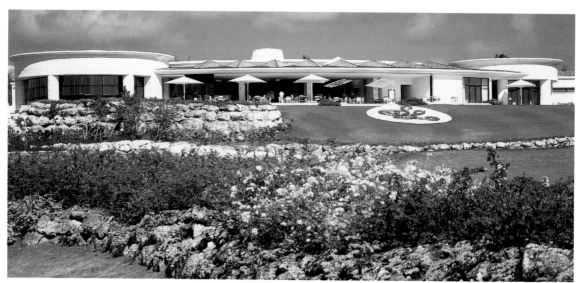

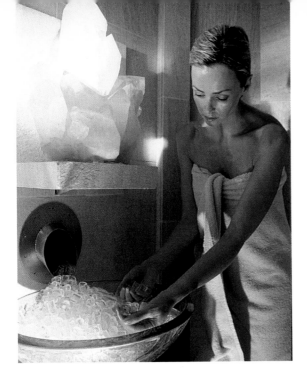

chamber lit by multicolored crystals in the ceiling. Then enter the really hot steam room. Finally, cool down in the Ice Cave, a refrigerated room where ice chips spill into a basin. Like the Romans, you are supposed to dump the ice over your head and chill out!

The Sandy Lane Hotel exudes the slow, tropical luxury of British colonial mansions. Reopened in 2002 with a new look, the hotel once again ranks among the world's best beach resorts.

The Ritual

Your personal journey at Sandy Lane is designed to transport you to a place where tension, fatigue, and stress melt away. The first step is a gentle welcoming ritual, which engages your senses. The sound of delicate Tibetan cymbals cleanses and clears your own personal space. Breathe the aroma of pure blended aromatic essential oils. Become grounded during the traditional foot cleansing by focusing on the feel of water and natural stones.

Elegance Redefined

Sandy Lane Hotel
Highway 1, Mahogany Road
St. James, Barbados
Phone: (246) 444–2000
Fax: (246) 444–2222
E-mail: reservations@sandylane.com
Web site: www.sandylane.com
Season: Year-round
General Manager: Colm Hannon
Spa Manager: Bridgette Laurayne
Spa Appointments: blaurayne@sandylane.com
Accommodations: 112 large suites with veranda or garden terrace. Marble bathrooms have multispray shower, Jacuzzi bathtub with a view. Resplendent in Porthault linens, Penhaligon soaps. Amenities include flat-screen TV with Internet access, DVD player, fax machine. Completely air-conditioned, ceiling fans.
Meals: Menu is a la carte, featuring local seafood and Bajan specialties. The main restaurant is L'Acajou; others are a beach-terrace restaurant, a pool cafe, and the Spa Cafe.
Facilities: The resort offers a private 18-hole golf course and tennis courts adjacent to the hotel and spa. The free-form pool near the spa is ideal for swimming laps. Cascading waterfalls add to the tropical ambience of the outdoor hydropool, which features underwater lounges. Unisex steam room, Ice Cave, fitness center with LifeFitness equipment and Lifecycles, motion studio, Pilates equipment. Eleven VIP treatment suites offer a private shower, bathroom, and changing facilities; nine suites feature private landscaped gardens.
Services & Special Programs: Massage, wraps and envelopments, rebalancing aromatherapy facial, Bajan synchronizing massage with two therapists, hydrotherapy bath, manicure, pedicure, makeup consultation, waxing, fitness evaluation, complimentary group exercise, yoga.
Rates: $$$
Best Spa Package: Four-hour ritual includes Purifying Herbal Linen Wrap with Volcanic Hot Stones, heated in an infusion of tri-dosha detoxifying herbs; Cleansing Express Facial and Relaxing Scalp Massage; exfoliation of the body with invigorating, soothing, or purifying ingredients; spa-inspired lunch. $550.
Credit Cards: Most major
Getting There: British Airways Concorde from London, regular flights from New York; US Airways via Philadelphia.
What's Nearby: Bridgetown (capital city), Barbados Museum & Historical Society in eighteenth-century British military prison, Speightstown (old whaling port), cricket matches.

GRAND LIDO SANS SOUCI RESORT—
CHARLIE'S SPA

Ocho Rios, Jamaica

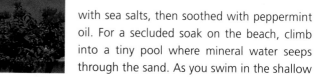

Legend has it that the natural mineral springs cascading into the spa pool at Grand Lido Sans Souci will fill the hearts of couples with the power of the passionate lovers who secretly bathed here in colonial times. Today at Charlie's Spa, aquacize in the pool and massage on a coral reef enchant hard-core fitness buffs as well as honeymooners.

The Grand Lido Sans Souci enjoys a private beachfront setting that's light-years away from the busy scene in Ocho Rios, yet close to north shore attractions like Dunn's River Falls. Locally owned and managed, the resort is part of the all-inclusive SuperClubs group, which provides lodging, meals and drinks, golf fees, and scuba-diving instruction in a one-price package. Here spa treatments are included too, on a limited basis.

Spa treatment rooms are housed in colorful wooden kiosks set into hillside gardens overlooking the sea. Ultimate stress relief comes in two gazebos set on coral cliffs, waves crashing below, where couples enjoy a secluded massage. Amid flowering hibiscus, bougainvillea, red tulip trees, palms, and exotic shrubs, a hot tub beckons. Look for spa mascot Charlie, a giant sea turtle, in his rocky grotto at check-in. A bar offers smoothies (or something stronger) while you wait for appointments on a tree-shaded terrace. Despite limited space, the well-trained Jamaican therapists provide a choice of twenty-five-minute back massage, body scrub, reflexology, or facial. And you can get a free pedicure and manicure in the salon. Anything else costs extra (if time slots are open).

Sybaritic escapes in the sea grotto start with a healthy sweat. From a sauna built into the rock, you relax on a table with the sea lapping below as your body is scrubbed

with sea salts, then soothed with peppermint oil. For a secluded soak on the beach, climb into a tiny pool where mineral water seeps through the sand. As you swim in the shallow bay, cool mineral water flows beneath warm salt water, creating a unique experience.

In French, *sans souci* means "carefree," so don't expect a structured program. Join a group doing aerobics to a reggae beat in the open-air beach pavilion, set out on a morning walk, or engage in yoga with a sea view. There is an air-conditioned cardiovascular and strength-training room with a few pieces of Cybex, Lifestep, and Schwinn equipment, but no trainers. A clothing-optional beach has its own bar and swimming pool.

Unlimited food comes with the daily tariff. You will be tempted to taste Jamaican specialties like jerk chicken, callalou soup brimming with local spinach and

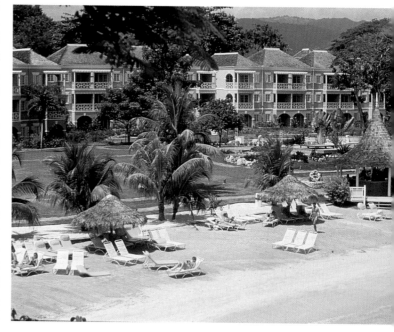

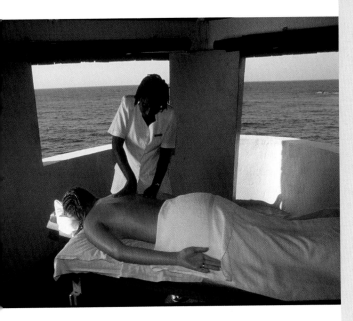

Grand Lido Sans Souci—Charlie's Spa
P.O. Box 103, Ocho Rios
Jamaica, West Indies
Phone: (876) 994–1353
Fax: (876) 994–1544
E-mail: reservations@superclub.com
Web site: www.superclubs.com

Season: Year-round

General Manager: Pierre Battaglia

Spa Director: Caroline Smith

Reservations: (800) GO–SUPER

Accommodations: 146 suites, including eight penthouses, all air-conditioned. Amenities include whirlpool bath in most suites, hair dryer, robes, direct-dial telephone, TV, minibar.

Meals: Japanese and Jamaican specialties mix with Continental cuisine in four restaurants. Unlimited selections and twenty-four-hour room service.

Facilities: Open-air treatments, natural mineral spring pool, two beaches, four tennis courts (lighted for night play), four swimming pools, three whirlpools, water-sports equipment, kayaks, sailboards, bocce, croquet, bicycling.

Services & Special Programs: Complimentary airport transfers, scuba diving with resort certification, waterskiing, golf course fee complimentary. Wedding coordinator.

Rates: $$$

Credit Cards: Most major

Getting There: Air Jamaica, Delta, or American Airlines to Sangster International Airport in Montego Bay; by car or van, the coastal road to Ocho Rios can be driven in about two hours. Airport transfers are complimentary; rental cars are available at the airport. Air taxi.

What's Nearby: Dunn's River Falls, rafting.

shrimp, or smoked marlin. Four restaurants and a twenty-four-hour beach grill offer lots of choices.

Grand Lido Sans Souci lives up to its name in the spacious suites. Some are terraced above the beach, others steps from tennis and water sports. For seclusion, eight penthouses offer sunbathing at treetop level. The resort's pink-beige plantation-style buildings are cheerfully accented with white gingerbread trim and balconies.

Entering the gates of Grand Lido Sans Souci is like returning to a tropical Eden where cares are left behind.

No-Worry (Sans Soucis) Skin Care

The signature skin-care line is Sans Soucis, made in Baden-Baden, Germany, by Biodroga. Known in Europe for antiaging treatments, Sans Soucis products are ideal for the Caribbean because their base of Baden-Baden mineral water gives them a light, nongreasy texture. Sun protection is particularly important here, and Sans Soucis uses new technology to screen out harmful ultraviolet rays.

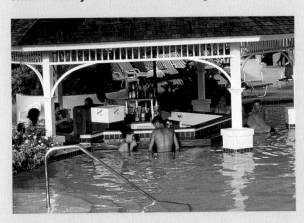

THE GOLDEN DOOR AT LAS CASITAS VILLAGE:
WYNDHAM EL CONQUISTADOR RESORT & COUNTRY CLUB

Las Croabas, Puerto Rico

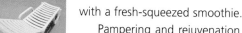

Secluded in a tropical golf resort, Las Casitas Village is a hotel that looks like a Spanish hacienda. Everything is small scale and personalized. A winding road through the scenic Arthur Hills Golf Course leads to the clifftop cluster of casitas. Palm-shaded and Spanish-tiled, a quiet courtyard contains a reception area, concierge, and an open-air breakfast bar that is complimentary to guests at the village. Settle into one of ninety pastel-colored suites without check-in formalities; your personal butler is on call to unpack, reserve a table at Le Bistro, and make spa appointments.

Stroll through gardens alongside a swimming pool to the Golden Door Spa. Housed in a three-story plantation-style villa, this Caribbean outpost of California's famed rejuvenation center creates a special sense of sanctuary. Zen-like elements of earth, water, and air surround you. Ascend the stairway to the Vitality Level for a workout in the Cybex cardiovascular and strength-training room or join an aerobics session in the Movement Studio. Scheduled throughout the day are Spinning, yoga, tai chi, stretching, and other exercise. Relax on the veranda overlooking the Atlantic

with a fresh-squeezed smoothie.

Pampering and rejuvenation take place on the top floor, the Tranquility Level. Ushered into a candlelit *niwa* (the Japanese word for resting place), you can take a traditional Oriental *ofuro* bath. Waterfalls relax shoulder muscles while you soak. Herbal tea and fruit, as well as cold water, are offered by your therapist.

What makes the entire spa so appealing is that it's integrated with its surroundings, reflecting the wonders of the rain forest and the bright turquoise sea. Many of the twenty-five private treatment rooms offer views of the gardens and sea. Outdoor sessions of yoga or tai chi on the lawn in front of the spa add new perspectives to this seaside retreat.

Swimming in the sea, however, requires a ferryboat ride to the resort's private island. This can be fun for kids but a bit noisy if you crave a place to read under the palms. The 500-acre resort provides action of every kind, from casino to shopping, championship golf to tennis, and offers a variety of restaurants. But you may never want to leave the village.

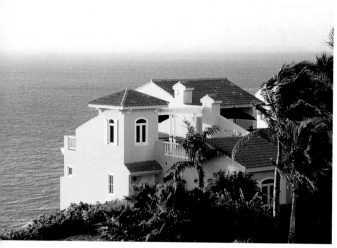

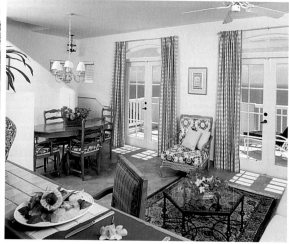

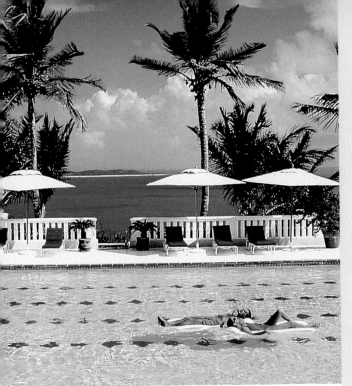

The Golden Door at Las Casitas Village: Wyndham El Conquistador Resort

1000 El Conquistador Avenue
Las Croabas, Puerto Rico 00738
Phone: (787) 863–1000
Fax: (787) 863–6758
Web site: www.grandbay.com
Season: Year-round
General Manager: Rob Gunthner
Spa Director: Joanne Diaz
Reservations: (888) 472–6229
Spa Appointments: (800) 468–8365
Accommodations: Ninety suites with one to three bedrooms in ground-level or split-level units, all air-conditioned. Each has fully equipped kitchen, living room, two TVs, VCR, multiline phones, stereo/CD player, and balcony. Other accommodations at the resort include more than 900 rooms and suites.
Meals: Golden Door cuisine served at the Spa Cafe for lunch, through room service at other times. Dinner in the village at Le Bistro features traditional French cuisine with Caribbean flair.
Facilities: The 26,000-square-foot Golden Door Spa provides a full range of therapies, exercise equipment, and strength-training units. Three freshwater swimming pools. Las Casitas Village has private swimming pool and hot tub. The marina offers fishing charters, sailboat rental. Golf and tennis. Camp Palomino provides day and evening programs for children.
Services & Special Programs: Local products derived from the rain forest and sea, as well as Golden Door signature treatments: herbal wraps, palomito salt glow, fango mud wrap, hydrotherapy bath. The Golden Door Spa Kurs combine a full body masque, a soak in a hydrotherapy tub, and a light moisturizing massage. Specialties include ayurvedic body treatments, facials, waxing. Personal fitness evaluation, exercise program.
Rates: $$$
Best Spa Package: Three-night casita accommodation for two, from $2,009 per person. Includes two spa treatments each or rounds of golf daily, spa drinks, one complimentary lunch for two, daily buffet breakfast, unlimited access to exercise facilities, tax. Also available: a Day of Beauty, $280, including three treatments and lunch. Gratuities not included.
Credit Cards: Most major
Getting There: Complimentary transfers from Luis Munoz Marin International Airport (sixty minutes).
What's Nearby: El Yunque National Rain Forest, historic Old San Juan, Vieques Island.

Smoothies Fight Sun Damage

Body-care experts at Essential Elements, known for its line of products for body and skin care, recommend this citrus smoothie as a healthy way to protect the skin from sun damage. Smoothies can be adapted to fit any nutritional need, they say. This one is revved up with vitamins and is as good as it sounds.

Citrus Smoothie
   1/2 cup milk
   1 cup cubed mango
   1 banana
   1/2 cup orange juice
   1 cup crushed ice
   1 tsp. honey
   2 slices orange, for garnish

Combine all ingredients, except orange slices, in blender. Blend until smooth. Garnish with orange slices. Serves two.

THE BODYHOLIDAY AT LESPORT

Castries, Saint Lucia

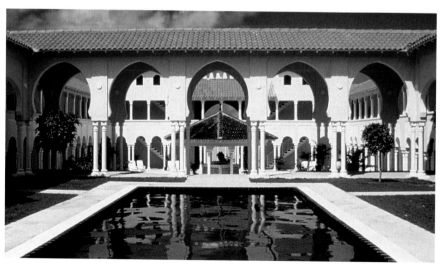

All-inclusive resorts have proliferated on the sunny Windward Islands, but few include spa treatments in the one-price-covers-everything package. At this laissez-faire spa, you are offered two daily treatments, plus a wide range of fitness and recreational activities, from tai chi to yoga, exercise classes, and meditation sessions. Superior guest rooms on a powder-soft beach and the peaceful spa pavilion add to a holistic holiday.

Tucked into a secluded cove near Saint Lucia's bustling capital and cruise port in Castries, this 20-acre resort is a tropical adventure with plenty of pampering. Designed like a plantation, colonial-style buildings spread out along the beach. The Oasis, a $3.5 million temple of well-being, sits atop a hill, isolated from beach sports and group games in the swimming pool. Here you can schedule workouts with a personal trainer, try the latest French skin care by Clarins, or simply do nothing. The lap pool is rarely crowded, and shaded lounges are perfect for reading and snoozing.

Built around an open-air courtyard, the Oasis resembles a colonnaded cloister, the hushed ambience broken only by bubbling fountains. The vista of the sea

has a tranquilizing effect. Complimentary services include a bubbling bath with herbs and sea algae, seaweed body wrap, and a circulation-boosting shower administered by high-pressure hose. There is a seawater pool for group exercise in the style of French thalassotherapy.

Planning a spa program starts with the resident nurse (called "sister" in the formal, British tradition still used by islanders) for a medical checkup. Once complimentary treatments have been scheduled, you're on your own to join aerobics classes and the daily program, which is listed on a bulletin board in the open-air pavilion where breakfast and lunch buffets are served. Sign up for instruction in archery, golf, fencing, and scuba diving. Outings include jungle walks, guided bike tours, and a visit to the hot springs at Mount Soufrière. You can play tennis day or night, go golfing, or use the putting green at no charge.

Because the resort is all-inclusive, reaching for your wallet is an exercise you can forget. Some extras, however, show up on your account when you depart on the resort's van for the airport. Treatments at the Clarins Salon are optional and not included in

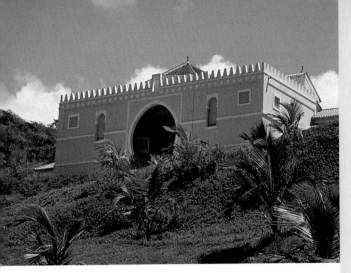

The BodyHoliday at LeSPORT
Cariblue Beach
P.O. Box 437 Castries
Saint Lucia, West Indies
Phone: (758) 450–8551
Fax: (758) 450–0368
E-mail: tropichol@aol.com
Web site: www.thebodyholiday.com

Season: Year-round

General Manager: Michael Bryant

Spa Director: Martha Willie

Reservations: (800) 544–2883; U.K. 44–870–220–2344

Accommodations: 152 rooms and suites in four-story buildings facing the sea. Luxury suites come with peaked-ceiling, four-poster bed draped in pink-stripped sailcloth. All rooms have bathrobes, hair dryer, telephone, TV, ceiling fans, air-conditioning.

Meals: Three meals daily, plus snacks. Breakfast buffet of fresh tropical fruit, juices, omelette to order, or continental tray delivered to room. Lunch buffet includes fried fish, stuffed chicken leg, rice, assorted vegetables, pizza. The Deli offers sandwiches and salads. Dinner can be steamed kingfish, veal scallop in champagne sauce, sea scallops with snow peas. Tao offers fusion cuisine and wines.

Facilities: The Oasis has hydrotherapy tubs, saunas, hot and cold plunge pools, Swiss needle shower, jet stream pool, whirlpool, fully equipped gymnasium, Clarins salon. Equipment for windsurfing, waterskiing, snorkeling, scuba diving, fencing, archery, golf, tennis; three swimming pools; putting green.

Services & Special Programs: Swedish, Thai, shiatsu and reflexology massages; marine baths and wraps; group exercise. Personal training. Clarins salon for hair and nail care, skin treatments. Couples massage instruction; golf and tennis training.

Rates: $$

Best Spa Package: Clarins anti–jet lag combination of massage, body wrap, and facial. Some spa services are complimentary, a few come with an extra charge.

Credit Cards: American Express, Diners Club, MasterCard, VISA

Getting There: Complimentary transfers from Hewanora International Airport (ninety minutes). Bring proof of citizenship; passport is best.

What's Nearby: Mount Soufrière (mud bath), the Pitons (rock climbing), Diamond Falls (hot springs), golf.

the BodyHoliday package. Parisian facials, hair and nail care, and stress-reducing massage and mud wraps are offered at prices that are a bargain if you're paying with dollars.

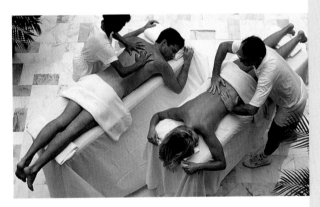

Beach Balm for Body and Soul

The sea is the origin of life. The plasma in our blood contains elements that match the composition of seawater. French scientists have shown that body fluids are naturally similar to seawater. Algae are rich in vitamins, mineral salts, and trace elements, which are vital for human health. Clarins incorporates seaweed and algae in skin-care products that nurture and protect. After exposure to sun, try an algae body wrap.

SOUTH AMERICA

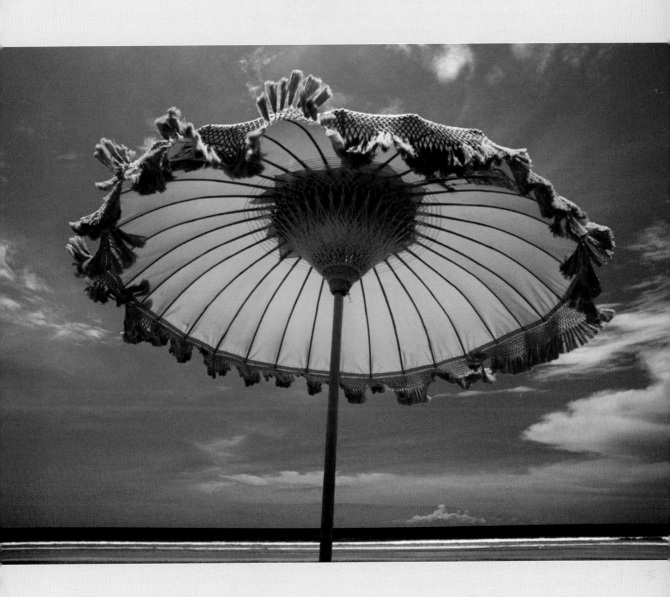

KUROTEL

Gramado, Brazil

High in the mountains of southern Brazil, an Alpine wonderland reminiscent of European resorts surrounds the Kurotel complex in the town of Gramado. Strolling the clean and flowery streets is like being in Bavaria. And in winter (the northern hemisphere's summer), the snow-covered slopes of Rio Grande do Sul could be in the Swiss Alps. Staying at the Kurotel is the best of both worlds.

Established in 1982, the Kurotel is based on a vision of a place devoted to total well-being, where modern medical technology and natural medicine's wisdom can be experienced together. The Kur Gramado (Gramado cure) focuses on preventive medicine, a concept that links lifestyle with prevention of illness. Created by an orthodox medical doctor, the program identifies existing health problems and contributing environmental factors, such as stress.

When you arrive at the hotel complex, your first impression is of a mountain chalet—red-tile roofs and long verandas overlook a flowering garden. Every Sunday afternoon, guests arrive to start the weeklong kur program. Greeted by Dr. Luis Carlos Silveira and his wife, Neusa, you learn that a high priority is placed on physical activity—walks in the woods and a Kneipp hydrotherapy course, gymnastics in the covered swimming pool, and one-on-one training in the gym. Hikes guided by staff members are scheduled daily—the region's dazzling landscapes are a major attraction.

Monitoring your progress, the team of psychologists, physiotherapists, and doctors use biofeedback equipment to help with control of emotions and stress level. A session on posture, which works on balance and breathing, helps you get to know your body.

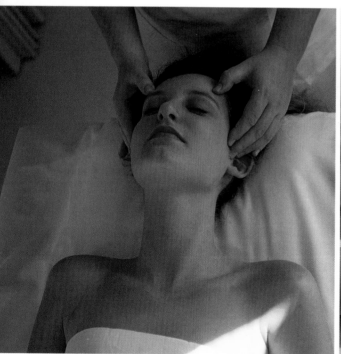
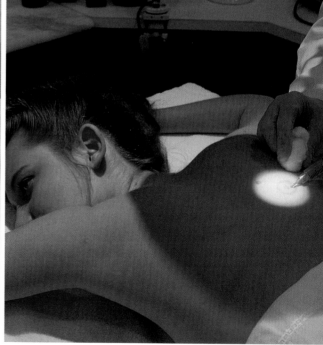

Natural therapies and scientific knowledge come together in the Kurotel Longevity Center. The spacious waiting room has a beamed ceiling, an open fireplace, and a juice bar offering herbal teas and fresh fruit. After a personal evaluation, a course of treatments is prescribed by the doctors. Facilities are comparable to those at European kur centers, with extensive use of baths, mud applications, and oxygen inhalation. For an advanced diagnostic checkup, there is a half-week program. (Everything is in English.)

Comfort also comes with the kur. Bedrooms are suite sized and decorated with antiques, country-style furniture, and luxurious draperies. Guests are a sophisticated mix of business, political, and social types from all parts of Latin America who speak several languages. If you feel the need to keep in touch with the office, you can stay in one of the business center suites fully equipped and staffed for international travelers. Meeting fellow guests in the lounge before a seated dinner, or in the Finnish sauna, or on hikes helps build a spirit of camaraderie.

From Kneipp to Cosmetics, Updating the Kur

Kur Gramado bases its philosophy of natural medicine on the healing water techniques developed in Bavaria by Father Sebastian Kneipp. For the first time in Brazil, the Kneipp water walk provides a natural exercise. Walking in water up to your calves strengthens body functions, according to the staff. The alternating warm and cold water, combined with the smooth stones underfoot, influences the kidneys and promotes excretion of residues. Kneipp treatments also call for the use of herbs and teas, which can also be found at the pharmacy in downtown Gramado. Completing the spa collection are all-natural kur cologne, skin moisturizers, and hair-care products developed and produced in Brazil.

Brazilian Longevity Center's European Alpine Kur

Kurotel
Rua Nacoes Unidas, 533
95670-000 Gramado
Rio do Sul, Brazil
Phone: 55–54–286–2133
Fax: 55–54–286–1203
E-mail: info@kurotel.com.br
Web site: www.kurotel.com.br

Season: Year-round

General Manager: Luis Carlos Silveira, M.D.

Spa Director: Neusa Silveira

Reservations: 55–54–286–2133 or (800) 272–3480

Accommodations: Suites and apartments with single or double beds, decorated in colonial or baroque style. All have private bathroom with marble-top basins, hair dryer, magnifying mirror, robes. Air-conditioning, TV, and phone are standard, and there is a CD/radio sound system. Apartments come with desk and easy chairs, comfortable sofa; four executive suites have office equipment.

Meals: Based on Swiss techniques, three high-energy meals and three snacks are served daily. The resident nutritionist adapted recipes with fresh ingredients from local farms, using herbs and spices from the hotel's own vegetable garden. Choices include soups, salads, seafood, chicken, rabbit, and beef, as well as shakes, juices, fruit, breads, and pies.

Facilities: Hydrotherapy baths and Kneipp water walk, galvanic baths, footbaths, respiratory inhalations, mud packs, indoor and outdoor swimming pools, gymnasium, exercise equipment, beauty salon. Medical clinic. Tennis court.

Services & Special Programs: Massage, underwater massage, fango with sea algae, reflexology, skin care, acupressure. Programs for stress management, antiaging, health evaluation, anti-cellulite, kinder kur.

Rates: $$$

Best Spa Package: Week-long Kur program includes medical evaluation, meals, lodging, and treatments. Prices vary with the season and start at $1,135 single occupancy, $993 double occupancy, plus 10 percent service charge.

Credit Cards: MasterCard, VISA

Getting There: From Rio de Janeiro, Sao Paulo, or Montevideo, by air to Porto Alegre (two hours). Rental car at airport. Transfers by private car on request ($120, round-trip).

What's Nearby: Atlantic Ocean resorts.

FOUR SEASONS RESORT CARMELO

Carmelo, Uruguay

Set on the Rio de la Plata, this peaceful haven is just a short hop from Buenos Aires or Montevideo. The combination of dramatic design, sports, and spa is unequaled in South America.

Melding Asian and Latin themes, bungalows and bilevel suites cluster amid pine and eucalyptus trees. Guest units are linked by walkway to the main lodge. Interiors feature a fireplace in a high-ceiling lounge with an entertainment center, as well as an upper gallery for sleeping. Designer touches include a double-basin bathroom in rose-colored marble with a deep soaking tub and separate shower and toilet.

The wooden spa building resembles an ancient inn. Entering a Zen garden, you change amid opulent teak furniture, a sculptured Buddha, and a painted Thai tree of life. An air-conditioned gym has the latest Cybex exercise equipment. Incense and flowers perfume an open-air courtyard where tea and juice are offered. Relax in an outdoor rain-forest shower, steam room, and sauna. Sounds are hushed; a splashing fountain, bird calls, and tinkling bells create an air of serenity.

Treatments are personalized with herbs from local farmers for body wraps and facials. Trainers from Thailand worked with aestheticians to develop the menu of treatments and salon services.

Sports top the resort agenda: Polo matches attract top Argentine and international players, and there are trail rides for guests; across the road is an 18-hole golf course and country club. At the airy main lodge, take tea

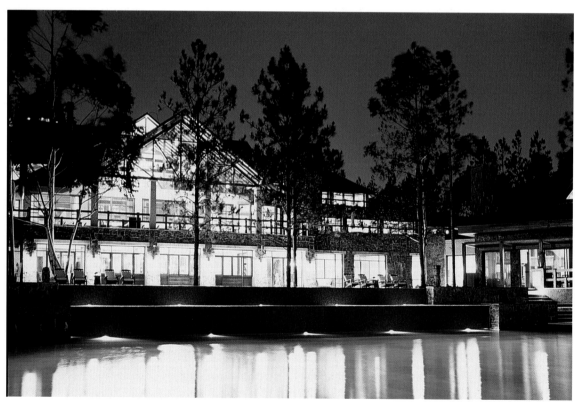

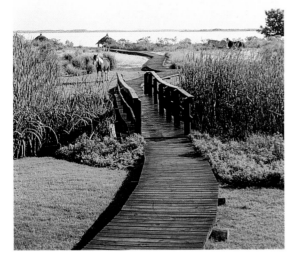

in a Thai sala, or read and check e-mail in the library. Meeting rooms terrace down to the vast swimming pool and restaurant. Balinese carvings and batik draperies enhance pan-Asian meals at Pura (meaning *temple*), where a spirit house floats in mosaic-tiled pool. Breakfast includes breads and croissants from the open-to-view bakery. Weekends there's a traditional barbecue—churrasco—on the pool terrace, with dancing under a sky glowing with lights of the city across the delta.

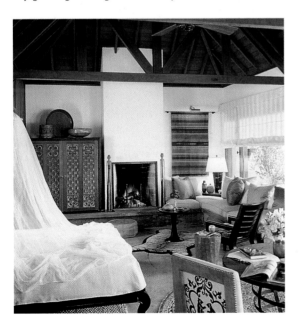

Four Seasons Resort Carmelo
Route/ruta 21, km 262
Carmelo, Colonia, Uruguay
Phone: 598–542–9000
Fax: 598–542–9999
E-mail: info@fourseasons.com
Web site: www.fourseasons.com/carmelo
Season: Year-round
General Manager: Peter Roth
Reservations: 54 (11) 4321–1690; (800) 332–3442
Accommodations: Twenty-four bilevel suites, twenty bungalows. Spacious quarters have fireplace, bathroom with heated floor, deep soaking tub, separate shower, twin vanity set in marble. Sleeping area features carved Chinese bed draped in netting. Completely air-conditioned. Amenities include robes, TV, CD player, phones, espresso machine.
Meals: Alternative cuisine menu based on Four Seasons healthy fare features seafood; organic produce of local farms; breakfast buffet of tropical fruit, fresh yogurt, and honey.
Facilities: Spa building has fitness center with cardiovascular and strength-training equipment, indoor/outdoor treatment rooms, studio for aerobics and yoga, lounge and juice bar, saunas. Swimming pool (heated) at main lodge; river beach. On-site horseback riding, polo, water sports, and an 18-hole, par-72 golf course. Nearby tennis, hiking.
Services & Special Programs: Massage, body wraps, aromatherapy, hydrotherapy; salon for hair and nail care. Concierge arranges local tours. Children's program.
Rates: $$$
Best Spa Package: Four Seasons Hotel Buenos Aires provides a three-night city package, three nights at the resort, and round-trip transfer by boat. Included are a choice of massage or golf, buffet breakfast daily, access to fitness center, plus tango lesson with champagne at Le Dome. Price per person is $1,000 based on double occupancy of room.
Credit Cards: Most major
Getting There: From Buenos Aires Ezeiza International Airport by boat and car (three hours); From Montevideo Airport by car or taxi via express route 21 (two-and-a-half hours); private planes land at Carmelo Airport.
What's Nearby: Buenos Aires by boat ($65 round trip), Carmelo, Colonia (historic zone).

SPAS AT SEA

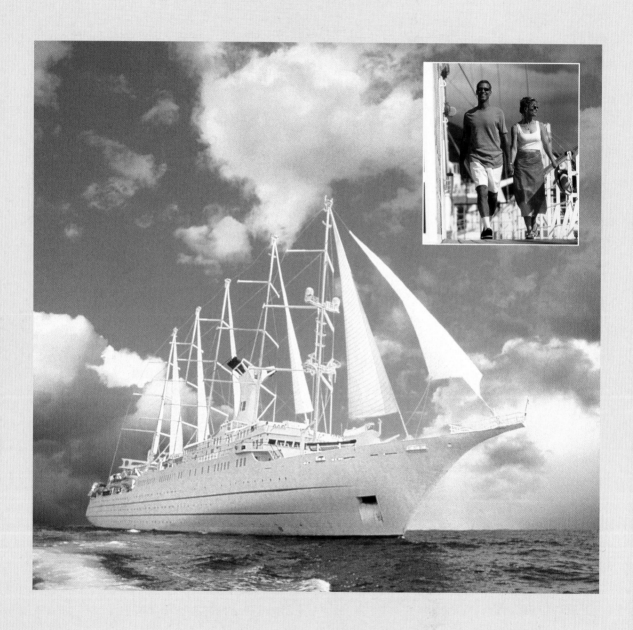

JUDITH JACKSON'S SEASPA—RADISSON
SEVEN SEAS MARINER

Radisson Seven Seas Cruises

Scents of mountain flowers, pine trees, fruit, and plants perfume Judith Jackson's SeaSpa aboard Radisson's *Seven Seas Mariner*. Personalized aromatherapy massages, facials, and baths are signature services designed to enhance your sense of well-being by reducing stress levels. In the hands of skilled therapists trained by Jackson, the experience reaches a higher level of relaxation, awakening the soul to a spirit of discovery.

Combining luxury and adventure, the *Mariner* cruises Asia, Australia, the South Pacific, the Caribbean, and South America. Accommodations for 700 passengers are all suites, ranging from 250 square feet to a two-bedroom 1,205-square-foot-master suite, all with private balcony. Ideal for long cruises, *Mariner's* big-ship amenities, attentive personal service, and no-tipping policy add up to a unique experience. On cruises through the Panama Canal, for example, this is one of the few ships to anchor in Gatun Lake at a private yacht club, allowing passengers to explore the rain forest and see the canal locks close up.

Judith Jackson's SeaSpa complements the *Mariner's* intimate design. With ten treatment rooms, it is located on an upper deck of the ship, brightened by natural light. The sauna and steam bath are available to passengers. On the pool deck are a jogging track, golf driving range, and fitness center. Unlimited access to the exercise equipment and scheduled classes lets you set your own schedule. Personal trainers are available to plan your exercise regimen.

Outpacing ships of similar size for comfort and spaciousness, and with its exclusive SeaSpa and stress-buster treatments, the *Mariner* charts exceptional cruise vacations.

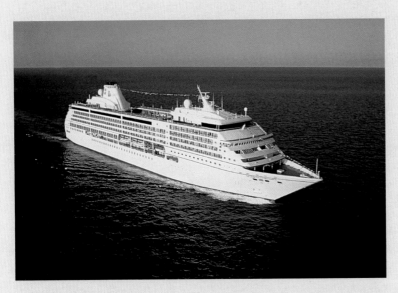

Stress-Buster Aromatherapy

**Judith Jackson's SeaSpa—
Radisson *Seven Seas Mariner***
Radisson Seven Seas Cruises
600 Corporate Drive
Fort Lauderdale, FL 33334
Phone: (954) 776–6123, (866)
359–8808, or (866) 314–3209
Fax: (954) 722–6763
Web site: www.rssc.com

SPA DU SOLEIL—MS *PRINSENDAM*

Holland America Line

With more ships cruising the world than ever, marine designers are competing to build the biggest and best spa at sea. Responding to passenger demand for enhanced spa services aboard their ships, the Holland America line teamed up with Steiner Leisure Ltd. in 2002 to create the Spa du Soleil aboard the MS *Prinsendam*.

With a 30-foot lap pool, ten treatment rooms, and separate sauna/steam rooms for men and women, the two-level Spa du Soleil sets new standards in comfort and elegance. In addition to the latest amenities and exercise equipment, the Roman-style decor of pillars, murals, and sculptures of goddesses is complemented by a soft color scheme, terra-cotta and mosaic tiling, and lots of natural light. What's special here are Steiner's personalized programs: Ionithermie, a cellulite reduction system that uses electrodes attached to targeted areas of the body; the Aphrodite suite, where you sink into a dry-float bed while getting a seaweed wrap; the Cleopatra bath suite; and the rasul mud chamber.

Spa du Soleil packs extraordinary elegance into compact spaces. Thanks to window walls, there is a feeling of being at sea that is energizing and relaxing. While on a treadmill, stepper, or bike, you have an expansive view of the sea as well as the lap pool and whirlpools. Awaiting a treatment in the quiet lounge, you can have herbal tea, Evian water, and fresh fruit.

Suites on the penthouse deck, closest to the spa, are among the most spacious afloat and have a private balcony. With built-in cabinetry, curved sofas, original art, soft lighting, and crystal vases filled with fresh flowers, the feeling of peace and tranquillity perfectly complements the spa experience.

Designed for a maximum of 758 passengers, the *Prinsendam* is the epitome of well-being afloat.

Unregimented, your days at sea provide the freedom to sample spa services and maintain a healthy regimen. Compared with the behemoths being built today for Caribbean cruising, *Prinsendam* turns back to an era of stylish informality and formal dining.

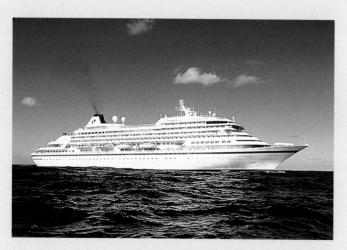

Classic Ocean Liner Elegance Creates Total Relaxation

MS *Prinsendam*
Holland America Line
300 Elliott Avenue West
Seattle, WA 98119
Phone: (206) 281–3535 or (800) 426–0327
Fax: (800) 628–4855
Web site: www.hollandamerica.com

STEINER SPA—CUNARD *QUEEN ELIZABETH 2*

Cunard Line

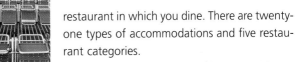

Surprisingly modern, this grand dame of the seas sailed into the new millennium in great shape. Thanks to the Steiner Spa, you can enjoy the latest in thalassotherapy treatments with fresh seawater as well as micronized marine algae. Featuring some of the most elaborate hydrotherapy facilities afloat, as well as exercise equipment and personal trainers, the *QE2* lets you ship out in style.

Crossing to Europe or America aboard this great liner is like a six-day resort vacation. All the elements of a spa program are at your disposal, as well as temptations like nonstop food, tons of caviar, and champagne.

Launched in 1969, *Queen Elizabeth 2* (usually called *QE2*) seems to get better with age. She underwent a major refit in 1999, after the company became part of the Carnival Cruise Corporation, and retains her high standards in first-class staterooms and suites, as well as in the Queen's Grill dining room. On cruises as well as crossings, you get the virtual run of the ship, but your stateroom or cabin category determines the restaurant in which you dine. There are twenty-one types of accommodations and five restaurant categories.

The indoor seawater pool is open 7:00 A.M. to 7:00 P.M. Adjoining the pool is a gym with Cybex, StairMaster, and LifeFitness exercise equipment, plus classes, all at no charge. The boat deck is for running or walking laps, but the open-air swimming pool on upper deck can be crowded when the ship is at full capacity of 1,740 passengers. A better bet is deep down in the hull, on deck six: The Steiner Spa boasts a room-size pool with bubbling jets for underwater massage. Sauna and steam room (coed) adjoin the pool and locker rooms; a $20 facility charge goes on your shipboard account. The receptionists schedule massage and other treatments. Seaweed body masques and facials are among services in ten private rooms. Try a multijet hydrotherapy bath, where you soak in freeze-dried algae, or clear your sinuses with seawater mist at inhalation stations.

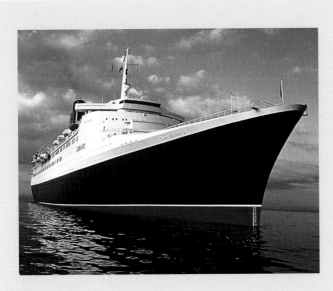

Traditions Updated with Thalassotherapy

Steiner Spa—Cunard *Queen Elizabeth 2*
Cunard Line
6100 Blue Lagoon Drive
Miami, FL 33126
Phone: (305) 463–3000 or (800) 728–6273
Fax: (305) 463–3010
Web site: www.cunard.com

WINDSPA—WINDSTAR'S *WIND SURF*

Windstar Cruises

Combining the adventure of yachting with the amenities of a luxury cruise ship, the 312-passenger *Wind Surf* is in a class by itself. Soothing and tastefully decorated staterooms, healthy gourmet dining, and the full-service WindSpa enhance cruises to romantic ports on the French and Italian rivieras, as well as in the Caribbean.

Framed by five tall sails, *Wind Surf* can dock in ports not accessible to big cruise ships. Distinctive itineraries on the Nice-to-Rome cruise during summer months include calls at Monte Carlo, Saint-Tropez, and Portofino. Caribbean cruises January through March start in Barbados. Standard cruises are seven days; year-end eleven-day sailings add ports.

Recreation ranges from aerobics to scuba. The ship's built-in marina lets you enjoy water sports right from the deck. Equipment for snorkeling, waterskiing, kayaking, and windsurfing is available on a first-come basis, at no charge. Scuba divers are charged $65 per tank. Excursions by Zodiac boat add to your sightseeing and shopping in ports. Or simply stake out a spot on deck and swim in the heated saltwater pool.

Wind Surf is for people who hate big cruise ships. With no formal evenings and a relaxed dress code consisting mainly of chic resort wear, the unregimented experience of the ship plus its extraordinary service adds up to a cruise adventure to cherish.

Ready for serious pampering? Head for the WindSpa on marina deck. Caring and courteous aestheticians provide stress-busting treatments and sun protection. This is one of the few ships to have a hydrotherapy tub for aromatherapy soaks. And there are eight rooms with oceanview portholes. So relax with a seaweed wrap or sports massage. Staffed and operated by Steiner, spa services are charged to your account aboard ship. Booking a package before sailing gets you priority on appointment times.

At sea the *Wind Surf* sails with all the stability of an America's Cup contender. This ship is built for comfort, and its length ensures smooth sailing. One of the most spectacular sights is her tall sails rising at sunset as she glides effortlessly toward the next port. It's instant karma.

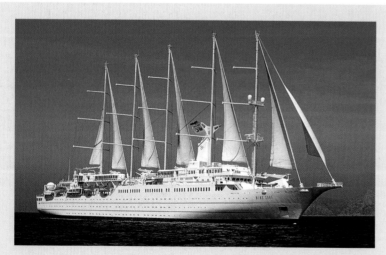

Sailing a Small Ship with a Big Spa

WindSpa on *Wind Surf*
Windstar Cruises
300 Elliott Avenue West
Seattle, WA 98119
Phone: (206) 281–3535 or (800) 258–7245
Fax: (206) 286–3229
E-mail: information@windstarcruises.com
Web site: www.windstarcruises.com

GLOSSARY OF SPA TERMS

Abhyanga-rhythmic: An herbal oil massage performed by two therapists, followed by a hot towel treatment.

Acupressure: A finger massage intended to release muscle tension by applying pressure to the nerves.

Aromatherapy: A massage with oils from plant and flower essences intended to relax the skin's connective tissue and stimulate the natural flow of lymph.

Ayurvedic treatments: Four-thousand-year-old treatments from India based on teachings from the Vedic scriptures, using oils, massages, and herbs.

Balneology: The traditional study and practice of water-based treatments using geothermal hot springs, mineral water, or seawater.

Bindi: Bodywork combining exfoliation, herbal treatment, and light massage.

Body polish: The use of large sea sponges to gently cleanse, exfoliate, and hydrate the body.

Complementary medicine: Complements to traditional Western medicine incorporating the ancient arts of acupuncture and Chinese herbal medicine.

Crystal healing: Healing energy believed to be generated by quartz and other minerals.

Drinking cure: A medically prescribed regimen of mineral water consumption.

Fango: A mud pack or body coating intended to promote the release of toxins and relieve muscular and arthritic pain.

Glycolic exfoliation: A process that uses a natural enzyme (found in citrus fruit) to break down the glue bond that holds dry skin on the face, soften lines, and smooth skin.

G5: A percussive hand massage to relax tense muscles.

Gommage: A cleansing and moisturizing treatment that makes use of creams applied with movements similar to those of an extensive massage.

Hatha yoga: A system of yoga that focuses on bodily control through the use of *anasas* (postures).

Herbal wrap: A treatment in which moisture, heat, and herbal essences penetrate the skin while the body is wrapped in hot linens, plastic sheets, and blankets. It is intended to promote muscle relaxation and the elimination of toxins.

Hot plunge: A deep pool for the rapid dilation of the capillaries.

Hot stone massage: Applied to chakra points, warm stones provide penetrating heat and are used for massage.

Hydrotherapy: Underwater massage; alternating hot and cold showers, and other water-oriented treatments.

Hydrotub: An underwater massage in deep tubs equipped with high-pressure jets and hand-manipulated hoses.

Inhalations: Hot vapors or steam mixed with eucalyptus oil inhaled through inhalation equipment or in a special steam room to decongest the respiratory system.

Kneipp kur: Treatments combining hydrotherapy, herbology, and a diet of natural foods, developed in Germany in the mid-1800s by Father Sebastian Kneipp.

Lomi lomi: A Hawaiian rhythmical rocking massage.

Mud wrap: A body treatment using warm mud to cleanse pores and lift impurities.

Naturopathy: Natural healing prescriptions that use plants and flowers.

Panchakarma: A type of massage therapy that uses warm, herbalized oils, and aims to restore balance to the body.

Paraffin wrap: The process of removing dead skin cells with hot oil and Japanese dry-brushing techniques, then applying melted wax infused with emollients.

Pilates method: Strength and flexibility training movements developed by Joseph H. Pilates during the 1920s.

Pizichilli: A purifying experience in which a continuous stream of warm, herbalized oil is poured over the body as two therapists perform a gentle massage.

Pressotherapy: Pressure cuffs used to improve circulation in the feet.

Pressure point massage: Massage and bodywork that use pressure on designated body parts connected to major nerves to relieve stress.

Qigong: Pronounced *chi kung*. A Chinese energy exercise that uses breathing and body movements recharge energy.

Rasul: Steam chamber for mud treatment.

Reflexology: Massage of the pressure points on the feet, hands, and ears, intended to relax parts of the body.

Reiki: An ancient healing method that imports universal life energy through the laying on of hands and mental and spiritual balancing. It's intended to relieve acute emotional and physical conditions.

Roman pool: A step-down whirlpool bath for one or two people.

Russian bath: A steam bath designed to flush toxins from the body.

Salt glow: A cleansing treatment that uses coarse salt to exfoliate the skin.

Scotch hose: A showerlike treatment with high-pressure hoses that alternate hot and cold water; intended to improve circulation through rapid contraction and dilation of the capillaries.

Seaweed wrap: A wrap using concentrated seawater and nutrient-packed seaweed. Minerals, proteins, rare trace elements, and vitamins are absorbed into the bloodstream to revitalize the skin and body.

Shirodhara: An ayurvedic massage in which warm herbal oil is dropped on the forehead ("the third eye") and rubbed gently into the hair and scalp.

Sitz bath: Immersion of the hips and lower body into hot water, then into cold water to stimulate the immune system. Also a Kneipp treatment for digestive upset.

Spa cuisine: Fresh natural foods low in saturated fats and cholesterol, with an emphasis on whole grains, low-fat dairy products, lean protein, fresh fruits, fish, and vegetables and an avoidance of added salt and products containing sodium or artificial colorings, flavorings, or preservatives.

Spinning: A group exercise class on stationary bicycles intended to provide aerobic conditioning by pedaling quickly at varied resistance levels.

Stress management: A program of meditation and deep relaxation intended to reduce the ill effects of stress on the system.

Sweat lodge: A Native American–inspired purifying ritual that takes place in a natural sauna made of rocks.

Swedish massage: A treatment that duplicates gymnastics movements, using stroking, kneading, friction, vibration, and tapping to relax muscles gently. It was devised at the University of Stockholm in the early nineteenth century by Per Heinrik Ling.

Swiss shower: A multijet bath that alternates hot and cold water, often used after mud wraps and other body treatments.

Tai chi: An ancient Oriental discipline of exercise and meditation based on movements intended to unite body and mind.

Target heart rate: The number of heartbeats per minute that an individual tries to attain during exercise, ideally 60 to 90 percent of the maximal heart rate. The American College of Sports Medicine recommends maintaining the target rate during exercise for twenty to thirty minutes three to five days per week.

Thalassotherapy: An ancient Greek system of water-based treatments using seawater, seaweed, algae, and sea air.

Vichy shower: A hydrotherapy treatment that involves lying on a cushioned waterproof mat and being showered by jets.

Watsu: An underwater treatment blending the techniques of deep tissue massage, acupressure, shiatsu, and yoga.

Yoga: A discipline of stretching and toning the body through movements or postures, controlled deep breathing, relaxation techniques, and diet. A school of Hindu philosophy advocating physical and mental discipline for the unity of mind, body, and spirit.

Zen shiatsu: A Japanese acupressure art intended to relieve tension and balance the body.

ABOUT THE AUTHORS

BERNARD BURT is an internationally recognized authority on the spa industry and a writer and leader in the field of spa vacations and fitness travel. His columns appear in *Healing Lifestyles & Spas, Spa Management Journal,* and *Pulse*, the magazine of the International Spa Association (ISPA). He has also written articles for leading magazines, such as *National Geographic Traveler*. The Board of Directors of the International Spa Association named Mr. Burt recipient of its Dedicated Contributor Award in 2001. The award honors his commitment to industry standards and his professional values.

PAMELA PRICE is a writer, editor, and radio personality who has visited more than 500 spas worldwide. Her articles have appeared in more than one hundred newspapers and magazines. She spent eight years at *Shape* magazine developing spa travel and cuisine features. She produced spa videos for the tourism boards of Switzerland and Italy and has produced and hosted several travel and health radio talk shows. In 1999 she served as an advisor for the *National Geographic Traveler* survey of American spas. Ms. Price is donating her royalties from *100 Best Spas of the World,* Second Edition, to Shelter from the Storm, a Palm Desert, California, organization that supports women and children suffering from domestic abuse.

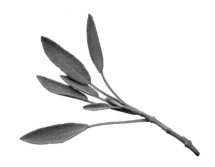

SPA NOTES